"Sat"

sat (sat) *adj.* abbreviation for the word "saturated" as it relates to hydrogen bonds in organic molecules called fatty acids.

"Fat"

fat (fat)   *n.* any of several white or yellowish substances, forming the chief part of adipose tissue of animals and also occurring in plants, that when pure are colorless, odorless, and tasteless, and are solid at room temperature.

"Rox"

rox (roks) *v.* slang for the colloquialism "rocks", defined as "to perform with greatness or to be great". Or as one contributor to urbandictionary.com sees it, "the most righteous word expressing awesomeness".

"Censored"

censor (sen'sər) *n.* 1 an official who examines books, news reports, motion pictures, radio and television programs, letters, etc., for the purpose of suppressing parts deemed objectionable on political, military, moral, or other grounds. 2 an adverse critic; faultfinder.
censored (sen'sərd) *adj.* suppressed or subject to censorship.

"Nutritional"

nutritional (nü trish'ən əl) *adj.* relating to the process, in animals and plants, involving the intake of nutrient materials and their subsequent assimilation into the tissues.

"Gem (s)"

gem (jem) *n., pl.* gems (jemz) something likened to (or prized as such) a precious stone because of its beauty or worth.

SatFatRox and Other Censored Nutritional Gems:
A Guide and Cookbook

By Juliana Comsa Norris

Publisher: SatFatRox.com
825 Gum Branch Road, Suite 129
Jacksonville, NC 28540
satfatrox@gmail.com

Cover and Schematic Artist George W. Cole
shotsofvinager@yahoo.com

Cover Design by Juliana C. Norris

First Edition: August 2014
Printed in the United States of America

Publisher's Note:
The author/publisher is not engaged in rendering professional advice or services to the individual reader. The ideas, procedures, and suggestions contained in this book are not intended as a substitute for consulting with your physician. The material in this book is provided for general educational purposes only and does not constitute medical advice or counseling, the practice of medicine or the provision of health care diagnosis or treatment. The author/publisher shall not be held liable or responsible for any loss or damage allegedly arising from any information or suggestion in this book. The recipes contained in this book are to be followed exactly as written. The author/publisher is not responsible for any adverse reactions to the recipes contained in this book.

No part of this book may be used in any manner whatsoever without written permission except as permitted under the U.S. Copyright Act of 1976, and in the case of brief quotations embodied in articles and reviews and with appropriate citing.

ISBN: 1499301146
ISBN-13: 978-1499301144

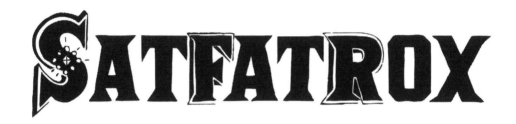

SATFATROX

AND OTHER
CENSORED NUTRITIONAL GEMS:

A Guide and Cookbook

Dear Brenda,
To sharing Akea
and all the good
it has brought us
both! Warmest &
Sincerest
agape Love!
Juliana

By
Juliana Comsa Norris

SatFatRox.com

For my girls, Abby and Nina

Mommy wrote you a book so you'll always know how to nourish yourselves.
Do not deviate from this path lined with palm shortening and coconut oil,
buckets of cocoa butter, quarts of coconut milk ice cream, and potatoes.
It is the path of your great health and happiness.

Acknowledgements

I wish to thank William King, Dr. Maurice Werness, and all of the other great minds that came together to create something unprecedented, revolutionary even. Akea has changed my life- my brain, my body - and the lives of so many dear to me, husband and children especially. We now exist in a realm of compassion and patience like we've never known before. Like the enzymes in each scoop, Akea itself is a catalyst for Nature's ultimate plan- balance. It has given me a clarity of mind and a focus that I didn't know I was capable of achieving. Never in my loftiest daydreams did I think I could churn out over 300 pages of coherent thought, the bulk of which have been written in the last 90 days.

Thank you to Dr. Uffe Ravnskov, Dr. Joseph Mercola, Dr. Peter Osborne, Dr. Tom O'Bryan, and Dr. Kelly Brogan, to name just a few for lighting my path on this journey of discovery and sound scientific knowledge. You have changed the course of my family's health and life, and in return, I will pay it forward to every human being willing to lend me an ear.

Thank you to George Cole, for your awesome artwork of turning me into a version of Holly I can only hope to resemble; to Sheree Alderman for her valuable time, input and turning on a dime. Thank you, Janice Khreis, for snapping a seren- dipitous family portait of us on our way to the Marine Corps Birthday Ball in November of 2012.

JKN: Over the past 10 months of brainstorming, podcast writing, recipe testing, and finally writing this book, as much as I tried to balance it all, I fell short many times. The business and my clients demanded my presence; the girls got what was left of me, and you acquiesced to seeing me a few hours a week, in passing, while being in charge of dinner most nights and grocery shopping the entire time. I know it's hard to be married to someone wearing a "mask of sanity", but at the end of the day, I hope the capriciousness makes for a laugh or two, and keeps you on your toes. Thank you for letting me linger in hyperfocus long enough to accomplish this feat and for being my sounding board and data gatherer, and formatting buddy. You're so good to me and we are lucky to have eachother and our beautiful little monkeys! I am now going to turn my "work space" back into the dining room, and get rid of the "Mop".

-Your Force of Nature

Contents

As in, it's extraordinarily good for you and irreplaceable for exceptional health. Saturated fats are *natural*. They are not trans fats, which are man-made and extraordinarily *not* good for you. Examples of saturated fats you should keep in your pantry and use intentionally, as opposed to incidentally: organic virgin coconut oil, organic palm shortening, organic red palm oil, cocoa butter, and palm kernel oil.

As in, it rules the body through its structural contributions to the trillions of cell membranes you have, 25 percent of your brain volume, and as the precursor to vitamin D (cholecalciferol) and all sex hormones- progesterone, testosterone, estradiol. Best source of dietary cholesterol: raw, whole eggs, from hens that pasture freely and are not fed soy. Soy will accumulate in the yolk, where the bulk of the protein in the egg can be found. I'm thinking if you're "allergic" to eggs, and you're buying them from the grocery store, you're more than likely allergic to the soy protein residues in the yolk. The solution is not to discard the yolk (a superfood), rather to find a new egg supplier.

As in, it's more addictive than cocaine, yet cheaper and more readily available than any other ingredient in processed food today. It's added to spaghetti sauce and salad dressing, and conventional recipes for baked goods call for ridiculous amounts of it. It is an indisputable contributor to heart disease, diabetes, psychiatric disorders, and even cancer. Sugar is extremely addictive but also immune system depressing, and inflammatory. Its consumption depletes our bodies of vitamin and mineral stores such as vitamin C, zinc, calcium, and magnesium. It will be the most difficult item to remove from your diet, but that's why you have this spectacular publication to guide you through.

Gem #4:   No Grains, No Pains   41

As in, ALL grains are indigestible by ALL mammals and therefore potentially inflammatory. Everyone's symptoms will vary, but signs of inflammation can be traced back to what you ate in the last 30 minutes and up to 6 weeks after the fact. Lacto-fermentation breaks down the prolamine sub-fraction of the endosperm into smaller amino acid chains, while sprouting can also reduce the gluten content. Rice, corn, oats, wheat, rye, barley, sorghum, and spelt are the most common grains and they all contain their own specific "gluten".

Gem #5:   Cow's Milk is For Calves   57

As in, if you're not a calf, you shouldn't be drinking the milk from a cow. The abundance of naturally-present hormones wreak havoc on our own hormone systems, the endocrine and reproductive systems, and the proteins found in milk increase body tissue acidity as well as contributing to a whole host of auto-immune conditions. Casein, one of the proteins found in milk, is very difficult to break down and consequently presents a slew of inflammatory possibilities to the body as a whole. If you are a new mother having problems nursing your baby, please do not resort to commercial infant formula as all of the manufacturers use copper (II) sulfate, also known as cupric sulfate. This "naturally occurring salt" is toxic and its acute toxicological symptoms mimic those of infant reflux and gastroesophageal reflux disease (GERD).

Gem #6:   Unfermented Soy is Unfit   91
             (For human consumption.)

As in, soy is not a health food, unless it's fermented and organic! 90 percent of the soy crops grown in the U.S. are of the genetically modified Roundup Ready variety, seeds that resist the application of the Monsanto herbicide Roundup. Meaning, soy crops won't die when they get copiously sprayed with Roundup! Meaning, you're eating Roundup! Avoid all unfermented soy and soy derivatives including: vegetable oil, soy flour, soy protein isolate, soy lecithin, tofu, soy milk, tofurkey, edamame, etc. Interestingly enough, Monstanto is also the creator of those Roundup Ready soybeans.

Gem #7:   Save the Olive Oil for Salads   103

As in, don't cook, grill, or bake with it! It is not heat stable, despite what it might say on the bottle or the fact that Rachel Ray pours it into a frying pan every chance she gets. Even low heat can damage and render it inflammatory to the body. Reserve the extra virgin, first cold pressed loveliness for your salads (and for dipping the biscuits and breads found in this book!)

Gem #8:   Fat, Friendly Flora and Lacto-Fermentation   105
            Facilitate Flushing (Way more than fiber alone.)

As in, it takes more than fiber to make this "Constipation Nation" regular. In fact, if you fill your diet with the fiber from 6 to 12 servings of whole grains a day, as recommended by your physician and the dietitian at the Health Board, while pairing that with the recommended "sparing" usage of fats and oils, you're more likely to create a cement-like plug in your colon than to promote healthy elimination. In the U.S., constipation is the number one reason patients present to their health care providers. Probiotics, lacto-fermented foods, and quality fat intake will get you flushing faithfully, while beans, potatoes and leafy greens give you plenty of fiber in your diet so you never have to turn to grains again.

Gem #9:   A Good Egg is a Raw Egg   115

As in, the healthiest way to eat an egg is 1. whole, and 2. raw. Cooking the egg denatures fragile proteins and, cooking the yolk oxidizes precious cholesterol and renders it inflammatory to the body. Put your fears of salmonella poisoning aside by purchasing local eggs laid by hens that truly roam free, while basking in the sun and eating lots of bugs. Better yet, keep your own hens for the absolute freshest eggs! If worse comes to worst, buy the organic version from the grocery store, but be aware that the Horizon brand has been accused in the past of lobbying to lower the standards of organic farming.

Gem #10:   Ideal Body Weight is a Result of Nourished Cells   121
            (You're not fat, you're inflamed and undernourished.)

As in, the *problem* is not obesity. The *symptom* is obesity. In the same way that the emaciation of an anorexic is not simply a need to "gain weight", the overabundance of body mass and physical volume must also be addressed on a systemic level in individuals who are "overweight". I believe if you have struggled with your weight, you are suffering from food allergies and sensitivities that have never even been fathomed by your health care provider, much less mentioned and addressed. And contrary to popular belief, increasing your physical activity is not going to address the root cause of your issue- malnutrition and systemic inflammation due to improper digestion of problematic proteins littering our food system. You're not overweight because you don't exercise enough! Packaged dehydrated meal replacements, bars, shakes, and the myriads of concoctions passing for "food" on the market today does nothing but rub salt in the wounds of those who need to be healed the most. The only way your body can be at its ideal weight is if your cells are nourished and all inflammatory substances in your diet are drastically reduced, if not eliminated. Only then will your body systems heal, and balance be restored.

Gem #11:   Spuds are Spectacular   135

As in, potatoes are a perfect food! They're full of fiber, magnesium, vitamin C, and contain more net usable protein than a cheese stick. They also have the highest satiety index rating more than twice that of its nearest competitor. The key is to eat only those grown organically, with their skins, baked or boiled, and in the presence of a high quality fat or oil (coconut oil or olive oil). Remember to not cook with olive oil, simply use it liberally in the potato salad recipes in the Cookbook part of this spud-tacular publication.

Gem #12: The Right Salt is Pink Salt   143

As in, the only salt that should be in your pantry is Himalayan Pink Salt, also known as Himalayan Rock or Crystal Salt. Over 50 percent of the mineral content of pink salt comes from over 80 different trace minerals. Our problem is that we equate the mineral sodium with the word "salt", and overconsumption of sodium is a huge issue in the Standard American Diet that has led to a whole host of health problems. However, since the body is unable to produce its own minerals, it is imperative that we obtain them from the foods we eat. When you crave salty foods, your body is demanding trace minerals, not just sodium and chloride. Pink salt your food without guilt, and begin savoring every last morsel.

Gem #13:   Artificial Sweeteners Kill   149
             (Brain cells at least.)

As in, they're called excitotoxins and they excite the nerve cells in the brain to death, while actually stimulating your appetite and contributing to numerous digestive and nervous system dysfunction. They kill your weight loss efforts. They kill brain cells. What more is there to say?

As in, chlorine in our water supply has been one of the most double-edged swords of the twenty first century. The fact that it's a poisonous gas that has the capacity, in the right dose, to kill all living things without discrimination (the bad and the good!), should be reason enough to remove it from the pipes before it even enters your house. The tragic less known part is that it contributes to hardening of the arteries leading to inflammation (the makings of heart disease), and the decimation of the good bacteria in the digestive tract.

As in, foods that are cooked at high temperatures as when being grilled on an open flame, deep-fried, broiled, and even browned, begin to form potentially carcinogenic substances called heterocyclic amines (HAAs), acrylamide being one of the most common. These substances are also present in certain canned (in aluminum cans) foods such as tomato paste and black olives; convenience foods like dehydrated soups and products containing soy protein isolates; and snack foods such as potato chips, donuts, and pretzels.

As in, the conventional amount of suggested protein consumption of 1 gram per pound of body weight is simply too much. If the protein is coming from an animal source such as meat or dairy, the metabolic process of digestion and processing results in the acidifying of the body's tissues and the potential for disease and dysfunction- the acid meadow. Pharmaceuticals (legal drugs), coffee, alcohol, refined foods, pasteurized dairy, and synthetic vitamins and minerals also negatively impact the body's alkaline-tending chemisty. Water has a neutral pH of 7. Coffee has an acidic pH of 1 to 2. Optimal body pH is between 7.35 and 7.45. When the body's pH deviates even slightly, chaos begins to reign and the acid meadow flourishes. Akea is an alkaline-forming food with a pH of 8.54.

As in, learn to identify your body's nutritional deficiencies through the hints it provides you via your cravings. Craving chocolate, salt, and fat, is not something you should be ashamed of! The right forms of all of those foods will provide fundamental vitamins, minerals, and brain food that can actually heal you. Honoring your cravings also means learning to differentiate between your body's cries for nutrients and your brain's withdrawal symptoms from inflammatory and addictive substances such as glutens, caseins, hypoxanthine, and artificial food additives.

Gem #18:   Herbs and Spices are Superfoods   199
             (And they're here to heal.)

As in, they actually have a place in your medicine cabinet in addition to your pantry! Preparing your meals with herbs and spices that have healing reputations and a plethora of antioxidants, bioflavonoids, and other organic compounds, will provide your cells with the raw materials to perform and heal at a level beyond our comprehension.

Gem #19:   Nuts and Seeds are Fragile   203
             (Handle them with care.)

As in, their high content of unsaturated fatty acids makes them extremely vulnerable to the damaging effects of oxygen and heat exposure. Milling them to make meals for baking is an unwise practice that contributes to inflammation while giving you a false sense of security that you're "having your cake and eating it too". Prepackaged seed meal like flax has the potential to become rancid long before it reaches your mixing bowl to make "gluten-free" muffins, only to add insult to injury when it's baked in a hot oven for 30 minutes. Do not bake with nuts, almond meal or flax meal. Purchase nuts still in their shells and eat them fresh, as soon as you crack them open.

Gem #20:   Your Skin is a Bigmouth (With no filter.)   207

As in, it gobbles up anything you spread on it because it is your largest organ, and it does not have a filtration system. Toxic chemicals in skin care products can and will be absorbed into your bloodstream, tissues, and organs where they will exert their effects without discretion or mercy. Thousands of questionable chemicals are used in the skin care industry, many even intended for use on children (mineral oil, creams, lotions and sunscreens!), and many of their effects can be as far reaching as those of oral pharmaceuticals.

As in, it's time for us to learn from cultures around the world that have mastered the art of living well, for a longer period of time. The vast majority of us don't need "an average of 2000 calories a day", every day! It's time we realized that the more we eat, even of good food, the more wear and tear we subject our body systems to and the faster they wear out. The phenomenal aspect to this is that when we actually *do* eat *good food,* we just naturally need less of it. This is the basis of super foods: foods that are relatively low in bulk and calories, yet loaded with vitamins, minerals, and phytonutrients to give us vibrant life, naturally.

Part II: The Foundation: Akea Fermented Superfoods and Probiotics

Part III: The Cookbook

Salads, Spuds, and Veggies:

Preface

I'm the type of individual that likes to do things right, the first time around. If I can't do it to my standards in the time I've been allotted, I'd rather put it off until I can. That's kind of an aggravation where issues such as organizing the mounds of paperwork on my desk, or writing a training manual for my office assistant are concerned. It seems to be one of my many quirks that people who interact with me on a daily basis have either learned to accept or at least pretend to not notice. I'm also an individual who has at least 11 different tasks, that all have "Priority 1" attached to them, floating through my mind at any given moment. Well, almost at any given moment. When I walk into an appointment with a client, the only priority on my list is them. I enter a degree of "hyperfocus" that makes me want to put everything else aside to help this ONE individual in my presence. Professionally, I'm the type of clinician who likes to get to the bottom of an issue. By identifying the root of a problem I can effectively help my clients conquer the pain, discomfort or annoyance for which they sought my services. And ultimately, facilitate an acquisition of knowledge about their own bodies that will help them address other concerns above and beyond that initial problem.

My advanced study of nutrition truly began about eight years ago when my eldest daughter developed eczema. She was just over a year old and the eight months that followed varied in degree of misery for her as I tried to figure out how to soothe it, how to keep her from scratching it, what soap to not use on her laundry, and on, and on. It was a most welcome day when I came across a naturopathic physician, two hours away from where we lived at the time, who calmly informed me within the first 3 minutes of my visit that it was something she was eating. She gave me a list of the "8 Most Allergenic Foods: Wheat, Corn, Soy, Dairy, Nuts, Fish, Shellfish and Eggs" and entrusted me with the task of eliminating them all- at the same time. As hopeful a day as it was, it was just as anxiety-promoting. After eliminating all of those foods for two weeks, I was to systematically add one at a time back into her diet to determine which one would cause a recurrence of her symptoms. The task would prove beyond challenging.

It took me longer than I thought or hoped, with the "experiment" lasting close to a year. There was never a moment that I didn't lie in bed at night racking my brain for what food I had introduced into her diet in close proximity to her initial outbreak but it finally came to me. When my breastmilk stores had depleted (dried up), six months after she was born, I tormented over which formula to feed her. She was on dairy for the next few months and then I resorted to soy, thinking that it had to be better than the "hormone-laced" cow's milk variety. One afternoon, she woke up from her nap frantic and wailing, complete with a fever and a raised rash on her chest, back, and belly.

I rushed her to Urgent Care where half way in to our 3 hour wait, she proceeded to throw up her entire lunch, roast beef, cheddar cheese, soy milk bottle and all from 6 hours prior. Thinking the carton of soy milk was possibly past its prime and had been the cause of the incident, I stopped giving her soy milk after that day. It wasn't until a few months later that I began giving her peanut butter, never once thinking the rash incident could have possibly initiated any future potential for immune reaction. But if she had a peanut allergy, her reaction would most likely have been anaphylactic in nature, which it wasn't. The only other ingredient in the peanut butter that could be implicated was partially hydrogenated soybean oil. Apparently peanut butter manufacturers have no qualms about using trans fats in one of the most common foods consumed by children but that's a whole other issue.

The day my eldest daughter woke up screaming from her nap with a fever and a rash, it seems her body had begun producing some antibodies to something she had been exposed to routinely. That something was soy. And the way her immune system attempted to purge the invasion of indigestible soy proteins, was through her delicate skin. After almost two years, we had finally figured it out and within a month of completely eliminating every last source of soy from her diet, her itching had decreased by 90 percent. Within 6 months, her discolored skin was completely healed. Come to find out though that I can't even tolerate it. It elicits irritable bowel symptoms in me and I can certainly do without those. Eight years ago, we became a soy-free family, and have never looked back. But shortly after that experience, I began stepping up my efforts to make sure I was building a solid biological foundation for both my children. With all the research I had done on soy allergies, I spent the next three years studying even more, pouring over books old and new. I would sit at my dining room table until midnight, a baby nursing on my breast and a toddler asleep on the family room floor (fed up with waiting for me to come to bed with her), and scour the web for the truth about how we REALLY should be eating.

I bought a grain mill attachment for my KitchenAid mixer so I could make my own organic whole grain bread. I started cooking only with coconut oil. I even went back to my college chemistry and biology textbooks to make sure I was fully understanding the logic behind the saturated fat and cholesterol controversy (there wasn't any). I bought soy-free chocolate chips, organic gummy bears, raw cheese, and grass-finished meat. I tried to eliminate all sources of "un-whole" foods in my pantry. I finally found sources, both online and in print, who were authorities on these subjects and whose documentation reflected significant consistencies between them. I began to feel more and more confident, after years of confusion, in the changes that I knew had to be made. I made some faster than others. I reneged on certain changes for a while, only to come back to them with greater resolve and conviction. I thought I had it all figured out.

Spending the last five years running a medical spa has made one thing increasingly clear to me. It has become undeniable that almost every person who has ever walked into my office was (and will be!) in need of some degree of nutritional counseling to address the root of the problem they are presenting with. Whether the primary reason for their visit was unwanted facial hair that seemed to sprout up out of nowhere on a female client, or chronic low back pain in a retired Marine, deficiencies in the diet play at least an 80 percent role. This realization ended up becoming quite a distraction considering that not many people expect to come in for laser hair removal and also get a nutrition lesson on what might be contributing to their post-nasal drip.

As a Certified Holistic Nutritional Consultant, Licensed Massage Therapist, Certified Laser Technician and Medical Laser Safety Officer, I have been exposed to an abundance of new clients, year after year, who didn't think their issues had an identifiable aggravating factor. For example, if you have chronic low back pain and have been sporting around 40 extra pounds around your midsection for the last 20 years, it is my ethical responsibility to make aware of the fact that eliminating that load will ease the burden on all of your anatomy, not just your lower back. Or if a mother brings in her acne-riddled teenager for a facial to try to calm his wounded skin, I would be remiss if I didn't bring up the impact of sugar and dietary sources of hormone- disrupting food products. These, of course, are just a couple of the more clear-cut examples of attempting to get to the root of a problem, but my day was consistently fraught with issues similar to these. I felt an anxiety set in if I didn't take steps to make this information known and readily available.

It wasn't until September of 2012 that my own health had hit a proverbial wall. What started off as a sore throat a few days after a non-cosmetic elective surgery, progressed to viral bronchitis, and within a few weeks, viral/allergic asthma. Now, I already knew that when I consumed dairy products, my post-nasal drip increased severely. I would feel as though I was about to "come down with something". I would get a sore throat, my sinuses would become congested, and I would start expectorating- all of the symptoms of the common cold or flu. I had also read on numerous occasions as I studied clinical nutrition for my certifications that there are certain foods that greatly increase the production of mucus in the body. Those foods are dairy products, white flour, and sugar. I resisted making changes in my diet for weeks partly because I just didn't have the energy to entertain the idea of finding a completely new way of feeding not only myself, but also my family (and partly because I loved dairy and white flour). I'm European! My mother baked bread three times a week, and made pizza completely from scratch. I couldn't imagine life without these foods. But I slowly, over the course of almost eight weeks, came to the realization that I was suffocating and drowning in midair.

As it turned out, certain foods that had made up a significant part of my current diet, and that I had been enjoying my entire life, had become instrumental in flooding my respiratory system with excess mucus. The gluten in wheat and the casein in dairy products had slowly trained my immune system to seek out and attempt to isolate those proteins from the rest of my body's tissues by surrounding them with mucous. The proteins, gluten and casein, in those foods resisted the actions of my digestive system, thereby preventing their complete and proper break down, and thus triggered the action of my immune system. I had never in my life been so sick, for such an extended period of time.

So in the last month of my illness, I turned back to the texts and resources I once used in my training to try and "heal myself". I began eliminating the pita bread I used to devour by the basketful at our local Mediterranean eatery, along with the pints of various Ben and Jerry's flavors I always stocked the freezer with, and the effects were alarming. After about 5 days of not eating those food groups, my symptoms lessened notably. But then I'd want to test out my theory and would load 2 tablespoons of butter on my baked potato. Within 20 to 45 seconds of the butter even being in my mouth, I would experience a bronchospasm. If you're not sure what one is, a bronchospasm occurs when the lungs make several aggressive, contracting attempts in close succession to clear themselves of debris and excess mucus. But the bronchioles, or airways leading to the lungs from the windpipe, are too swollen and irritated from all of those unproductive coughs, to allow air back into the lungs. So basically, the lungs can't get anything out and any air the person does take in through their mouth, ends up in their stomach. And then the dry heaves begin. Imagine feeling like you're going to throw up but can't breathe all at once. It's a terrifying feeling if you're experiencing it firsthand, and I can only imagine how much more so if it's happening to an asthmatic child before your very eyes.

Each and every time I "cheated" with either wheat or dairy products, the writing on the wall became bigger and bolder. The post-nasal drip, the phlegm in the back of the throat, the stuffy nose the next morning, the gas and bloating within a few short minutes of the first bite or spoonful, and most notably of all, the bronchospasms. All would return in such close proximity to my consumption that to deny the connection would have been daft. After 6 long weeks of suffering, it had been enough of a foundation-shaking experience that I was determined to put an end to it as soon as I was able.

In November of 2012, our entire household stopped eating wheat and dairy products. No more organic sour cream or butter, and no more whole wheat pita bread either. We had switched to rice bread instead and still enjoyed our oatmeal, rice pasta and organic corn tortilla chips- all of which clearly stated on the packaging that they were "gluten-free". I began suggesting rice bread to my nutrition clients so much so that our grocery store would be out of stock every second time we went to stock up. I decided I would try my hand at making my own and began scouring the internet for "gluten-free" recipes for bread and pancakes and cream puffs. Any recipes I did come across, I had to tweak since they contained some type dairy ingredient such as butter or skim milk powder.

I shopped Amazon.com for a new inventory of flours such as tapioca and brown rice, along with some mysterious powder called xanthan gum (an absolute must in gluten free baking), and conveniently placed my most used products on auto ship. I even started shopping the "gluten-free" aisle of the grocery store and was relieved to find "gluten-free" cake mix. All the while, my symptoms seemed to become less and less noticeable. My "gluten-free" brown rice bread was delicious and appeased my husband and both my daughters. I was even able to make my Thanksgiving stuffing with it, without sacrificing a bit of the flavor or texture of the old wheat bread version.

Thus began the preliminary planning stages of a "gluten-free" cookbook that would also have some traditional recipes I grew up with that didn't have any questionable ingredients in them to begin with. After all, if all you had to do to be "gluten-free" was shop the grocery store aisle by the same name and make your own bread, this was going to be a pretty straightforward endeavor. So I spent the next six months working on recipes using the "safe" foods that from my general knowledge were free of "gluten"- rice, oats, corn. I still wasn't sure what the difference between regular oatmeal and "gluten-free" oatmeal was but I figured I'd spring for the $6 bag of "gluten-free" just to be on the safe side.

In April of 2013, it took a week of twice-daily, organic granola consumption to reveal yet another foundation-shaking fact. By the end of the week, I had personally gone through an entire cereal box, and noticed along the way a steady increase in my mucus production. In my house, we call it "being phlegmy". I couldn't understand what had triggered it and was a bit discouraged at the potential for my hypothesis being disproved. Studying the ingredients list of the granola box, I came across an ingredient called barley malt extract. Call me foolish but, even though I had seen the ingredient before, and even though I knew that barley was on the forbidden list for gluten-intolerant individuals, I simply hoped it was just some kind of "natural" flavoring agent much like vanilla extract, and that it certainly couldn't have any amount of gluten in it, otherwise, why would they put it in something labeled "gluten-free"?

I proceeded to Google what barley malt extract was and whether or not it contained gluten, never once thinking about the veritable Pandora's Box I was about to open. Along with a site belonging to a "Glutenfreedietitian".com, I also came across Dr. Peter Osborne's website, GlutenFreeSociety.org and proceeded to watch, in complete dismay, his video presentation "Gluten For The Layman". In this presentation, Dr. Osborne, a Sugarland, Texas chiropractic physician and Diplomat of the American Clinical Board of Nutrition (DACBN), discusses all grains. What's a grain? Wheat, rye, barley, corn, rice, oats, to name but a few. He also describes the difference between gluten sensitivity and gluten intolerance, as well as all of the diseases that can be caused by gluten intolerance, including the most studied, Celiac disease, as well as in my case, asthma.

Turns out, all grains contain a form of gluten specific to that grain. And if you're sensitive to gluten- you're sensitive to *all* gluten! So if you see a box on the shelf that says "Gluten Free Oats", you've just witnessed "loophole marketing". The only gluten the FDA deems problematic enough to warn consumers against is wheat gluten. As long as a product contains less than 20 parts per million (ppm) of gliadin, the gluten found in wheat, the manufacturer can label the product "gluten-free". So, not only did barley malt extract contain gluten, barley gluten to be exact, but apparently, so did oats- oat gluten to be exact. And rice contains rice gluten, and corn contains corn gluten, and you get where I'm going with this. My entire approach had to completely shift. I, along with every site I had previously tried a recipe from, had been "duped" into thinking that solace could be sought from the big bad gluten monster by baking my cake with rice flour. If I gave people recipes made with corn starch and rice flour, touting them as "gluten-free", I would be playing just as large a part in the "loophole marketing" as the manufacturers who certainly knew better!

You can't tell me that "A Leader in Gluten Free" hasn't come across this news in over 30 years of being in business. But according to their site, their:

> …family has been committed to providing the very best in Gluten Free flours, cereals, baking mixes and grains for our friends on Gluten Free diets. So you could say we know a thing or two about what it takes to make a wide variety of the best products available. You see, we thoroughly batch test every Gluten Free product in our quality control laboratory upon delivery, during production and after packaging…

> To assure the integrity of all of our Gluten Free products, we adhere to a standard of no more than 19 parts per million of gluten. We've even built a separate Gluten Free packaging division complete with specialized machinery to make sure that our products maintain their purity--just as nature intended. By going to these lengths, we're able to ensure that folks with wheat allergies, celiac disease and gluten intolerance can trust that our products are safe to consume.

Finally, the explanation I had been searching for to justify that $6 bag of oatmeal:

> Fortunately, our Gluten Free Oats are guaranteed pure and delicious, free of all gluten contamination. To ensure that they stay just as gluten free as the day their seedlings sprouted from the earth, we test each batch in our quality control laboratory when they arrive from the farm and once again after they are packaged in our dedicated gluten free facility. So if you want the very best quality product, look for the 'Gluten Free' symbol on the packaging-- it's your guarantee that it has passed our lab testing and is of the highest quality.

I'm embarrassed for them, to tell you the truth.

So, let's cut to the chase. The problem is that it's not just *my* digestive system that can't break down those proteins. We are all affected unproductively to some degree by these foods. And as I have discovered over the last year, it wasn't just my respiratory system that had been affected. Lifelong problems concentrating, mood swings, intermittent digestive issues, fluctuating weight and body shape, along with annoying skin issues, all began to dramatically improve once I began consistently abstaining from my newly identified dietary enemies. More and more research is surfacing about foods that humans, in general, should be avoiding. Just because you don't have Celiac Disease, or aren't anaphylactic to peanuts and shellfish, that doesn't mean you have a green light to eat everything the food industry dupes the FDA and USDA into allowing them to market.

In retrospect, over the 35 years of my life, I clearly had some degree of gluten and dairy intolerance. I was diagnosed with IBS when I was 16, my brother with ulcerative colitis when he was 15. Both of those disorders folks are inflammatory bowel conditions. I'm sure there were many other symptoms that we, along with our parents, experienced, and chalked it all up to anything from laziness to personality quirks. It seems so strange to most people when they realize the majority of inflammatory diseases start in the gut with an immune-mediated reaction which then progresses into systemic inflammation and even full-blown autoimmune diseases. To truly be effective at managing or hopefully overcoming physiologic dysfunction, it needs to be addressed on all levels. We MUST isolate and focus on when and where this process starts.

My personal health crisis had led me to explore yet another nutritional field of study, the gluten and casein contribution to inflammation. Especially because it didn't matter if my clients' issues were related to muscle tension and joint pain; acne; wrinkles and fine lines; or coarse, unsightly facial hair, every single one of those issues could dramatically improve if the sufferer's diet was optimized. Hard to believe that ALL of these problems could possibly be rooted in nutrition, but they are. Back in my office, I found myself spending a considerable amount of "extra time" I didn't have jotting down pointers for the client that would give them a starting point. These notes were intended to "whet their appetite" to research more on their own as they embarked on the journey to take control of the underlying causes of the initial problem they had come to see me for. Frustratingly, it was wishful thinking on my part. There was just way too much information to be relayed in fifteen minutes, or even an hour! Not to mention the anxiety all this information had precipitated could be read all over the person's face (no matter how excited they were about this "wealth of knowledge" they had been exposed to).

The fact of the matter remains: we chase our tails, day in and day out, trying to figure out how to eat, what to eat- to be healthy, happy, skinny, and free of pain. We become frustrated with each new "discovery" about how to stay healthy, happy, and skinny, since it just so happens to contradict the last new "discovery" five years ago of how to do the same. We fall prey to every new product on the market with the words, "Cholesterol Free", "Low Fat", "Natural" and "Gluten-Free" on its sleazy packaging. We don't know how our bodies work. We can't distinguish truth from marketing ploys. We're confused about which fats are "healthy" and which ones should be used as motor oil. We don't know what grains are and we think eggs are dairy products. We know sugar is bad for us so we try to replace it with pesticides and coal tar derivatives. We let history repeat itself and delude ourselves into thinking we can outsmart nature. And all those little annoyances you feel the need to take care of at your local medical spa, cosmetics counter, dermatologist's office, and gym (yes I said it, obesity is not caused by lack of exercise), are all due to capitulating to faulty nutritional dogma. We're in rough shape inside and out. And sending lawyers, guns, and money, is only going to make the fan stinkier.

After almost two years since my personal health crisis temporarily derailed me, I have carved out the path that my family and I will happily not deviate from. I finally gave the grains to my chickens. Bid goodbye to even the raw goat cheddar and tossed he organic gummy bears in the trash bin. We don't eat any grains, soy, or dairy products. We even gave up meat in the summer of 2013. The last thirty six years of my life have culminated in these pages. This is it. This is having your chocolate chip cookie and not feeling like a blimp afterward. This is soaking up your runny yolk with a fresh-baked garlic and herb biscuit; country fried potatoes without heartburn and atherosclerosis. It's realizing why when you crave chocolate, you'd better eat chocolate (the whole food kind!)

I've allowed my *Grain Brain* to procrastinate long enough and hope this guide finally gets you on the right path to lose your *Wheat Belly,* learn *The Whole Soy Story,* so you *Don't Drink Your Milk* and finally free yourself from the *Sugar Blues.* Because it really has been *The Great Cholesterol Con* over the past fifty years, that has led us to seriously examine *Nutrition and Physical Degeneration.* Consider the path cleared of soybean speed bumps and pasteurized potholes. Free from irrational, unfounded fear of cholesterol and "salt", but also void of damaged pourable oils, mishandled nuts and seeds and their respective "meals".

For every woman who has walked into my office with coarse, unsightly facial hair, this book is for you. For every child with eczema whose skin is eating them alive, this book is for their parents. For every child whose asthma chokes them into despair, this book is for their parents too. For every Marine who spends 3 hours in the gym, six days a week so they can try to "make weight", this book is for them. For every person who wants to finally eat right but doesn't know where to start, this book is for you. Don these Censored Nutritional Gems and begin to share them. You will see your life and the lives of those whom you hold dear begin to sparkle with happiness, clarity of mind, and unequivocal good health. The gag order has been lifted: saturated fat rocks and cholesterol is king- always has been, always will be.

Part I

The Guide:
21 Censored Nutritional Gems

Introduction:
Unearthing the Censored Nutritional Gems

We are in the midst of a huge paradigm shift. What we've been told and what has been preached by those we entrusted our health to in the medical community about heart disease, cancer, weight loss, and nutrition in general, for the past 50 some odd years is finally being challenged, and rightfully so.

Here we are in this era with access to quality information, coming from unbiased experts from around the world. Physicians, clinical nutritionists, chemists, biologists, scientists worthy of Nobel Peace Prizes, and research warriors- individuals who pour over books, professional publications, reference texts and numerous other publications- give us perspectives and information that, even though may be logical and seem like the most prudent way to approach these subjects of health and nutrition, have for one reason or another been suppressed, censored even.

It is the censoring of this information that many believe has contributed so abundantly to the pathetic state of our health as a population. We've been doing what we've been told; staying away from butter, and not eating egg yolks and eating 6 to 12 servings of whole grains a day, and to what benefit? We're in the worst shape, literally and figuratively, in the recorded history of mankind. We tried to pull the sugar out of our diets over a hundred years ago by replacing it with saccharin, which was discovered while experiments with coal tar derivatives were being conducted at Johns Hopkins University. Yet somehow we are perfectly on course by the year 2050 to have 33% of our population diagnosed with Type II Diabetes.

According to current statistics from the Centers for Disease Control and Prevention (CDC), 1 in 3 Americans will die from cardiovascular disease, in one form or another, each year. It is the leading cause of death in America today and "people of all ages and backgrounds can get the condition". So, don't think because you're 25, you're not on the hit list. That's a pretty sad fact that one third of deaths each year are due to a condition that the CDC maintains 80% of which could be prevented if people would just change what they ate, exercised on a regular basis and stopped smoking. Basically, something has to change. The modern method of staying "healthy" just isn't working.

So, if ever there was a perfect time to alter the course of your longevity by learning what you're made of, how your body works, and how what you eat, think and do, can help you live exceptionally, that time is now! You're about to unearth a collection of *Censored Nutritional Gems* that will help you take control of your wellness- right here, right now. Put your thinking cap, *and apron*, on and get ready to be liberated!

1
SatFatRox

Has anyone ever told you you're not eating enough fat? That's a new one, isn't it? I tell my clients that all the time because they're not. And you're not. The vast majority of us in the Western world are not eating enough *fat*. Fats are naturally solid at room temperature. How much of that kind of fat are you eating daily? Oh, you're getting plenty of *oil*- rancid, damaged, inflammatory oil. And you're probably also getting what you think is "naturally" solid at room temperature in the forms of hydrogenated and partially oils. But the stuff your cell membranes and brain are made of, the stuff that your sex hormones and happy brain chemicals are synthesized from- you're not getting nearly the right amount of those on a daily basis. And in order to get enough of those RIGHT fats, you must consume fatty foods that are naturally solid at room temperature- saturated fat.

We're going to examine this issue of "not getting enough" in just a bit, but let's first identify where you would find saturated fats as a whole. From the website of the Weston A. Price Foundation for Wise Traditions in Food Farming, and the Healing Arts, www.WestonAPrice.org, "... saturated fats, such as butter, coconut oil and palm oil, and meat fats like beef tallow and suet tend to be solid at room temperature." Saturated fats are termed so because of their greater number of hydrogen atom bonds than their unsaturated counterparts. It's what makes them very stable or resistant to damage, in the presence of oxygen and heat. It's what differentiates them from the pourable or liquid at room temperature oils, which are unsaturated (examples would be olive oil, canola, soybean deceptively known as vegetable oil, sunflower oil, and any other oil pressed from a nut or seed, or legume.) Again from westonaprice.org,

> According to conventional nutritional dogma also known as the teachings of the allopathic or Western medical community, these traditional fats are to blame for most of our modern diseases--heart disease, cancer, obesity, diabetes, malfunction of cell membranes and even nervous disorders like multiple sclerosis. However, many scientific studies indicate that it is processed liquid vegetable oil--which is laden

with free radicals formed during processing--and artificially hardened vegetable oil--called trans fat--that are the culprits in these modern conditions, not natural saturated fats we've been led to believe.

In the interest of really gaining a clear understanding of this topic, let's define the terms fatty acid, triglyceride, fats, and oils. Fats and oils are made up of substances called triglycerides and triglycerides are formed when three fatty acid molecules are attached to a glycerol molecule. Glycerol is an alcohol, specifically a sugar alcohol or polyol. Other examples of polyols are the non-nutritive sugar substitute xylitol, along with sorbitol and mannitol.

Now, if we take an even closer look, chemically speaking, fatty acids are actually chains of carbon atoms with hydrogen atoms as "arms", and a "tail" of a glycerol molecule. The important thing to remember is that those fatty acids are organic molecules and they are found in both plants AND animals in varying proportions. It is the way the carbon atoms are connected to one another in that chain that deems a fatty acid saturated or unsaturated. If the carbons in the chain are all connected by something called a *single* bond, it means that every carbon atom shares *one* pair of electrons, or as it would appear in Figure 1A, one electron "in front" and one electron "behind". The other two available electrons on the carbon are attached to, or "saturated" with, hydrogen atoms- two to be exact- one on the "left", and one on the "right".

Figure 1A. Author-created

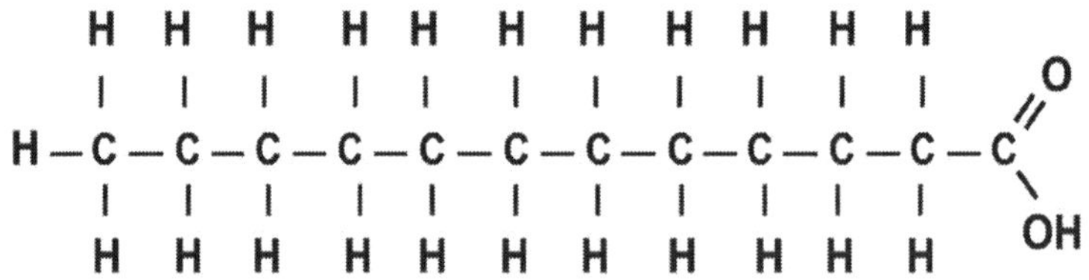

Saturated Fatty Acid

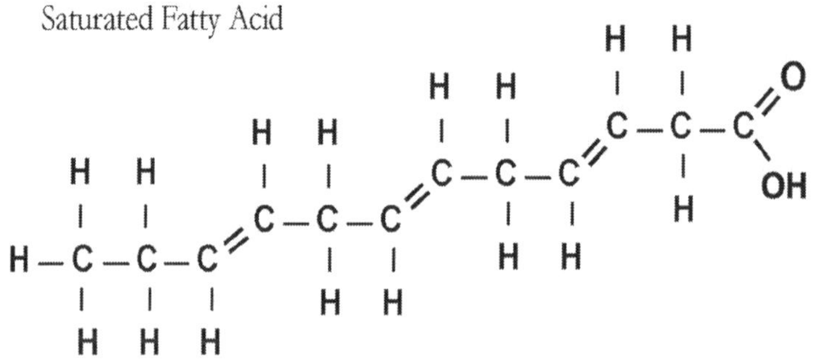

Polyunsaturated Fatty Acid

Conversely, if the chain of carbons contains two carbons bonded to each other via something called a *double* bond, it means they share *two* pairs of electrons and those are called UN-saturated bonds. So a saturated fat is composed of mostly saturated fatty acids and unsaturated oils are composed mostly of unsaturated fatty acids. When we say that saturated fatty acids are saturated with hydrogen atoms, that's because instead of sharing that second pair of electrons in their outer shell with another carbon, that pair of electrons is shared by two hydrogen atoms. Notice also how, in the diagram, the saturated fatty acid has a "straight" structure, where the unsaturated one has more of a zigzag pattern? It's that zigzag pattern that can lead to parts of the fatty acid being disrupted by situations such as exposure to heat, when the other fatty acid molecules begin to collide with one another. Or when free radicals like oxygen atoms "bounce" against the fatty acid and can again change the overall structure by changing the direction of one of the branches. So, it is the sound chemical structure of the saturated fatty acid that lends to the stability of the substance in the presence of oxygen and heat.

You've probably heard the terms mono- and poly- associated with unsaturated oils such as olive oil and canola oil (boo, hiss). Mono-unsaturated means that the particular substance is made up chiefly of fatty acids with only ONE double bond somewhere in that chain of carbons. An example of a mono-unsaturated fatty acid would be the omega-9 oleic acid found in olive oil and walnuts. *Polyunsaturated* means that there is more than one double bond occurring somewhere along the chain. An example of such a compound would be the omega-3 essential fatty acid, linolenic acid (alpha linolenic or ALA).

The truth is that both saturated and unsaturated fatty acids are naturally occurring and required for life. The unspoken part is that unsaturated fatty acids must be treated with the utmost respect so that they don't become damaged, and consequently, something not found in nature. The body is designed to recognize, utilize, and benefit only from substances occurring in nature, so it only makes sense that if you introduce a damaged oil into the body, you're going to sound an alarm (or 5). The two saturated fatty acids in Figure 1B on the next page are lauric and stearic. Note how they lack any double-bonds between their carbons.

Such is also the case with man-made substances such as partially hydrogenated oil, or trans-fatty acids. These are made from pourable oils through a very highly involved process that results in the "straightening" of the chemical structure of the oil so that it resembles a saturated fatty acid and maintains a state that is solid at room temperature. It even acquires a much higher melting and smoking point than the naturally occurring saturated fat. But guess what? You can't fool the body. It recognizes that the new substance is not one of the tools it normally depends on to heal and function, and instead, an inflammatory reaction is triggered as it tries to dilute the toxicity of the imposter and minimize any possible harm it could do to the tissues. Figure 1C illustrates an original unsaturated fatty acid before and after hydrogenation.

Figure 1B Author-created

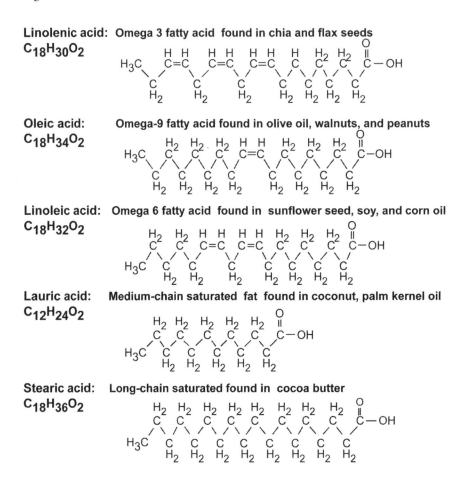

Humans need saturated fats because we are warm-blooded and our bodies do not function at "room temperature". Our bodies maintain a temperature of about 98 degrees and that's pretty tropical considering some folks like their rooms at around 70 degrees. Saturated fats provide the appropriate stiffness and structure to our cell membranes and tissues. When we consume a lot of liquid unsaturated oils, our cell membranes do not have structural integrity to function properly, they become too "floppy," and when we consume a lot of trans fat, which is not as soft as saturated fats at body temperature, our cell membranes become too "stiff." This is where the confusion lies in mainstream information sources.

Figure 1C. Source: www.indiana.edu/~oso/Fat/trans

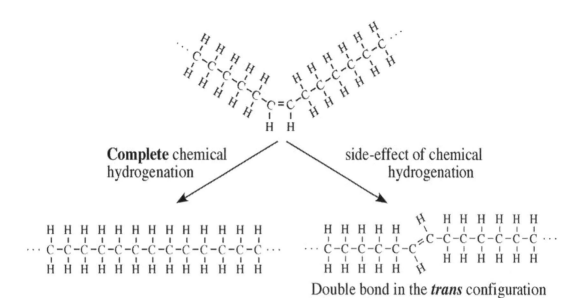

Complete chemical hydrogenation

side-effect of chemical hydrogenation

Double bond in the ***trans*** configuration

People too often confuse man-made trans fats, also known as hydrogenated or partially hydrogenated oils, with naturally occurring saturated fats. They are not the same thing! And contrary to the accepted view, which is not scientifically-based, saturated fats do not clog arteries or cause heart disease. In fact, the preferred food for the heart is saturated fat; and saturated fats lower substance called Lp(a), which is a very accurate marker for proneness to heart disease.

Saturated fats play many important roles in the chemistry of the body. They strengthen the immune system and are involved in inter-cellular communication, which means they have the ability to protect us against cancer by "alerting" the cells around them when they detect a cell not functioning as it should. They help the receptors on our cell membranes work properly, including receptors for insulin, thereby protecting us against diabetes. The lungs cannot function without saturated fats, and saturated fats are also involved in kidney function and hormone production. Perhaps one of the most significant responsibilities of saturated fats, especially considering the tragic psychological state of our population, is the role they play in the functioning of the central nervous system or CNS.

If you're not familiar with the components of the nervous system, they include the brain, spinal cord, and all of the nerves branching out from the spinal cord. The spinal cord is actually a bundle of nerves that leaves the brain and runs down the length of our spine, within which it is safely housed. The spinal cord serves to mediate communication between the brain and every single part of the body via nerves. Nerve cells, also known as neurons, can vary in length from less than 1 millimeter, as those found in the brain itself, and as long as 3 feet, like the sciatic nerve that runs from the spinal cord all the way to the big toe. Nerves are conduits of electrochemical power that allow communication between the brain and the rest of the body's organs and muscles, and back again. Those very nerve cells are "insulated" with a sheath made of saturated fat that facilitates faster conduction of messages, or impulses, up and down the nerve, back and forth between the brain and the specific area the nerve innervates. And not only are saturated fats required for the nervous system to function properly, but over half the fat in the brain is of the saturated variety! That says a lot since the brain is 60 percent fat.

Considering the degree of importance of the responsibilities outlined above, you would think that saturated fat would have a "minimum daily consumption recommendation" on a nutrition label vice a "maximum". Numerous physicians, clinical nutritionists, and lipid chemists even advise we consume at least 50-60% of our total daily calories from fats and oils- with the majority of those calories coming specifically from saturated fats! That would mean if you're eating a 2000 calorie a day diet, you should be consuming at least 55 grams of the stuff! Chew on that for a minute while we consider the maximum recommended daily intake of saturated fat per the guidelines of the USDA.

* Percent Daily Values are based on a 2000 Calorie diet. Your daily volumes may be higher or lower depending on you calorie needs.

	Calories	2,000	2,500
Total Fat	Less than	65g	80g
Sat fat	Less than	20g	25g
Cholesterol	Less than	300mg	300mg
Sodium	Less than	2,400mg	2,400mg
Potassium		3,500mg	3,500mg
Total Carbohydrate		300g	375g
Dietary Fiber		25g	30g
Protein		50g	65g

Calories per gram
Fat 9 · Carbohydrate 4 · Protein 4

Notice how on a typical nutrition label the recommended daily amount of saturated fat amounts to 20 grams out of a total fat suggestion of 65 grams, for a 2,000 calorie a day diet. Now, if you were following the advice of those numerous physicians, clinical nutritionists, and lipid chemists, your total daily fat intake would be more like 110 grams per day!

Add to this equation how verboten fat has been in general over the last 50 years, and I'm sure most of the people in the Western world, who believe they're eating "healthy", would be nowhere near noshing on 65 grams of any fat in a day, saturated or otherwise. So, let's suspend disbelief for a moment to assume that we *are* getting the right amount of "satfat" by following the USDA recommendations. What would you have to eat in one day to get to the amount of 20 grams of saturated fat? One whole egg contains 1.5 grams. One tablespoon of butter contains 8 grams, and one chicken breast, with the skin, contains about 7 grams. But wait! You stay away from butter and only buy skinless chicken breast, so you're only getting about 1.5 grams from that "heart-healthy" version. If you did eat one whole egg, along with 2 tablespoons of butter, and one skinless chicken breast, *every day*, you're still only racking up 19 grams of saturated fat- less than half of what the true experts on fats and oilsactually suggest! Are you eating 2 tablespoons of butter and one whole egg every day? *Quod erat demonstrandum*! And even if you are, you still need to double-up!

Human beings have been consuming saturated fats from animal products, raw milk products and the tropical oils for thousands of years. The last hundred years of modern processed vegetable oils, not the consumption of saturated fats, have brought with them the epidemic of modern degenerative diseases. Saturated animal fats not only carry the vital fat-soluble vitamins A, D and K2, which we need in large amounts to be healthy, but they also facilitate the body's ability to actually process and absorb those fat-soluble vitamins.

How that relates to our food is that if something is composed mainly of saturated fatty acids, its physical state of matter at room temperature is going to be solid or semi-solid. An example of a solid saturated fat would be cocoa butter- it looks a like a chunk of white chocolate actually. Coconut oil is an example of a saturated fat that can vary in its solidity in that, at a temperature of about 76 degrees Fahrenheit, it is liquid, at 72 degrees Fahrenheit is semi-solid but still spreadable, but at 65 degrees Fahrenheit, it's pretty solid. It's also a fantastic superfood that we will be using consistently in our cooking.

Coconut oil and palm kernel oil are nature's richest sources of the medium chain saturated fatty acid, lauric acid, which is widely known as a natural anti-fungal, anti-viral, and anti-microbial agent, and of which, only mother's milk has a higher concentration. Palm kernel oil comes from the seed of the palm fruit, not to be confused with red palm oil, which is actually pressed from the fruit itself, and yet another fantastic, highly-saturated oil that can be used for cooking and baking. Conversely, an unsaturated fatty acid substance would be pourable even at temperatures nearing 45 to 60 degrees Fahrenheit, so considerably colder but still fluid. We actually refer to them as oils, as opposed to fats. Examples would be olive oil, almond oil, soybean goop, peanut oil and pretty much any other oil pressed from a seed, nut or legume (remember that peanuts and soybeans are legumes, not vegetables).

The reason bonds are so important, not just in cooking but also in our diets overall, is that unsaturated bonds are relatively reactive and chemically unstable. So situations like extreme increases in temperature or prolonged exposure to oxygen can basically change the structure of that original molecule and possibly damage it or oxidize it, and that can make it inflammatory to the body if that damaged fatty acid is consumed. Excessive inflammation is bad. Eating damaged oils leads to excessive inflammation. Saturated fat resists damage from heat and exposure to oxygen. It's what our brains are made of. Deprive the body of dietary saturated fat, and you deprive the brain of its ability to function and heal itself. Starve your diet of saturated fat and suffer the wrath of cognitive disorders like dementia and Alzheimer's; emotional disorders like anxiety and depression; reproductive and endocrine disorders; and on, and on, and on.

Censored Nutritional Gem #1: SatFatRox

Suggested reading:

The Cholesterol Myths: Exposing the Fallacy that Saturated Fat and Cholesterol Cause Heart Disease, Uffe Ravnskov, MD

Know Your Fats: The Complete Primer for Understanding the Nutrition of Fats, Oils, and Cholesterol, Mary G. Enig, Ph. D

The Coconut Oil Miracle, Bruce Fife, ND

Saturated Fat May Save Your Life, Bruce Fife, ND

Cholesterol and Saturated Fat Prevent Heart Disease - Evidence from 101 Scientific Papers, David Evans

Eat Fat Lose Fat, Mary Enig, PhD and Sally Fallon

Fats That Heal, Fats That Kill, Udo Erasmus, PhD

The last word on saturated fat goes to…

Elizabeth Walling, a freelance writer specializing in health and family nutrition. She is a strong believer in natural living as a way to improve health and prevent modern disease. She enjoys thinking outside of the box and challenging common myths about health and wellness. Find her article (reprinted below with permission) and download her ebooks, *The Nourished Metabolism*, and *Love Your Body*, on her website, www.LivingTheNourishedLife.com.

More Coconut Oil Benefits: Lauric Acid

The benefits of coconut oil truly reach far and wide, but certain components of this tropical oil stand out for their valuable contribution to good health. Lauric acid, a medium-chain fatty acid found mainly in coconut oil, is one of these prized substances. Pure coconut oil contains about 50 percent lauric acid, and is the most abundant natural source of lauric acid available.

How the Body Uses Lauric Acid

When lauric acid is present in the body, it is converted into monolaurin, a monoglyceride compound which exhibits antiviral, antimicrobial, antiprotozoal and antifungal properties. It acts by disrupting the lipid membranes in organisms like fungus, bacteria and viruses, thus destroying them.

The compound monolaurin is an effective treatment for candida albicans and fungal infections like ringworm and athlete's foot. Monolaurin also specifically targets bacterial infections as well as lipid-coated viruses like herpes, the measles, influenza, hepatitis C and HIV. Researchers in the Philippines have even begun studies to prove the effectiveness of lauric acid against HIV/AIDS because of its strong antiviral properties. Plus, lauric acid is basically non-toxic, which gives it a distinct advantage over modern pharmaceutical drugs that are typically used to fight viruses, bacterial infections and fungal infections. Without a plentiful source of lauric acid, the body cannot produce monolaurin, and all of these important benefits are lost. Many people who regularly consume coconut oil experience less sickness.

Breast milk is the only other natural source that contains such a high concentration of lauric acid, which could explain the drastic decrease of infections of all types in breast-fed babies.

A Missing Element in Today's Diet

The lauric acid content of foods and infant formulas has been rapidly decreasing over the years. Manufacturers and consumers alike have turned from using coconut oil and have replaced it with cheap vegetable oils, obliterating lauric acid intake in the process.There is no recommended daily allowance (RDA) for lauric acid, but as a guideline, Dr. Mary G. Enig suggests adults and growing children can benefit from an intake of 10 to 20 grams of lauric acid per day. It's interesting to note that nursing babies consume up to 1 gram of lauric acid per kilogram of body weight per day.

You can get about two grams of lauric acid from one tablespoon of dried coconut, and quality coconut milk will contain about three and a half grams per two ounces. But coconut oil by far contains the best concentration of lauric acid - about seven grams per tablespoon. Renowned coconut oil experts like Mary Enig and Bruce Fife recommend the average person eat about three tablespoons of coconut oil each day. This amount will not only provide protection against bacteria and viruses, but it will also increase your metabolism and improve the condition of your skin and hair, in addition to many other benefits.

To reap the full benefits of using coconut oil, choose a high-quality source that offers coconut oil in its best form: organic, cold-pressed and extra virgin.

References:

McCullough, Fran. (2003). The Good Fat Cookbook. Published by Simon and Schuster Adult Publishing.

Murray, Michael. (2005) Encyclopedia of Healing Foods. Published by Simon and Schuster Adult Publishing.

2
Cholesterol is King

It's time to discuss that dreaded, naughty C-word. It's enough to make us cringe and conform to any demands those entrusted with our care make on our diets. How bad is your bad and how high is your good? And what do all those letters mean anyway: HDL, IDL, LDL, VLDL? Do you really even need it? And why does all the stuff that's high in it taste so darn good? I'm talking about cholesterol, a word with enough shame attached to it that its mere untterance scares us into a confessional.

We cross our fingers when we leave the lab after having blood drawn, hoping the results don't earn us too vicious a tongue-lashing from our doctor when we return to discuss them, Please don't be over 200, pretty, pretty please! Praying our LDL is low enough and our HDL is high enough, but never really understanding the connection between the various "types" and what makes one bad and the other good. You just know that it's in your blood, some people have more of it and some have less. I'm certain I've never heard someone not having enough of it. Here's a question for you: has your doctor or primary care manager ever told you what your body even does with the stuff? Considering that your very own liver produces cholesterol, wouldn't you think that there has to be a reason for this? There must be, at the very least, a use for it, if not a demand? The next time you visit your primary care manager, ask them this simple question, "Why does my very own liver- my body's main detoxification organ- produce cholesterol?" And when they can't give you an answer, you can give them this book.

The liver is the site of cholesterol production via a process known as the mevalonate pathway. As the body's demands and needs for cholesterol increase (because the body demands and needs cholesterol), the liver and intestine theoretically have the ability to synthesize sufficient amounts of cholesterol to meet those needs through the mevalonate pathway. Hannah Yoseph, MD, author of *How Statin Drugs Really Lower Cholesterol, and Kill You One Cell at a Time*, describes mevalonate as cell food, much in the same way as glucose is brain food. Through a series of steps and enzyme actions, the details of which are beyond the scope of this guide, mevalonate is eventually converted to cholesterol after taking the form of numerous intermediates called isoprenoids. Isoprenoids are a caegory of non-steroidal compounds that are essential for normal activity in the cell. Notice how I'm trying to emphasize the word "normal"? Meaning, if you prevent the cell from being able to make substances such as dolichols, heme A, ubiquinone, and isopentenyl-adenosine, all of which are isoprenoids, you prevent the cell from being able to function normally. Once all of those substances are progressively synthesized, one last enzymatic action results in the production of cholesterol. And it is that freshly-synthesized, unoxidized, cholesterol that then must feed into several other pathways to form steroid hormones, vitamin D, bile acids, and other lipoproteins. Which, at the risk of sounding like a broken record, *are all essential for cells to function normally.*

Alrighty then! Now, let's discuss the acronyms: HDL, IDL, LDL, and VLDL. These are all lipoproteins. Though you're probably most familiar with HDL and LDL, which we've been told also answer to the names "Good" and "Bad" respectively, there are a couple more that you should know of. I'm thinking IDL would be christened "Ugly" and that would leave VLDL as "Voldemort: Le Dark Lord", or more aptly, "He Who Shall Not Be Mentioned", since they never have the courage to scold you about how high it is, let alone bring it up in conversation.

I know that the terms cholesterol and lipoproteins are used interchangeably many times, especially by healthcare professionals who failed organic chemistry or "passed" because the professor was left with no choice but to grade on a curve, but they're not the same thing at all. Not even a tiny bit. HDL stands for High Density Lipoprotein, that's the "good" guy (they say). LDL stands for Low Density Lipoprotein, that's the "bad guy". VLDL stands for VERY Low Density Lipoprotein. That would be the "Dark Lord". And IDL stands for Intermediate Density Lipoprotein. A lipoprotein is a substance made up of approximately equal amounts of lipids and proteins. *What's a lipid?* The word lipid is actually an umbrella term for a whole host of compounds found in both plants and animals that do not interact cooperatively with water but that do have the potential to provide energy in the form of calories.

But saying that lipids are fats would actually be backwards. Fats and oils are types of lipids. But so are waxes. Then you have a separate category of substances that have some of the same qualities as lipids but cannot be used as sources of energy, and those are called lipoids. That piece of information will play an important role later on but for now, commit to memory the fact that a lipoprotein is a combination of a lipid and a protein and when you add all those L's together after you left the lab, you get what's called your *total lipoprotein profile*. Please note that I did not utter the C-word at all in this paragraph. Until now. Cholesterol is NOT a type of fat. Fat is used for energy, it has calories. Cholesterol is not a fatty acid like the omega-3-6-9s. Cholesterol is not saturated or unsaturated. It has no caloric value, meaning your body cannot and does not use cholesterol as a source of energy.

You've seen words like waxy and fatty describing cholesterol and what thoughts come to mind beyond, *Well of course it clogs your arteries, it's fatty and waxy and sticky, much like taffy.* It doesn't come in the form of good, bad, or ugly, as the confused, inflamed, (and I'm certain, constipated) physician's assistant tried to tell me when I picked up my dreaded numbers in November of 2013. However, it is possible to turn it into something bad and ugly when you expose it to heat or the damaging actions of free radicals.

When you heat cholesterol above a certain temperature, it oxidizes. Oxidized cholesterol creates unnecessary inflammation. That same poor physician's assistant also tried to tell me that cholesterol is the same as a lipoprotein. It isn't. There is only one cholesterol, with one chemical formula, no matter where it's found in the human body, in animals, or in our food- and it is not a lipoprotein. Where ever did we get the idea that lipoproteins are the same as cholesterol? Probably the same place we got the idea that it and saturated fats clog arteries. Either way, the truth is about to set you free. Lipoproteins are transporters of cholesterol throughout the body. Why would lipoproteins do a ridiculous thing like that? Because it's their job. Because cholesterol is not responsible for all the evil in the world as it has been accused for the last fifty years. And because cholesterol is not water-soluble, so it needs a method of transportation through a water-based liquid (your blood).

In organic chemistry, when a compound or substance ends in the letters –ol, like xylitol, sorbitol, or methanol- that substance is referred to as an alcohol. Some other examples of alcohol molecules you might be familiar with are ethanol, which is the alcohol that occurs naturally in wine, beer and spirits. Then we have isopropyl alcohol, also known as "rubbing alcohol". Glycerol is the alcohol molecule that holds the three fatty acid groups in triglycerides together. (Remember that a triglyceride is just the word for the chemical form that most fat exists in when it's found in the food we eat as well as in the body.) Alcohols are some of the most common organic compounds pertaining to life, and by organic, we mean that the molecular structure of that compound is made up of one or more atoms of the element carbon.

So just what is cholesterol? Basically, it's an alcohol. Specifically, one of high molecular weight, which along with other extremely important substances in the body called steroids, can be categorized as a lipid. Glycerides, fatty acids (both saturated and unsaturated), lipoproteins, and non-glycerides such as sphingolipids and waxes also fall under that category. So, it's the fact that cholesterol falls under that broad "lipid" umbrella that has confused many of us into accepting the idea that could clog arteries. More recently though, cholesterol has actually been referred to as a "lipoid", and that underscores the fact that cholesterol is not only a steroid in its own right, but also the precursor (or starting point) for other steroids in the body. Steroids act as anti-inflammatory agents and are necessary for homeostasis- the ability or tendency of an organism or cell to maintain internal equilibrium by adjusting its physiological processes. A homeostatic imbalance would be any situation where the body has to adjust business as usual to accommodate for the disturbance in the force. If they're not dealt with quickly, homeostatic imbalances become opportunities for dysfunction, which can then lead to dis-ease and dis-order.

Yet another one of cholesterol's extremely important roles in the body, as a primary constituent of cell membranes, is due largely in part to its chemical structure. Being an alcohol of high molecular weight decreases cholesterol's solubility in water. Here's why: one molecule of cholesterol is made up of 27 atoms of carbon, 45 atoms of hydrogen, and one hydroxyl or OH group, where ethanol (drinkable version is called ethyl alcohol which is a mixture of ethanol and water), is composed of only 2 atoms of carbon, 5 atoms of hydrogen and one hydroxyl group. Even if you don't understand the core of that info, just look at the numbers and employ more than and less than. The reason this is so important is that alcohols of low molecular weight are highly soluble in water and have the propensity to become one homogenous solution or mixture. That's why you can mix pomegranate juice with vodka (which is ethyl alcohol) and not have it look like oil and vinegar. But if you look closely when you pour alcohol into a glass of water, you're going to notice a shimmer almost as the alcohol enters the water and then slowly mixes with it. That shimmer would be much more noticeable the higher the molecular weight of that alcohol. Why? Because with increased molecular weight, alcohols become less soluble in water.

So cholesterol is a naturally-occurring, organic compound and it is found in most animal tissues because it is an integral component of cell membranes. Our bodies and those of all animals are made up of billions of tiny little things called cells and every single one of them is surrounded by a cell membrane. Think of the cell membrane as the continuous bubble surrounding a castle in the clouds (humor me), both above it and below it. Its purpose is protection- from the "elements", from "invaders", but built strategically with drawbridges and gates to allow certain visitors to enter and keep out the ones who bring down property values. That cell membrane is made of three main things: a type of lipid called a phospholipid which is comprised of both unsaturated and saturated fatty acids (but a higher percentage of saturated fatty acids!); protein channels that act as "gates"; and guess what else? Cholesterol. Now imagine instead of cholesterol, our membranes contained the low molecular weight alcohol, ethanol. You'd end up with "leaky cell syndrome", unable to control what entered or what departed.

A couple other characteristics of a high molecular weight alcohol are that its or melting point, density and viscosity is also higher. So, they're denser, less runny, they're not as miscible, meaning they don't dissolve well in water and that makes them the perfect structural material for building protective walls like our cell membranes. They have to be that way because they have to guard one of the most important structures inside the cell, the nucleus- command central of the cell. The nucleus is not membrane-bound, and that does not bode well for its contents, our DNA. Every virus and parasitic organism would love to gain access to our DNA (our genetic code). Our DNA does everything from telling a cell to behave in a certain way or exhibit a certain trait; it can turn a cell against the very body it lives in and even instruct that cell to self-destruct. The long and short of it: We must protect this house. "This house" being each and every one of our cells. And the way we do that is by making sure the cell membrane can repair itself when necessary by having ready access to its constituents- both unsaturated and saturated fatty acids, amino acids (the building blocks of proteins), and cholesterol.

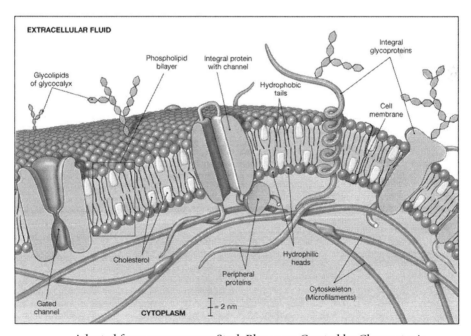

Adapted from source: www.StudyBlue.com; Created by Classmates in
Biology & Chemistry 2083 2011-12 with Professor Krosnick at Southern
Arkansas University

While standing guard in the cell membrane, cholesterol can become "wounded". The correct term for wounded cholesterol is actually oxidized cholesterol. But once the cholesterol in a cell membrane has been oxidized by substances like free radicals and other toxins, it must be replaced. But how? In chariots called lipoproteins! A lipoprotein functions as a transporter of cholesterol in the blood. Cholesterol has to be transported to and from the cells by these carriers. It's carried *away* from the cell by HDL "chariots", to be disposed of after it's been wounded, and a fresh batch is delivered to replace the damaged and oxidized. High density lipoproteins (HDL) remove the damaged cholesterol and drop it off in the gallbladder, where it is converted to bile salts, which are then "dumped" into the large intestine to be excreted out of the body through the feces (provided there actually is movement occuring in the large intestine. See chapter 8 if you're a citizen of the Constipation Nation).

So HDL is touted as a hero because it is indirectly removing cholesterol from the body. But "that" cholesterol should be removed because it has served its purpose and must be replaced. Enter the dreaded LDL. Did you know that a cell has the ability to actually increase the number of LDL receptors in its membrane in an effort to "catch" more fresh cholesterol to meet increasing cell demands? Low-density lipoproteins carry fresh cholesterol to the cell to replace what HDL carted away and to provide the cell with life-supporting raw building materials. How is that a bad thing? If your LDL count is off the charts, it's because the cholesterol in your cell membranes is being damaged at an abnormally high rate. An elevated LDL level means the body is trying to maintain the homeostatic balance of protecting the contents of your cells by delivering fresh cholesterol from its production center, the liver. Taking a statin drug to lower LDL blocks the enzyme in the liver that produces cholesterol, by disrupting the mevalonate pathway.

Now that your LDL has nothing to carry to your cells to help them out, LDL levels drop by way of negative feedback! But the reality is that the cell has just been deprived of the raw material it depends on to not only keep its contents secure, but also to repair and divide. No cell division means death. LDL makes its way throughout the body dropping off cholesterol everywhere its benefits are required, including the walls of damaged arteries and other blood vessels. It combines with vitamin C to "spackle" cracks and ruptures caused by inflammation. So, to borrow from Meyer Texon, M.D., a well-known pathologist at New York University Medical Center; saying that cholesterol contributes to narrowing of the arteries because it can be found in the plaques on thickened arterial walls is like saying white blood cells are to blame when we find pus in an infected cut on the skin. We don't blame the white blood cells for filling the wound with pus. That "gunk" is what's left of the used-up white blood cells or macrophages while they fought off and engulfed the bacteria trying to enter the body through the broken skin. Let's stop blaming cholesterol when all it's here to do is heal us and help us function!

Dr. Uffe Ravnskov's book, *The Cholesterol Myths: Exposing the Fallacy that Saturated Fat and Cholesterol Cause Heart Disease*, gives us a scientifically sound explanation of exactly what the title describes. According to *The Cholesterol Myths*, some of the other essential responsibilities that cholesterol has in the body is as precursor to hormones that help you deal with stress and protect against heart disease and cancer. Cholesterol is required to make all sex hormones in the body, including androgen, testosterone, estrogen, progesterone, and DHEA.

Cholesterol is also the precursor of vitamin D, which is vital for bone development and strength, proper functioning of the nervous system (your brain, spinal cord, and all of your nerves), mineral metabolism, muscle tone, insulin production, reproduction, and immune function. That, in and of itself, is an impressive list of responsibilities and without cholesterol in the presence of sunlight, your body can become deficient in vitamin D. It's extremely important that I reiterate this very established fact: the body cannot produce its own vitamin D without *cholesterol* in the presence of sunlight. We hear about it all the time. People go to the doctor and are old they're vitamin D deficient, not vitamin D *precursor* deficient.

As I was doing research for this book, this omission became more and more prevalent in several locations but rather sadly in a book that I had hoped would be consistent and forthright, *Why Do I Still Have Thyroid Symptoms When My Lab Test Are Normal?* The author, Datis Kharrazian, DC, DHS, MS, MNeuroSci, FAACP, DACBN, DABCN, DIBAK, CNS, educates the reader most thoroughly in the realm of understanding the function and dysfunction of the thyroid gland, specifically hypothyroidism, or Hashimoto's. It's a wealth of information that could very well change the course of someone's health and I wholeheartedly appreciate and value Dr. Kharrazian's holistic, integrative approach to healing the body. Although Dr. Kharrazian does a commendable job educating the reader about the well-documented hazards of gluten (more accurately gliadin) and more recently casein, to the thyroid, it is his discussions on vitamin D, throughout the book, that illustrates my point so vividly.

When addressing the detrimental effect of vitamin D deficiency in Hashimoto's, Dr. Kharrazian never once implicates a potential shortage of its precursor, cholesterol, as a root cause of the deficiency. Instead, he blames our diets for lacking in vitamin D-rich foods like liver, organ meats, lard, butter, and egg yolks. He recognizes the impact of the issue, vitamin D deficiency, by maintaining:

A vitamin D deficiency is associated with numerous autoimmune conditions, including Hashimoto's, and autoimmune rates have been skyrocketing in recent years. Adequate vitamin D helps keep the immune [system] balanced so it does not swing out of control into an autoimmune disease... Many factors are involved with the promotion of vitamin D deficiencies, which include a lack of sunlight exposure and inadequate consumption of vitamin D rich foods such as oily fish. Gastrointestinal inflammatory disorders reduce the absorption of vitamin D. Ethnicities with darker skin and individuals with obesity are more at risk for vitamin D insufficiencies. Also, as individuals become older, they become less efficient in photo production to use sunlight to process vitamin D.

Nowhere in his landmark book (that I have recommended to many clients, and will continue to do so!) will you find any link between cholesterol and vitamin D production. One other source that is just as guilty, albeit certainly more biased where the subject is concerned, is the National Institutes of Health Office of Dietary Supplements website. Directly from the site:

Vitamin D is a fat-soluble vitamin that is naturally present in very few foods, added to others, and available as a dietary supplement. It is also produced endogenously when ultraviolet rays from sunlight strike the skin and trigger vitamin D synthesis. Vitamin D obtained from sun exposure, food, and supplements is biologically inert and must undergo two hydroxylations in the body for activation. The first occurs in the liver and converts vitamin D to 25-hydroxyvitamin D [25(OH)D], also known as calcidiol.

The second occurs primarily in the kidney and forms the physiologically active 1,25-dihydroxyvitamin D [1,25(OH)2D], also known as calcitriol. Vitamin D promotes calcium absorption in the gut and maintains adequate serum calcium and phosphate concentrations to enable normal mineralization of bone and to prevent hypocalcemic tetany. It is also needed for bone growth and bone remodeling by osteoblasts and osteoclasts. Without sufficient vitamin D, bones can become thin, brittle, or misshapen. Vitamin D sufficiency prevents rickets in children and osteomalacia in adults. Together with calcium, vitamin D also helps protect older adults from osteoporosis.

Where, pray tell, is this hugely significant detail on a government site designed to "educate the public"? I actually lost all hope in the source after reading the very first sentence, considering that vitamin D isn't a vitamin after all. If you want to make sure you're getting enough vitamin D, try this simple solution: cook two freshly-laid eggs in coconut oil, on low/medium heat, making sure to leave the yolk as runny as possible. Put them on a plate and if it's not raining outside, eat them while sitting on your front step, patio, deck, etc. Take your time (about 15 minutes should do it). Repeat every single day of the week.

Lastly, most of us are familiar with the neurotransmitter (brain chemical) serotonin, but you may not realize just what paramount a role cholesterol plays in the proper functioning of serotonin receptors in our brains. Serotonin is the body's natural feel-good chemical involved in appetite, sleep, learning, mood, behavior, depression. Mark A. Mintun, M.D., professor of radiology and of psychiatry at Washington University at St. Louis led a team that studied 46 people with active depression and compared them to 29 individuals who were not depressed. The scientists focused on levels of the 5-HT2A receptor, a type of serotonin receptor. They were surprised to find that volunteers with depression had fewer serotonin receptors throughout their brain compared to the 29 non-depressed participants. Receptor levels in the hippocampus were significantly lower among the depressed individuals. The hippocampus, a region in the brain, plays a key role in mood regulation and long-term memory.

Low cholesterol levels have been linked to aggressive and violent behavior, depression, and suicidal tendencies. According to researchers at Macalester College, the absence of serotonin has been associated with greater aggressive behavior. They say that serotonin levels have been correlated with higher levels of irritability, impulsivity, aggression, disordered eating, and sleeping problems. What ails America? Depression, disordered eating, sleeping problems, aggressive behavior. We are starving our brains, our cells, our immune systems. We can't thrive without it and life can be really cruddy if you rob your diet of it.

Censored Nutritional Gem #2: Cholesterol is King:
It rules the kingdom that is your body through healing mechanisms and sound infrastructure.

Suggested Reading:

The Cholesterol Myths: Exposing the Fallacy That Cholesterol and Saturated Fat Cause Heart Disease, Uffe Ravnskov, MD

How Statins Really Lower Cholesterol and Kill You One Cell at a Time, James B. Yoseph, Hannah Yoseph, MD

Cholesterol is Not the Culprit, Fred A. Kummerow, PhD with Jean M. Kummerow, PhD

The Big Fat Cholesterol Lie, Jackie Storm, PhD

Know Your Fats: The Complete Primer for Understanding the Nutrition of Fats, Oils, and Cholesterol, Mary Enig, PhD

Cholesterol Clarity: What The HDL Is Wrong With My Numbers? Jimmy Moore with Eric C. Westerman, MD

The Cure for Heart Disease, Dwight Lundell, MD and Todd R. Nordstrom

The Great Cholesterol Con: The Truth About What Really Causes Heart Disease and How to Avoid It, Malcolm Kendrick, MD

The last word on Vitamin D goes to...

Chris Masterjohn, armed with a PhD in Nutritional Sciences and a mission to spread the truth about dietary cholesterol via his website, www.cholesterol-and-health.com, writes:

> Since cholesterol is a precursor to vitamin D, inhibiting the synthesis of cholesterol will also inhibit the synthesis of vitamin D. Since sunlight is required to turn cholesterol into vitamin D, avoiding the sun will likewise undermine our ability to synthesize vitamin D. And since vitamin D-rich foods are also rich in cholesterol, low-cholesterol diets are inherently deficient in vitamin D. Vitamin D is best known for its role in calcium metabolism and bone health, but new roles are continually being discovered for it, including roles in mental health, blood sugar regulation, the immune system, and cancer prevention. Yet standard modern advice -- take cholesterol-lowering drugs, avoid the

sun, eat a low-cholesterol diet -- combined with a recommended daily intake of vitamin D that is only a tenth of what many researchers believe to be sufficient all seems to pave the way for
widespread vitamin D deficiency.

Indeed Chris, indeed.

The last word on cholesterol goes to :

Dr. Uffe Ravnskov, MD, PhD

Born 1934 in Copenhagen, Denmark.
Graduated 1961 from the University of Copenhagen with an MD.
1961-1967 various appointments at surgical, roentgenological, neurological, pediatric and medical departments in Denmark and Sweden.
1968-79 various appointments at the Department of Nephrology, and the Department of Clinical Chemistry, University Hospital, Lund, Sweden; 1975-79 as an assistant professor at the Department of Nephrology.
1973 PhD at the University of Lund. A specialist in internal medicine and nephrology.
1979-2000 a private practitioner. Since 1979 an independent researcher.
Honoured by the Skrabanek Award 1999 given by Trinity College of Dublin, Ireland for original contributions in the field of medical scepticism.
Honoured by the 2007 Leo-Huss-Walin Prize for Independent Thinking in Natural Sciences and Medicine.

On August 31st, 2014, in an address to his newsletter subscribers, Dr. Ravnskov makes his masterpiece, *The Cholesterol Myths: Exposing the Fallacy That Saturated Fat and Cholesterol Cause Heart Disease,* free to the public.

My first English book *The Cholesterol Myths: Exposing the Fallacy That Saturated Fat and Cholesterol Cause Heart Disease* is now for free.

Due to a conflict with the publisher its publishing was stopped six years ago. However, last year I saw that both new and used copies are still sold from amazon. I was told that ten different publishers sold it and one of them told me that they got the book from Ingram Content Group. I told Ingram that they were allowed to publish it provided that I got a reasonable fee, but they did not answer.

I also ordered a copy to see if it has been changed but amazon answered that I was not allowed to buy it. I therefore asked one of my friends to buy a new copy. They sent a used copy (I found the name of the previous owner in the book) claiming that it was new. The price including shipping and handling(!) was $95.50!

I have therefore decided to offer the whole book for free on the web and it is now available on www.Ravnskov.nu/CM. Please inform your family, friends and the public!

My book is a detailed description of the fraudulent way the cholesterol campaign was started with almost 300 references to the scientific literature. It may be a little difficult to read for lay people. If so, I recommend my other books in English, *Fat and Cholesterol are Good for You!* and *Ignore the Awkward! How the Cholesterol Myths Are Kept Alive*

Dr. Ravnskov is a:
Member of International Science Oversight Board
Member of the editorial board of Cholesterol
Member of the editorial board of Journal of Lipids
Director of THINCS, The International Network of Cholesterol Skeptics

www.Ravnskov.nu/Uffe

Notes

3
Sugar is the Root of all Nutritional Evil

What the avant garde of endocrinology tells us today, the sorceress [natural healer] in what we called the Dark Ages knew by instinct or learned by experiment. Generation after generation, century after century, the people turned to the natural healers…Natural healers believed the universe was governed by law and order of which every petal of every plant was a part…When physicians were few, practicing savage male rituals like bloodletting and lopping off extremities, the natural healer was able to cure people by combining the healing power of plants with the laying on of hands and common sense advice about diet, fasting, and prayer… The words holy, whole, healthy, and hale all stemmed from the same root. A whole food was holy, blessed by the nature spirits, and intended to protect the health of man. Sugar was obviously not a whole food like a green plant or an amber grain… If it had any history, it was an alien history. Judgment was therefore suspended unless and until a sorceress from Cheltenham could consult with a sorceress from Barbados. Meanwhile, it was brought from afar by lackeys of the church and state who-in the eyes of the natural healers had an unblemished record for having brought nothing but death and taxes, toil and trouble, wars and pestilence.

It may seem odd to start a chapter with such a lengthy passage from another author's work but it spoke to me (loud and clear). For weeks I struggled with how best to convey the harm and hazard that sugar has inflicted on humanity, and that it continues to inflict to this day- with no hope of winding down. It is the above passage from William Dufty's, *Sugar Blues*, first published in 1975, that I hope will whet your appetite to learn more about those hazards, and will feed your resolve to remove it from your diet forever. In recanting the history of cane sugar Dufty turns the clock back to approximately 325 B.C., when an admiral in the service of Alexander the Great explored the East Indies and described the sweet nectar as a "kind of honey" growing in canes or reeds. Sometime after 600 A.D., the Persians began cultivating sweet cane. It would be the school of medicine and pharmacology at the University of Djondisapour, described by Dufty as "the pride of the Persian Empire", that would be credited with researching and developing a process for "solidifying and refining the juice of the cane into solid form that would last without fermenting."

The Persian Empire rose and fell, as empires always do. When the armies of Islam overran them, one of the trophies of victory was the secret for processing sweet cane into medicine… It wasn't long before the Arabs took over the saccharum business.

When Muhammed sickened with fever and died, his kalifa or successor set out, with the faith that moves mountains, to subjugate the whole world with an army of a few thousand Arabs. With military campaigns among the most brilliant in the world's history, he came within an ace of succeeding…Within 125 years, Islam expanded from the Indus River to the Atlantic and Spain, from Kashmir to Upper Egypt. The conquering caliph had ridden to Jerusalem with a bag of barley, a bag of dates, and a water skin.

One can read stories about a successor, Omattad Caliph Walid II, who mocked the Koran, wore fancy outfits, ate pork, drank wine, neglected his prayers, and developed a taste for sugared drinks…Arab armies of occupation took with them the rice grains from Persia and the cuttings of the sweet cane that the Persians had found in India…Islam soon discovered many new diseases and, perforce, divorced science from religion.

In the Koran, the sacred book of Prophet Elijah Muhammad, sugar is not mentioned. But the heirs of the Prophet are probably the first conquerors in history to have produced enough sugar to furnish both courts and troops with candy and sugared drinks.

An early European observer credits the widespread use of sugar by Arab desert fighters as the reason for their loss of cutting edge. Leonhard Rauwolf is the German botanist who gave his name to the plant *rauwolfia serpentina*… Rauwolf made voyages in the lands of the Sultan through Libya and Tripoli. His journals, published in 1573, contain timeless military intelligence:

"The Turks and Moors cut off one piece [of sugar] after another and so chew and eat them openly everywhere in the street without shame… in this way [they] accustom themselves to gluttony and are no longer the intrepid fighters they had formerly been…The Turks use themselves to gluttony and are no more so free and courageous to go against their enemies to fight as they had been in former ages." This may be the first recorded warning from the scientific community on the subject of sugar abuse and its observed consequences.

Is sugar really that bad for me? you ask. Yes. I'm sorry that doesn't give you much hope, I'm sure, but sugar, and not just the refined fine white powder that bears a striking resemblance to some other highly addictive refined white powder- yes I'm talking cocaine- is actually more addictive than the illegal drug that has destroyed the lives of so many people around the world. "Research studies indicate that sugar may be similar to morphine and heroin in its ability to increase opioids in the brain that produce pleasure. This increase in opioids is a major part of the physiology that fuels your addiction and the craving for sugar…"

If sugar addiction came with no other consequences other than brain pleasure-center stimulation, some might consider its crimes somewhat pardonable. Sadly, its addictive nature only serves to bombard the body with sugar's widespread deleterious effects, facilitating systemic disturbances throughout, that over time lead to physical degeneration and ultimately, untimely death. Sugar causes rapid increases in insulin levels; the loss of important minerals; hormonal disruptions; increase susceptibility to food allergies; paralysis of the immune system; as well as a host of psychological dysfunctions. Alcoholics are especially sensitive to sugar's destructive euphoria, as Dr. Kathleen DesMaisons explains in her revolutionary book about healing sugar sensitivity, *Potatoes not Prozac :*

- The brains of alcoholics are different from other brains. This special configuration is inherited.

- There are people who are sensitive to carbohydrates and have a more powerful blood sugar response to eating them.

- When needed, the brain releases opioids (natural painkilling chemi cals), and these can affect your choices of what you eat.

- Sugar acts like an opioid drug, such as morphine and heroin, in the brain.

Her working hypothesis- as a clinician whose educational training was non-traditional and interdisciplinary- was based on listening to people's experiences and conceptualizing a theory that involved all relevant scientific categories and disciplines:

- There is an inherited biochemical condition called sugar sensitivity that has predictable and specific effects on the brain and on a person's behavior. The foods a sugar-sensitive person eats and when they eat them will affect them profoundly.

• Sugar has the same painkilling and euphoria-stimulating effect in the human body as opioid drugs do. These drug effects of sugar are heightened in sugar-sensitive people. Sugar addiction, like drug addiction, is real and can open the gate to other addictions.

• Changing what sugar-sensitive people eat and when they eat it can have a powerful effect on their well-being and behavior.

When we say "sugar", we're talking about any industrially manufactured or extracted caloric substance that tastes sweet, has calories coming from carbohydrates and whose form is not found in nature. Corn syrup, of the high fructose variety or not, disaccharides, dextrose, dextrin, maltodextrin, sucrose, maltose, all of these substances are produced via human involvement in a lab or through a very involved process of either extraction from the original source (fructose and lactose) and/or refining. So, they're neither natural nor whole. And yet, it's not illegal, at all! It's what we try to coax good behavior out of our children with. It's what helps the medicine go down. Yes, of course, one drug chased with another drug. Sugar has extremely detrimental effects on our bodies both visible and on a microscopic level. It wreaks havoc on all systems.

Over the past week I have come to the realization that people with the kindest of intentions end up bringing discomfort and suffering into the lives of those who don't have the heart to refuse their kind gestures. Those sweet individuals who give your kids lolli-pops at the bank, and cookie samples in the grocery store, and bring treats loaded with diabetic-coma-inducers to school when it's their snack week are truly just trying to be nice. They're not thinking of anything but the gesture. That's the problem. This entire book with all of its months ofhyper-focus, and late nights of my children asking when I'm going to come and tuck them in, and people asking hopefully, "Is your book ready?", is meant to gently, but definitely, rid your life of the most inflammatory, deadly, fleecy wolf we've ever exposed our taste buds to.

It will drive you insane. It will turn you into a person you no longer recognize (both mentally and physically- just watch an episode of *The Next Great Baker* to see people unraveling before your very eyes). It will destroy relationships and lives, all while leaving you yearning for just one. More. Bite. Nothing has ravaged humanity as unequivocally as the white, addictive, sensual powder called sugar. And we seem to be powerless against its seductive demeanor, with the sweetest, kindest folks being its biggest advocates spouting all sorts of excuses granting you permission to indulge:

How could something so yummy be that bad for you?
Come on, live a little!
Everything in moderation!
A little bit won't hurt!
It's St Patrick's Day!
Kids are supposed to eat candy!
It's the Marine Corps Birthday Ball!
It's Family Day!
You're on vacation!
It's Mardi Gras! It's his birthday!
It's Easter!   Once in while!
It's Halloween!
It's Grandma's birthday!
It's Christmas!
It's Hanukkah!
It's Valentine's Day!
It's our year-end school celebration!
It's Mother's Day!
It's Administrative Professional's Day!
It's Father's Day! It's Memorial Day!
It's Independence Day! It's President's Day!
It's New Year's Eve!
It's New Year's Day!
It's…it's nothing, just eat it, what the heck is wrong with you?
You really need a reason??

I'm sure we could come up with 365 "special events" that need to be commemorated with something whose first ingredient is sugar. And if somehow a day dawns that Hallmark hasn't deemed significant enough to make a greeting card for, there's always I made it just for you! It's organic and fat-free! Yes, I get it – it's all that and a freakin' bag of chips. The problem is that it makes us sick. All of us! It's been almost three weeks since I baked with a natural sweetener (I made chocolate chip cookies). For the most part, as you'll see when you turn to the cookbook section of the book, I only use wildflower honey, organic molasses or organic maple syrup. Once in a blue moon, I'll use Rapadura Whole Unrefined Sugar, or organic confectioner's sugar (without cornstarch!), but even with those natural sweeteners, the amount in my recipes is a fraction of what a conventional recipe calls for, and the remaining "sweetness" is provided by high quality powdered stevia.

Regardless, when the family eats natural sweeteners, we get a little gassy and notice the nose starts running if we don't load up on the probiotics and oil of oregano. Now heaven forbid I make a frosting with refined sugar, even organic; we're all up a creek. The histamine production goes into overdrive. We all get phlegmy, irritable, guilt-ridden, bloated, foggy, remorseful, and finally; convinced. Convinced that the next time we want something "sweet", we'll put more of our organic raw cacao powder in our Akea shakes in the morning. I'm calling it the "7-Stages of Sugar Consumption", (not to be confused with Dr. DesMaisons' Seven-Step Program, learn more at www.RadiantRecovery.com). And the sooner you realize that it is an addiction, the sooner you'll begin taking the necessary steps to distance yourself from this "abuser", forever.

I think the thing I hate most about sugar is the fact that it so shamelessly makes my children sick. It makes my eldest daughter exhibit every "cold symptom" in the book. Her sinuses become congested; her post-nasal drip increases- she starts coughing and expectorating as a result; her nose gets runny- and then it gets chapped as a result. The list goes on. In fact, as I write these words, it's almost midnight and I can hear her at the opposite end of our house coughing and trying to blow her little nose, without any success, unfortunately, because her sinuses are so inflamed that nothing has any intention of flowing freely. It wasn't I who was the provider of her poison this time around. No, it was a sweet, well-meaning friend who brought my two little sweeties two little chocolate muffins this afternoon, baked without gluten, but with coconut oil, and organic sugar. Remember how I mentioned that I hadn't used a natural sweetener to bake with for almost three weeks? That's because I had been working on the Banana Muffin/Bread recipe and the naturally-occurring fructose in the bananas, coupled with a teaspoon of powdered stevia, made the addition of a separate natural sweetener completely unnecessary.

One thing you have to realize when it comes to immune system function is that the longer you go without upsetting it, the more violent the reaction the next time it's faced with an opponent. My daughter had gone almost three weeks without consuming any honey, molasses, maple syrup, etc. The only sweet stuff that she had eaten came from whole fruit- bananas, strawberries, and blueberries in her Akea smoothie every morning. For a snack a few times a week; a grapefruit, an orange or, an apple with Coconut Peanut Butter had been the only fructose she had taken in. That is, until the little chocolate muffin beckoned her, when she didn't have the heart to refuse a friend who had baked something special for her, "the same way your mom would make it". It has now taken almost 6 days for her symptoms to subside- symptoms of a "cold", yes, but don't forget that the symptoms of a cold are the exact symptoms of any immune-mediated reaction. I blame sugar. Even the organic kind.

Psychologically-speaking, Dr. DesMaisons describes:

Being born sugar sensitive means that pretty early on you get wacky. Even as a child, you can start being moody, impulsive, mouthy, withdrawn, stubborn, dramatic, or reactive. As your diet stays off-kilter, these early responses set in as behavior patterns. People think this is your personality. You buy into this, and as you grow older the behaviors expand to include all-or-nothing thinking, self-absorption, grandiosity, helplessness, and a feeling of being "lees than," despite outward appearances. You develop the Dr. Jekyll/Mr. Hyde dichotomy…

Endocrinologically, and subsequently bio-psychologically, William Dufty sums it up perfectly:

The difference between life and death is, in chemical terms, slighter than the difference between distilled water and the stuff from the tap. The brain is probably the most sensitive organ in the body. The difference between feeling up or down, sane or insane, calm or freaked out, inspired or depressed, depends in large measure upon what we put in our mouth. For maximumefficiency of the whole body- of which the brain is merely a part- the amount of glucose in the blood must balance with the amount of blood oxygen… When all is working well, this balance is maintained with fine precision under the supervision of our adrenal glands.

When we take refined sugar, it is the next thing to being glucose so it largely escapes chemically processing in our bodies. The sucrose passes directly into the intestines, where it becomes "predigested" glucose. This in turn is absorbed into the blood where the glucose level has already been established in precise balance with oxygen. The glucose level in the blood is thus drastically increased. Balance is destroyed. The body is in crisis.

The brain registers it first. Hormones pour from the adrenal casings and marshal every chemical resource for dealing with sugar: insulin from the endocrine "islets" of the pancreas works specifically to hold down the glucose level in the blood in complementary antagonism to the adrenal hormones concerned with keeping the glucose level up. All this proceeds at emergency pace, with predictable results. Going too fast, it goes too far...

All this is reflected in how we feel. While the glucose is being absorbed into the blood, we feel "up". A quick pick-up. However, this surge of mortgaged energy is succeeded by the downs, when the bottom drops out of the blood glucose level. We are listless, tired; it requires effort to move or even think until the blood glucose level is brought up again. Our poor brain is vulnerable to suspicion, hallucinations. We can be irritable, all nerves, jumpy. The severity of the crisis on top of crisis depends on the glucose overload. If we continue taking sugar, a new double crisis is always beginning before the old one ends...

After years of such days, the end result is damaged adrenals. They are worn out not from overwork but from continual whiplash. Overall production of hormones is low, amounts don't dovetail. This disturbed function, out of balance, is reflected all around the endocrine circuit. The brain may soon have trouble telling the real from the unreal; we're likely to go off half-cocked. When stress comes our way, we go to pieces because we no longer have a healthy endocrine system to cope with it. Day-to-day efficiency lags, we're always tired, never seem to get anything done. We've really got the sugar blues.

If you need any more convincing, you really need to pick up that book for yourself, ASAP. So what's the answer? If it's more addictive than cocaine, how do you cut it out? As Dr. Leo Marvin's book puts it in the movie *What About Bob?*: Baby Steps. You bought this book. This book isabout removing the inflammatory substances from your diet. Sugar is the most inflammatory of them all, but also the most addictive. Start nourishing your body on a cellular level with high quality fats, whole, raw vegetables, minimally with fruit, whole pastured eggs, and with a high quality fermented whole food supplement (see chapter 10). As you'll see in the next two chapters, gluten from grains and proteins from cow's milk are next in line inflammation-causing substances. You must remove them both from your daily diet in order to give your immune system the reprise it needs to start healing you.

The baby step part of that is going to come by cooking and baking with the recipes in the cookbook part of this book. You'll notice that I have included recipes for all sorts of desserts including, Chocolate Chip Cookies, Chocolate Chunk Muffins, and Banana Bread. These recipes were crafted without the use of refined sugar, and with considerably less natural sweetener than any conventional recipe you'll come across. A couple of them don't even call for honey, only the natural sweetness from the fruit inherent to the recipe. Additionally, the high quality fats and blend of flours used will slow down the processing and subsequent absorption of any naturally-present sugars, due to their higher-than-grain protein and fiber content. It is important to note that even natural sweeteners like honey, maple syrup, molasses, and even fruits, contain sugar. We now understand that they too must be limited in their consumption, or at the very least consumed in the presence of fat, fiber and protein to reduce their potentially disruptive effects on the body.

When you begin nourishing the body on a cellular level, you will notice a dramatic decrease in your cravings for sugar and other refined carbohydrates, and possibly even some fruits. Try not to spend too much time questioning or second-guessing yourself, just marvel a bit and ride the wave. Restoration of balance (homeostasis) is upon you and healing and recovery from malnutrition will soon follow. The question about fruit should be answered more thoroughly. All fruits contain a combination of naturally-occurring sugars (sucrose, maltose, fructose, glucose, etc.) which should be limited to no more than 25 grams per day to maintain optimal health. According to highly reputable sources such as Dr. Patrick Quillin, a clinical nurse specialist (CNS), and also a registered dietician (RD), who as of the April 2000 publication date of his article Cancer's Sweet Tooth, in Nutrition Science News, had worked with more than 500 cancer patients as director of nutrition for Cancer Treatment Centers of America in Tulsa, Oklahoma, sugars are the preferred fuel for cancer cells:

> Understanding and using the glycemic index is an important aspect of diet modification for cancer patients. However, there is also evidence that sugars may feed cancer more efficiently than starches (comprised of long chains of simple sugars), making the index

slightly misleading. A study of rats fed diets with equal calories from sugars and starches, for example, found the animals on the high-sugar diet developed more cases of breast cancer. The glycemic index is a useful tool in guiding the cancer patient toward a healthier diet but it is not infallible. By using the glycemic index alone, one could be led to thinking a cup of white sugar is healthier than a baked potato. This is because the glycemic index rating of a sugary food may be lower than that of a starchy food. To be safe, I recommend less fruit, more vegetables, and little to no refined sugars in the diet of cancer patients.

The "glycemic index" or GI is a classification system of dietary carbohydrates based on the relative rise in blood glucose after the administration of the food in question as compared to a standard glucose challenge (GI of 100). To illustrate Dr. Quillin's point even more clearly, the article, *International tables of glycemic index and glycemic load values: 2008*, by Atkinson et al. in the December 2008 issue of Diabetes Care can frustrate even the most logical of us: a Snickers bar has a glycemic index of 50, but a baked russet potato has a GI of 111. Vanilla cake made from packet mix with vanilla frosting (Betty Crocker) has a GI of 42, yet a parsnip has a GI of 52. One can clearly see how fat can reduce the normally rapid uptake of almost 10 teaspoons of refined sugar (38 grams to be exact, less than 1 gram of fiber) from a piece of cake so dramatically, it gives you the impression that a parsnip (3.6 grams of sugar, 3.6 grams of fiber) would be an inferior choice. But as the American Diabetes Association also confirms on their website:

> The GI of a food is different when eaten alone than it is when combined with other foods. When eating a high GI food, you can combine it with other low GI foods to balance out the effect on blood glucose levels.

> Many nutritious foods have a higher GI than foods with little nutritional value. For example, oatmeal has a higher GI than chocolate. Use of the GI needs to be balanced with basic nutrition principles of variety for healthful foods and moderation of foods with few nutrients.

Is there anything else besides fat that can lower the glycemic index of a food? So glad you asked! A 2002 study at St. Michael's Hospital in Toronto, Canada, concluded that 1 gram of *beta-glucan*, a polysaccharide found in the bran of oats and barley, consumed concurrently with a 50 gram serving of carbohydrate predictably reduced the GI of said food by 4 units, thus deeming beta-glucan "a useful functional food component for reducing postprandial glycemia." The optimal daily dose of Akea contains 1 gram of fermented oat beta-glucan. But to reiterate the sugar-cancer connection, Drs. Mercola and Pearsall, in their 2006 book, *Sweet Deception*, also bring the following important point to light:

> In early 2005, cancer finally passed heart disease as the number one cause of death in the United States. Many scientists and medical specialists have proposed that sugar intake can lead to cancer by the following mechanism: The cells of your body naturally produce waste products called free radicals. Your body compensates with enzymes to neutralize the toxic effects for these free radicals. These protective enzymes require the proper mineral balance in order to be effective, and since sugar drains the minerals of your body, your enzymes are not nearly as effective as they could be. This leads to a buildup of free radicals, which then can cause a decrease in the availability of oxygen to your cells that can lead to cancerous cell mutations. This correlates with research done by Otto Walberg in the 1920s that showed that cells became cancerous when 35 percent of the oxygen was removed from their environment.

Serving Size 100g	Total sugar (g)	Fructose (g)	Sucrose (g)	Glucose (g)
Apple (raw, peeled)	10.10	6.03	0.82	3.25
Avocado, California	0.30	0.08	0.06	0.08
Banana	12.23	4.85	2.39	4.98
Blueberries, raw	6.89	-	-	4.88
Watermelon	6.20	3.36	1.21	1.58
Cherries, sweet	12.82	5.37	0.15	6.59
Grapes, American variety	16.25	-	-	7.20
Grapefruit	6.89	1.77	3.51	1.61
Mango	13.66	4.68	6.97	2.01
Orange, most varieties	8.50-9.35	-	-	1.97
Papaya	7.82	3.73	0.00	4.09
Peach	8.39	1.53	4.76	1.95
Pineapple, most varieties	8.29-10.32	1.94-2.15	4.59-6.47	1.70-1.76
Plum	9.92	3.07	1.57	5.07
Pomegranate	13.67	-	-	-
Raspberries, raw	4.42	2.35	0.20	1.86
Strawberries, raw	4.89	2.44	0.47	1.99

Source: USDA National Nutrient Database for Standard Reference

How many servings of fruit you can consume per day to stay within the healthy limits discussed above really depends on the fruit itself. Looking at the table on the page 37 gives you an idea of just how much sugar you're taking in when you brag about eating a whole bag of apples at work (JKN).

Remember that all sugars will have stimulating effects on the endocrine system and the pleasure centers of the brain, and all sugars will upset the natural glucose-oxygen balance of the blood if not consumed judiciously in the presence of high quality fats, protein and fiber, and greatly reduced in quantity and frequency of consumption altogether. The parting fact that gives this chapter its name has to do with how a crop native to the tropics ever made it onto the lips of Europeans and eventually, Americans. Once more from *Sugar Blues:*

> After the rise of Islam, sugar became potent political stuff. Men would sell their very souls for it. The same fate that had crippled Arab conquerors was now to afflict their Christian adversaries. En route to wrest the Holy places from the grip of the Sultan, the Crusaders soon acquired a taste for the sauce of the Saracens. Some of them wanted only to languish in the land of the infidels until they could get their fill of fermented cane juice and sugar candy. European rulers discovered that their ambassadors at the Egyptian court were being corrupted by the sugar habit and won over by bribes of costly spices and sugar…

Since the last major crusade had ended almost 100 years earlier, it was in a diplomatic position paper submitted to pope Clement the V, in 1306, that an appeal for renewal of the Crusades would outline a strategy to defeat the Arabs and bring home some sugar:

> In the land of the Sultan, sugar grows in great quantities and from it the Sultans draw large incomes and taxes. If the Christians could seize these lands, great injury would be inflicted on the Sultan and at the same time Christendom would be wholly supplied from Cyprus. Sugar is also grown in the Morea, Malta, and Sicily, and it would grow in Christian lands if cultivated there. As regards Christendom no harm would follow.

> In the face of serpentine assurances such as this, Christendom took a big bite of the forbidden fruit. What followed was seven centuries in which the seven deadly sins flourished across the seven seas, leaving a trail of slavery, genocide, and organized crime.

I don't know if this information will deter you from continuing to celebrate the sweetness that is sugar. I don't know if you'll think twice about allowing your children to go door-to-door peddling this legal drug in the form of cookies, caramel corn, and various other confectionaries, all in the name of fundraising and character building. I'm not sure if when you get a stuffy nose or feel like the weight of the world is on your shoulders that you'll associate your malaise to the handful of funsize candy bars you grabbed off a coworker's desk on your way out of the office. What I am sure of is that I feel I have exposed you to enough information so that you can never say, *No one ever told me.* As a family, we have suffered sugar's wrath long enough, and are relieved to say that we're an ace away from kicking the habit entirely, honey and all. It feels emancipating to say the least.

Censored Nutritional Gem #3: Sugar is the Root of all Nutritional Evil

Suggested reading:

Sugar Blues, William Dufty

Sweet Deception: Why Splenda, Nutrasweet, and the FDA May Be Hazardous to Your Health,
Drs. Joseph Mercola, DO and Kendra Degen Pearsall, ND

Lick the Sugar Habit, Nancy Appleton, PhD

Bittersweet: The History of Sugar, Peter Macinnis

Sugar and Slaves: The Rise of the Planter Class in the English West Indies, 1624-1713, Richard S. Dunn

Potatoes not Prozac, Kathleen DesMaisons, PhD, Addictive Nutrition

Depression of the glycemic index by high levels of beta-glucan fiber in two functional foods tested in type 2 diabetes, Jenkins et al., European Journal of Clinical Nutrition (2002) 56, 622-628. doi:10.1038/sj.ejcn.1601367, PubMed Id 12080401

4
No Grains, No Pains

It should come as no surprise to see the 83 year old Bob Moore sporting what cardiologist William Davis would call, a "wheat belly". That jovial bearded man, synonymous with "Whole Grains from the Heart", has spent the last thirty years turning Bob's Red Mill into an employee-owned company with $153 million in annual sales, according to the Winter 2013 edition of the George Fox Journal. Compare that small fortune with the 2012 annual revenues of Novato, California-based super foods importer Navitas Naturals at a paltry 20 million, and you can easily see why so many Americans are sporting both a "wheat belly" and a "grain brain".

Navitas imports, packages and sells organic raw foods from around the world. Stuff like raw organic cacao powder, maca, chia, and acai- you know, the stuff we all snack on to deliver a serious dose of vitamins, minerals, antioxidants, and other healing substances to our depleted, malnourished bodies. Not. Our pantries are actually stocked with "Gluten-Free Muesli", and "All Natural Gluten-Free Cornstarch", and "Gluten-Free Chocolate Cake Mix". All with Bob Moore's grandfatherly presence and warm smile reassuring us that what's written on the package is gospel.

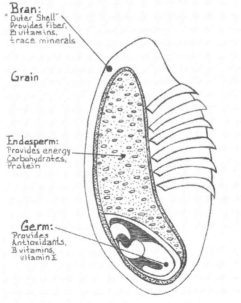

Artist: George Cole

It's time to set the record straight, once and for all, about the whole grain pain that has been inflicted on all of us for far too long. In terms of plant anatomy, a grain is defined as such if it contains three things: the bran (the hard outer layer), an endosperm (contents which, when milled, amounts to the bulk that is "flour"), and the germ or embryo (provides nourishment for the grain to grow, develop, and eventually sprout into grass). It is within the endosperm of every grain that a potentially problematic protein can be found. I say potentially because if you're a bird, you have nothing to worry about. If you're human, that's a different story. Try as we might to paint a picture of wholesomeness and numerous benefits that eating grains might provide, the truth of the matter is that our digestive system simply can't break down those proteins into small enough "pieces" to not trigger the action of the immune system. In order to truly understand the significance of this chapter we're going to have to "squirrel" away from grains and discuss the immune system for a wee bit. It will all tie together, I promise.

Our immune or lymphatic system is the body's defender and, to an extent, detoxifier/purifier. Its job is to identify what doesn't belong and to act in a protective manner. So, when it is presented with a protein foreign to the body itself (often times referred to as an antigen), or something in the body that has been damaged, such as a "used up" cell, it attempts to rectify the situation through a number of processes, all meant to either lessen the toxic load on the body or to isolate and destroy the offending suspect. For example, phagocytosis is the process where specialized white blood cells called macrophages (macrophagocytes), residing in every tissue of the body, engulf apoptotic (dead) cells and foreign proteins, and also produce immune effector molecules such ascytokines. Through their ability to clear pathogens and instruct other immune cells, these cells play a paramount role in protecting the body, but can also contribute to the development of inflammatory and degenerative diseases. Did you get all that? It means they can cause over-activity of the immune system, which can then lead to the immune system turning on other tissues or organ systems within the very body it is meant to protect.

To better illustrate this idea, consider the two types of immunity in the body: non-specific and specific. Non-specific has also been termed natural, native, or innate immunity, and is a system in place prior to the body being exposed to an antigen or protein. It also lacks discrimination among antigens, meaning it can confuse antigens that are similar in structure, and can further be enhanced after each exposure to those antigens through effects of cytokines. Specific immunity is also known as acquired or adaptive immunity. It is induced and enhanced by an antigen, and is able to finely discern between antigens, as the hallmarks of the specific immune system are memory and specificity. The specific immune system "remembers" each encounter with a protein or foreign antigen, so that subsequent encounters stimulate increasingly effective defense mechanisms. The specific immune response also amplifies the protective mechanisms of non-specific immunity, directs or focuses these mechanisms to the site of antigen entry, and thus makes them better able to eliminate foreign antigens. That means it can enlist the action of non-specific immune processes to more effectively get the job (protecting the body) done. Now, back to the subject at hand!

Proteins are made up of building block-type molecules called amino acids. There are hundreds of amino acids in nature but only 20 of them are present in all life on earth. We'll discuss proteins and amino acids in more detail in chapter 16, but for now, just commit to memory that the proteins we eat must be digested, or broken down into their single chain amino acids so that our cells can actually use them, and so that the immune system won't shift into overdrive to attempt to protect us from them. We established what it takes to be considered a grain and now we discuss the contents of the endosperm of all grains, gluten. Gluten is actually a generalized term for a type of protein composed of two primary subfractions: prolamines and glutelins.

The prolamine gliadin, is found in wheat, and has been the most studied subfraction of gluten due to its role in celiac disease, also known as leaky gut syndrome. It is only gliadin that is being referred to when you see food packaging labeled as "gluten-free". The USDA allows a product that tests at fewer than 20 parts per million (ppm) of gliadin to be labeled entirely free of gluten. Why is gliadin the only gluten deemed problematic enough to merit labeling? Because all of the research done almost sixty years ago, was on gluten sensitivity as it related to celiac disease. And since the total percent of gluten (gliadin) in wheat is the highest out of all the grains (69 percent of the protein in wheat is gliadin), the squeaky wheel just happened to receive all of the grease. Even though studies as new as 5 to 30 years ago regarding the inflammation potential of corn and rice have been published, they have been largely ignored and allowed to settle at the bottom of the proverbial pile.

The problem is that all grains contain an endosperm, and consequently a type of prolamine specific to that grain, inside the endosperm. The chart on page 52 contains the most common grains and the amount of their specific prolamine content compared to the total amount of protein in the grain. We can see that rice seems to be the least concentrated with its prolamine, orzenin, and corn is the second highest in terms of "gluten" content, with 55 percent of its total protein coming from the prolamine *zein*. The relevance of this information as it relates back to the immune system makes complete sense to me but as I read these last few paragraphs to my husband, he requested I "break it down some" for him (and possibly others!)

Grain	Prolamine	% Total Protein	Grain	Prolamine	% Total Protein
Wheat	Gliadin	69	Millet	Panicin	40
Rye	Secalinin	30-50	Corn	Zein	55
Oats	Avenin	16	Rice	Orzenin	5
Barley	Hordein	46-52	Sorghum	Kafirin	52

Source: www.GlutenFreeSociety.org

If an individual is sensitive to "gluten", as evidenced through innate, non-specific immunity, and as would be the case of people carrying any subsets of the gene HLA or human leukocyte antigens, they could potentially be predisposed to not just celiac disease, but to other autoimmune diseases as well. And because the non-specific immunity lacks discrimination among antigens (proteins), it lumps all the other antigens that are similar in structure (zein in corn, avenin in oats, orzenin in rice, etc.) to gliadin in the same ill light, and reacts in just the same alarming manner to all of them.

Now, let's say the individual doesn't carry the HLA subset gene for gluten, but for one reason or another their digestive system is unable to completely break down the proteins contained not just in grains, but any food in general, like dairy or peanuts. What happens then? That's when specific or adaptive immunity deploys, induced by the "antigen" that is that partially digested protein. Even though the specific immune system is able to finely discern between antigens, its reaction is enhanced with repeated exposure so that if it becomes overwhelmed, it calls on the reinforcements of the non-specific immune system. And thus begins a brutal, drawn-out war between the immune system and the rest of the body, as it treats what should be nourishing it, as something that is poisoning it.

Immune-mediated reactions are classified as symptoms indicating the exposure of the immune system to something it deems it must protect the body against. We're going to be dealing with this exact issue again in the next chapter when we discuss Censored Nutritional Gem #5, *Cow's Milk Is For Calves*. These symptoms include fever, headache, increased histamine (chemical messengers of the immune system) production resulting in increased mucus production (which then results in sinus congestion, sneezing, and post-nasal drip, etc.), itchiness of eyes or skin, and even rashes or various other eruptions. Now consider the drug aisle of a grocery store or the shelves stocked with over-the-counter drugs in a pharmacy. How many are devoted to either allergy relief or cold and flu drugs? My guess is two thirds because the other third is stocked with digestive aids, mostly for constipation but a few in honor of

Montezuma's Revenge as well. Have you ever noticed that many of the allergy medications can also be used for the symptoms related to a cold or the flu- runny nose or congestion, sneezing, coughing, fever? So, are you "catching a cold" or have you been exposed to something your body's immune system doesn't recognize, can't process, and is therefore working overtime to isolate and try to dilute by surrounding it with mucus produced by all those histamines?

Nine out of ten clients who walk through the doors of my office are either on a prescription allergy medication, blood pressure or blood sugar medication, cholesterol-lowering drug, thyroid regulating drug, or antidepressant. Eight out of those nine have never been informed by their physicians that there could be a connection between their diet and their symptoms and disorders. Considering that there are over 200 medical conditions associated with gluten sensitivity including but not limited to: anxiety, acne, arthritis, asthma, irritable bowel syndrome, ulcerative colitis, depression, dementia, chronic constipation, ADHD, diarrhea, type 1 diabetes, even schizophrenia(!), you would think that more primary care managers might take note and pass the information down to their patients. But they don't. So my clients look at me like I have 3 heads when I tell them that the uneven skin tone (melasma) they've come to me to lase off their face could be an indicator of thyroid dysfunction. Because they've already been to see their doctor about it and there's "nothing wrong" with their thyroid!

The long and short of it is this: the only way to ensure that the problematic proteins in grains are rendered harmless to us is to subject them to a process called lacto-fermentation, for a *long time,* whereby friendly microorganisms "predigest" them into single-chain amino acids, or even double chains called dipeptides, that will not trigger the action of the immune system. Or to sprout them nearly into the grasses that would normally be produced if the grain was planted in soil and watered. Then and only then, will you remove the inflammatory potential associated with their consumption, even though most gluten practitioners will tell you to avoid them altogether. As sensitive as I am to grains and dairy, even quinoa, there is one product that contains fermented quinoa, millet, amarynth and buckwheat, which I can consume without any symptoms whatsoever, and that's Akea. I've devoted an entire part of the book to it and we'll discuss it at length later on but for now, have a look at the ingredients lists below from a couple "gluten-free" mixes available from Bob's Red Mill, purveyors of fine "gluten-free" fare.

Gluten-Free Chocolate Cake Mix Ingredients:
Evaporated Cane Juice, Unsweetened Cocoa, Garbanzo Bean Flour, Potato Starch, Tapioca Flour, Whole Grain Sorghum Flour, Fava Bean Flour, Baking Soda,

Xanthan Gum, Sea Salt (magnesium carbonate as flowing agent), Cream of Tartar

Gluten-Free Pizza Crust Mix Ingredients:
Whole Grain Brown Rice Flour, Potato Starch, Whole Grain Millet Flour, Whole Grain Sorghum Flour, Tapioca Flour, Potato Flour, Evaporated Cane Juice, Xanthan Gum, Active Dry Yeast, Sea Salt (magnesium carbonate as flowing agent), Guar Gum

Remember, every grain has a "gluten" specific to it- whether that grain is wheat, or oats, and yes, CORN. Corn is a grain folks, not a vegetable. Not a fruit. And when you decide to clean up your diet and remove the processed foods and cut out your carbs, what are you really removing- grains, pasta, bread, cereal, cookies, muffins, crackers, pizza, donuts, Poptarts. You may be cutting out the carbs (and the refined unsaturated oils, and the artificial flavors, etc), but it's the inflammatory proteins within those innocent carbs that are contributing immensely to your weight-gain.

Visit www.GlutenFreeSociety.org and subscribe to Dr. Peter Osborne's free e-Newsletter, and get some daily help navigating the waters of gluten intolerance and sensitivity. Not everyone who is gluten intolerant has Celiac disease.

Censored Nutritional Gem #4: No Grains, No Pains

Suggested Reading and Websites:

www.GlutenFreeSociety.org, Peter Osborne, DC, DABCN

www.TheDr.com, Thomas O'Bryan, DC, DABCN

www.KellyBroganMD.com, Dr. Kelly Brogan, Holistic Psychiatrist specializing in women's health.

Grain Brain: The Surprising Truth about Wheat, Carbs, and Sugar--Your Brain's Silent Killers, David Perlmutter, MD and Kristen Loberg

The No-Grain Diet: Conquer Carbohydrate Addiction and Stay Slim for Life, Joseph Mercola, DO with Alison Rose Levy

Wheat Belly: Lose the Wheat, Lose the Weight, and Find Your Path Back to Health, William Davis, MD

Take Control of Your Health, Joseph Mercola, DO

Your Hidden Food Allergies Are Making You Fat, Roger Deutsch and Rudy Rivera MD

5
Cow's Milk is For Calves

I've never liked milk. For as long as I can remember, the mere smell of it turned my stomach. I used to tell my friends' moms that I was allergic to it when I was over at their houses for play dates so they wouldn't think I was being ungrateful when they offered me a glass. I was up a creek if crackers and cheese were served, or when the ice cream came out. See, I could definitely look past the fact that the creamy, delectable, yumminess was made from that stuff I couldn't stand. In fact, I could binge on it like nobody's business if it was combined with sugar and salt! Only I couldn't indulge at those play dates because I was "allergic to milk". Out of the mouths of babes?

Equally as controversial as saturated fat and cholesterol is the subject of humans consuming the milk of other mammals, specifically, that of a cow (common name for milk products is dairy, and just so we're 100 percent clear, eggs are not dairy products). Truth be known, the best part of dairy, as long as it's not pasteurized (!!), is the saturated fat and cholesterol. That's where it starts and that's where it ends. Alright, so there are some fat soluble vitamins in there too, but only if the cows are pasture-fed (eating green grass, and no grains or silage), and if the cream is not pasteurized, otherwise it's all negated. Why shouldn't it be pasteurized? That's a can of worms I'm not going to open too widely, but I'll refer you to a little book by someone named R. Pearson, *Pasteur: Plagiarist, Imposter: The Germ Theory Exploded*, if you need convincing that pasteurization is of no health benefit (on the contrary). An interesting point: the sale of raw butter is actually illegal in the Land of the Free. Just like cocaine. And heroin.

In researching this book my goal was to present as concise an explanation regarding nutrition taboo as possible. I wanted to provide you with the stories behind why the subject at hand is taboo to begin with, along with whether or not there is a purpose or essential role for the forbidden substance in the body. For example, if a food has been largely demonized by the mass media or government agencies, I wanted to grant you access to the other side of the story so that your consumption decisions are truly informed. On the other hand, does a food touted as promoting health have the potential to offend the body on a chemical level in any way, shape, or form? If so, I wanted to give you a heads-up of how that food does offend the body because, everywhere you look, you find contradiction and potential for frustration.

Case in point, I was astounded at how over half of the fifty-odd books I used as references for *SatFatRox* presented with quality information that I could verify from academic texts, but were then loaded with rhetoric, about other subjects, that still pandered to conventional paradigms! My ADHD kept luring me to inform you of those discrepancies, inaccuracies, and omissions of scientific facts, but I reeled it in and resigned myself to enlightening you about those instances via future blog posts on www.SatFatRox.com. I'm foreshadowing here but just humor me (*Whitewash*, page 216, "we get our vitamin D from the sun").

So here's my take on the white stuff from a cow: it has all the right ingredients and nutrients to take a newly birthed calf from a birth weight of about 80 pounds, to a weaning weight of about 418 pounds in 7 to 8 months- that's a fivefold weight increase. Over the next 16 months, it nearly triples its weaning weight by eating only green grass (theoretically). So, a cow is considered to be full grown at the age of two years and varies in weight, depending on the breed, from 1000 to 1500 pounds at that full grown age. Once that calf is weaned, its rate of growth slows significantly. Do you think that calf ever comes back to the udder for Sunday dinner when it's full grown? It doesn't. It drinks its mother's milk for 8 months and never goes back. because if it did, it would weigh a helluva lot more than 1500 pounds as an adult. Cows know that milk is only for babies because it lays down a solid foundation for physical development and maturation. Calves, lambs, horses, pigs, and other mammals also know not to wander over to the sheep and try out that species' milkshake. Why is it so hard for humans to understand this?

A human baby takes about 24 months (wishful thinking weaning age) to triple its birth weight which, on average, is 7.5 pounds (CDC, Births: Final Data for 2012). Full grown age (physically, unfortunately not mentally) is 18 years, with a full grown weight varying from 100 to 150 pounds (let's assume I'm talking about women here). From about 23 pounds at the age of 2, to about 125 pounds at the age of 18 yields a five-fold weight increase. The reciprocal is true when we talk about cows. What does all this mean and what does it have to do with the price of tea in China? It means that all the growth factors naturally present in cow's milk (note that I'm not about to begin discussing the synthetic ones that are administered to commercial dairy cows to keep their production profitable), which are meant to increase the birth weight of a calf by five times in 8 months, will almost guarantee a "fully-grown" human's resemblance to that of a cow, if that human has been either weaned on cow's milk or worse, bottle-fed cow's milk formula (the ills of which we will be discussing at the end of this chapter).

So, does milk really "do a body good"? Good question- what kind of milk and what kind of body? *Cow's milk.* Only if you're a baby cow, and drinking it right from the udder, udderwise, if it's pasteurized it'll kill ya. *What about goat's milk?* I'll get to that in a minute but quid pro quo for a second here, why are you drinking milk? *Because it's good for me? It gives me calcium.* The misconception that the best way for humans to take in calcium is via cow's milk is just that, a misconception. Oh, it's true that cow's milk isloaded with the stuff, more than three times the amount of calcium than in human milk, per 100 grams. So what? Does that mean that more is better? Can we pause for a minute and consider the idea that maybe the nutrient composition of every species' milk is masterfully formulated for that species (there are over 5000 mammalian species on earth, by the way, why aren't we milking pigs)? Just because cow's milk is "brimming" with calcium, doesn't make it a superfood (unless you're a calf).

Perhaps the bigger dilemma we're faced with, aside from whether or not we, as humans, should be drinking cow's milk because "it gives us calcium", is just how much dietary calcium we really need anyway. Considering a "perfect" world where all infants are nursed by their mothers until wishful-thinking-weaning-age of around two years (yes, I know there are cases where this simply isn't possible, we'll get to that soon enough), and that during that time, human breast milk is providing the babe with all of the calcium their rapidly growing body needs, what perfect food will we consumer afterwards to meet the body's metabolic needs and also stave off osteoporosis? Well, what perfect food does the cow eat after it is weaned? Broken record time: grass. Green grass. Theoretically, that cow can get every last ounce of nutrition her body needs from green grass, calcium inclusive! I say theoretically because if you haven't heard, commercial dairy cows are fed copious amounts of anything *but* grass. Yes, they're still standing and breathing and "alive", if you call what they're doing living. But they're not thriving. Because they're not getting their calcium from green plants!

If you're going to insist on drinking baby food, I'm going to insist it comes from a goat- preferably raw, and most definitely fermented, if you can go that extra mile, to optimize its digestion even further. If you need it to supplement an infant's diet, goat's milk is significantly closer in chemical makeup to human milk than cow's milk is to human milk. Blending it with coconut milk (along with an organic fermented superfood supplement I know of), and a few milliliters of organic extra virgin olive oil, will provide a far superior substitute than cow's milk or any infant formula on the market today. I came across the website, www.MtCapra.com, which focuses on the healthful effects of goat's milk. According to an editorial on the site by Texas Osteopathic Physician Dr. Thomas R. Cooke, who "for over thirty years, has been caring for patients in culture of holistic treatment, practicing a preventative illness approach, while teaching and encouraging patients the importance of wellness care", goat's milk pretty much trumps cow's milk for superiority where consumption by humans is concerned (note that I will have to clarify something in reason number four). From the article

Benefits of Goat Milk vs Cow Milk:

1. Goat's milk is less allergenic.

In the United States the most common food allergy for children under three is cow's milk. Mild side effects include vomiting, diarrhea, and skin rashes and severe effects can be as serious as anaphylactic shock! Needless to say it is a serious condition. The allergic reaction can be blamed on a protein allergen known as Alpha s1 Casein found in high levels in cow's milk. The levels of Alpha s1 Casein in goat's milk are about 89% less than cow's milk providing a far less allergenic food. In fact a recent study of infants allergic to cow's milk found that nearly 93% could drink goat's milk with virtually no side effects!

2. Goat's milk is naturally homogenized.

If you were to place a glass of fresh raw cow's milk and a glass of fresh goat's milk in the refrigerator overnight, the next morning you would find that while the goat's milk looks exactly the same, the cow's milk has separated into two distinct 'phases' of cream on the top and skim milk on the bottom. This is a natural separation process that the dairy industry does away with through an extremely damaging process called homogenization, whereby the fluid milk is forced through a tiny hole under tremendous pressure which destroys the fat globule cell membrane and allows the milk and cream to stay homogeneous or suspended and well-blended. The problem is that once the cell membrane of the fat globule has been broken, it releases a superoxide (which is a free radical) known as Xanthine Oxidase. We've all heard that free radicals cause a host of problems in the body not the least of which is DNA mutations which often lead to cancer. Goat's milk has smaller fat globules and that in part, allows it to stay naturally homogenized.

3. Goat's milk is easier to digest.

Goat's milk has smaller fat globules as well as higher levels of medium chain fatty acids, reminder that medium chain fatty acids are types of saturated fatty acids that can be found abundantly in both coconut oil and human breastmilk. This means that during digestion, each fat globule and individual fatty acid will have a larger surface-to-volume ratio resulting in a quicker and easier digestion process.

4. Goat's milk rarely causes lactose intolerance.

All milk contains certain levels of lactose which is also known as 'milk sugar.' A relatively large portion of the population suffers from a deficiency (not an absence) of an enzyme known as lactase which is used to, you guessed it, digest lactose. This deficiency results in a condition known as lactose intolerance which is a fairly common ailment. (Lactose intolerance and cow's milk allergy (CMA) are two distinct conditions. CMA is due to a protein allergen, while lactose intolerance is due to a carbohydrate sensitivity.)

Goat's milk contains less lactose than cow's milk and therefore is easier to digest for those suffering from lactose intolerance. Now the interesting aspect to consider is that goat's milk isn't much lower than cow's milk (contains about 10% less than cow's milk) and yet, countless lactose intolerant patients are able to thrive on goat's milk. Although the answer for this is unclear, it has been hypothesized that since goat's milk is digested and absorbed in a superior manner, there is no "leftover" lactose that remains undigested which causes the painful and uncomfortable effects of lactose intolerance. [I beg to differ and will explain why shortly.]

5. Goat's milk matches up to the human body better than cow's milk. This matter is both an issue of biochemistry as well as thermodynamics. Regarding the biochemistry of the issue, we know that goat's milk has a greater amount of essential fatty acids such as linoleic and arachidonic acid than cow's milk as well as significantly greater amounts of vitamin B-6, vitamin A, and niacin. Goat's milk is also a far superior source of the vitally important nutrient potassium. This extensive amount of potassium causes goat's milk to react in an alkaline way within the body whereas cow's milk is lacking in potassium and ends up reacting in an acidic way.

Thermodynamically speaking, goat's milk is better for human consumption. A baby usually starts life at around 7-9 pounds, a baby goat (kid) usually starts life at around 7-9 pounds, and a baby cow (calf) usually starts life at around 100 pounds. Now speaking from a purely thermodynamic position, these two animals have very significant and different nutritional needs for both maintenance and growth requirements. Cow's milk is designed to take a 100 pound calf to a weaned weight of 525 pounds in 7 months, eventually, that cow will weigh about 1200 pounds. Goat's milk was designed and created for transforming a 7-9 pound kid into a weaned kid of 35 to 55 pounds at 2 months, and human milk to transform a 7-9 pound infant into a weaned 2 year old of 25 to 35 pounds. This significant discrepancy, along with many others, is manifesting on a national level as obesity rates sky rocket in the U.S.

One very important thing to realize is the fact that a cow does not filter her female hormones (e.g. estrogen) from her milk, and our ingestion of her naturally-occurring hormones wreaks havoc on our own hormone regulation systems, the endocrine and reproductive systems. Goats and humans however, do filter their hormones from their milk. There are no estrogens passed from mother to kid/infant in goats and humans, and the intake of dietary estrogens, be they from soy or cow's milk, plays a huge role in many disorders in the Western world originating from something called estrogen dominance.

Regarding Dr. Cooke's Reason #4: let it be known that the vast majority of mammals eventually stop producing lactase, shortly after they are weaned from their mother's milk. It's a natural progression as we grow from babies to toddlers and no longer depend on mommy's milk to nourish us. The logical inference of this is in response to the fact that other mammals are never again going to encounter milk sugar for the remainder of their lives once they've been weaned. The vast majority of humans also stop producing lactase between the ages of 5 and 7. Logic, once again, would suggest that we should not be encountering milk sugar for the remainder of our lives. Dr. Cooke admits, "This deficiency results in a condition known as lactose intolerance which is a fairly common ailment." Of course it's fairly common, normal even! We're all lactose intolerant to some degree or another because we're all mammals, and mammals shouldn't encounter milk, and consequently milk sugar, after they are weaned! But guess what else we're encountering besides milk sugar? Twice the amount of casein found in human milk.

Casein is already a difficult protein to break down, that's what makes it prized in industrial applications. According to the website of a carpenter's glue manufacturer, "Caseins are still valued by manufacturers for their durability, water resistance and non-toxicity." Visit www.NationalCasein.com for all your commercial adhesive needs. If that wasn't enough to dissuade you from consuming increased amounts of it,

the destructive effects of pasteurization make the casein considerably more difficult to digest. The heat involved in pasteurization destroys the naturally-occurring enzymes that would normally aid [the calf's] digestion of the milk, all while disrupting the structure of all other proteins present, rendering them something not normally found in nature (denatured). So, not only is pasteurized milk indigestible by a calf's digestive system (it can actually kill it), but the human digestive system has no idea what the heck to do with a substance that has entered the body via the same way "food" would, but that it simply cannot
recognize or even break down.

Remember that the digestive system's function is to use the enzymes and acids in our gastric juices to splice proteins (and fats and carbohydrates) into their individual building blocks called amino acids (and fatty acids and saccharides, respectively). Only single amino acids (peptides) and double amino acids (dipeptides) are able to safely leave the gut and travel to the cells, without "crying wolf" to the immune system. If a chain of amino acids longer than a dipeptide manages to slip between the cells of the intestinal wall, you're about to trigger an immune-mediated response. And that triggers a little ditty called inflammation. So, proteins are what trigger immune action, and they can enter the body through our mouths, not just from those dreaded trees, grasses and pollen [sarcasm intended]. Why then can human infants tolerate goat's milk without a problem? Because goat milk lacks the casein content that cow's milk is rich in. Lactose has nothing to do with it, thank you very much.

For all those folks out there insisting that our ancestors were perfectly healthy drinking milk thousands of years ago, you're half right- they did indeed partake in it. But according to the writings and observations of the Greek physician Hippocrates (the Father of [Modern] Medicine), cow's milk could cause rashes and gastric problems. My thoughts are that what they were most likely nourishing themselves with, without digestive backlash, was goat's milk; raw or not pasteurized, and/or lacto-fermented. We'll discuss lacto-fermentation more in chapter 8, but for now, a few other (major) issues with cow's milk.

From Joseph Keon's book, *Whitewash: The Disturbing Truth About Cow's Milk and Your Health*, the following is an excerpt to help you understand why, and just how many, symptoms can manifest in response to the inability of the digestive system to break down proteins:

> With an allergy to cow's milk, symptoms persist even when lactose is removed. That is why when people who have been improperly diagnosed

as "lactose intolerant" may seek out "lactose-free" or reduced lactose dairy products and then become frustrated when their symptoms persist.

Cow's milk contains at least thirty proteins that can elicit an allergic response; the most common include casein, B-lactaglobulin (BLG), a-lactalbumin (ALA), bovine y-globulin (BGG), and bovine serum albumin (BSA). When they are ingested, allergenic proteins may cause the production of local and circulating antibodies. Reactions can be immediate (manifesting in minutes or a few hours) or delayed (24 to 72 hours). Symptoms can last from days to weeks. Food allergy symptoms can include skin rash, hives, swelling, wheezing, congestion, diarrhea, constipation, vomiting, nausea, watery eyes, runny nose, buildup of mucus, earaches and ear infections, headaches, skin discoloration, joint swelling, asthma, ulcerative colitis, inability to focus, colic, chronic fatigue, swelling of the throat, intestinal bleeding, anaphylactic shock, and death.

In children, the most common symptoms include irritability, skin rash or eczema, asthma, and earaches.The delayed onset of the symptoms makes diagnosing foodallergies challenging. It also explains why people often don't attribute their condition to the food they've eaten.

Common Symptoms of Food Allergies			
General	Respiratory	Cardiovascular	Neurologic
Chronic fatigue	Rapid breathing	Chest pain	Blurred vision
Excessive sweating	Coughing	Tachycardia	Dizziness
Frequent urination		Palpitations	Headache/Migraine
Sleep disturbances			Poor concentration
Behavioral	Gastrointestinal	Muscular	Dermatologic
Anxiety	Bloating	Cramps	Eczema
Irritability	Diarrhea	Myalgia (Myofibrosis)	Hives
Nervousness	Dry mouth	Muscle spasm	
Emotional instability	Intestinal obstruction		
	Nausea/Vomiting		

Source: Keon, J., WhiteWash

Regarding acne, he continues:

While people have made anecdotal associations with certain foods, including dairy products, for years, one dermatologist took the connection more seriously. Dr. Jerome K. Fisher of Southern California spent a decade studying 1,008 of his own patients in an attempt to determine what stimulated their acne. His conclusion, which he presented to the American Dermatological Association in 1965 in a paper entitled, *Acne Vulgaris: A Study of One Thousand Cases*, was that it was the milk in their diet. Dr. Fisher found that as their milk consumption increased, so did the severity of his patient's acne; conversely, as they cut back on their intake of dairy, their condition improved.

Compared to the general population, those suffering from acne drank up to four times the amount of milk, as much as four quarts per day. Although some physicians have cited the natural change in an adolescent's hormones as a cause of acne, Dr. Fisher came to believe that the greater influence was the effect of drinking cow's milk. The reason is that cow's milk is loaded with naturally-occurring hormones and growth factors. One of these compounds, the female hormone progesterone, is broken down into the male hormone androgen. Androgen activates the production of sebum, a wax-like product secreted by the sebaceous glands on the face. When the sebum hardens it blocks the pilosebaceous canal and appears as a blackhead on the surface of the skin. It is the body's effort to rid itself of this hardened sebum that leads to inflammation and the dreaded red blemishes on the skin…[that] fill with blood and lymph fluids…

But what about estrogen dominance and the hormone link to cancer?

Bioactive hormones from cow's milk present another possible cancer risk factor. A glass of milk contains a variety of hormones and growth factors- as many as fifty-nine, including as many as eight pituitary hormones, six thyroid hormones, seven hypothalamic hormones, seven steroid hormones, six thyroid hormones, and eleven different growth factors. Among these are the steroid hormones estradiol, estriol, progesterone, and testosterone. How these components might promote the growth of breast or prostate cancer is uncertain, but the potential link surely warrants caution. Since cancer is essentially the unregulated growth of mutated cells, it would seem prudent to eliminate any unnecessary exposure to growth-promoting compounds.

Ganmaa Davaasambuu, a physician with a Ph.D. in environmental health, a working scientist at Harvard University and a fellow at Radcliffe Institute for Advanced Study said, "Among the routes of exposure to estrogens, we are mostly concerned about cow's milk," the source of between 60 and 80 percent of all estrogens consumed. She points out that estrogen levels in milk are so high because of the modern practice of milking cows throughout their pregnancy, when estrogen levels increase significantly. Milk derived from a cow in late-stage pregnancy can contain as much as thirty-three [33!] times more estrogen (estrone sulfate) than milk from a cow that is not pregnant.

If you're thinking at this very moment, that there's not a snowball's chance in Hades that you could give up cheese, allow me to give you some insight into that emotion. What makes the issue of partially-digested cow's milk proteins so dangerous is their ability to resemble the body's own opiate-like brain chemicals, endorphins, by fitting directly on opiate receptor sites of cells in the brain. Milk (and grain proteins!) have been studied and shown to yield "active peptides" which are present in the digestive tract after a meal, and since we're unable to break them down into those single or double chain amino acids, several effects can occur. Regular traffic of peptide information passing from food digests into the bloodstream can have mixed opiate agonist-antagonist activity (meaning they can promote an action or sensation in the brain or halt it), basically able to produce dysphoria (a state of unease or generalized dissatisfaction with life) and even psychotic symptoms. As opposed to endorphins, the body's own feel-good brain chemicals, these peptides are termed exorphins, and are addictive. Loukas and associates identified the structures of two such cow's milk-derived exorphins that elicit opioid activities, referred to as casomorphins. These two peptides carry information by finding and binding to brain receptors which ordinarily respond to endorphins.

Exposing the brain to these peptides basically sends the message: go to sleep, feel bad, but go back for more. One of the casomorphins is a 7-chain peptide fragment from partially digested alpha-casein, and the other, a 5-chain peptide fragment from partially digested beta-casein. Take-home message: you can't imagine giving up cheese because it's as addictive as heroin. Approximately. One last excerpt from Keon's, *Whitewash*, helping parents who want to remove the inflammatory foods from their children's diets, and then you can just pick it up from SatFatRox.com and read the whole book for yourself:

First, some people find this change requires great dedication and vigilance. It means more than directly eliminating all dairy, wheat, oats, barley, and rye (all of which contain gluten) from the diet… because many commercially prepared foods include casein and/or gluten in some form.

Second, the gluten- and casein-free diet (GFCF) protocol is not something one can do half-heartedly. Some parents hope they can only make certain dietary modifications and still produce dramatic results, but the evidence indicates this is simply not the case. You need comprehensive exclusion of the potentially offending proteins to see a recovery or improvement.

Third, parents should be aware that removing casein and gluten from their child's diet can result in symptoms of withdrawal. Speaking from Dr. Robert Cade's office, Malcolm Privette cautioned that some children will exhibit "classic" withdrawal symptoms, including sweating and dilated pupils. They may even express rage after being deprived of the food source of the opiates. These compounds have been giving the child an exaggerated sense of pleasure. Parents need to be prepared for such reactions- which can be good indications that you are going to see behavioral improvements…

You will not only need to eliminate the obvious products- including milk, cream, butter, sour cream, buttermilk, and yogurt- but will also need to be aware of other casein-based ingredients, including ammonium caseinate, calcium caseinate, potassium caseinate, and sodium caseinate.

Now, replace "child" in the above paragraphs with "you". The possibility that you're going to go through withdrawals when you give up dairy (and gluten!) is well-documented. Be prepared. To arm yourself, refer to chapters 1 and 2, and front-load your diet with quality fats and un-oxidized cholesterol to give your body the raw materials to begin synthesizing your own endorphins quickly and efficiently, while also referring to chapter 3 to help combat sugar sensitivity and its effects on your serotonin and beta-endorphin levels.

Let's return for a moment to the deleterious effects that chronic inflammation can have on the body, and the subsequent disorders it can lead to, with the help of California Chiropractic Physician (DC) and Diplomat with the American

Clinical Board of Nutrition (DACBN) Dr. David M. Marquis, who has written commanding piece on how excessive inflammation negatively impacts every body system. From his widely publicized article, *How Inflammation Affects Every Aspect of Your Life*:

> Your gut is made of an incredibly large and intricate semi-permeable lining. The surface area of your gut can cover two tennis courts when stretched out flat. Its degree of permeability fluctuates in response to a variety of chemically mediated conditions. For example when your cortisol is elevated due to the stress of an argument or your thyroid hormone levels fluctuate due to burning the midnight oil your intestinal lining becomes more permeable in real time.
>
> Then you sit down to eat and partially undigested food, toxins, viruses, yeast, and bacteria have the opportunity to pass through the intestine and access the bloodstream, this is known as leaky gut syndrome, or LGS.
>
> When the intestinal lining is repeatedly damaged due to reoccurring leaky gut syndrome, damaged cells called microvilli become unable to do their job properly. They become unable to process and utilize the nutrients and enzymes that are vital to proper digestion. Eventually, digestion is impaired and absorption of nutrients is negatively affected. As more exposure occurs, your body initiates an attack on these foreign invaders. It responds with inflammation, allergic reactions, and other symptoms we relate to a variety of diseases. You can probably begin to see how diseases develop.
>
> So you might ask, what's the harm of inflammation and ongoing allergic reactions? It may sound relatively harmless, but this situation can and often does lead to numerous serious and debilitating diseases. Since your immune system can become overburdened, these inflammatory triggers are cycled continuously through your blood where they affect nerves, organs, connective tissues, joints, and muscles.
>
> The presence of inflammation is what makes most disease perceptible to an individual. It can and often does occur for years before it exists at levels sufficient to be apparent or clinically significant. How long it has been smoldering really determines the degree of severity of a disease and often the prognosis assuming the inflammation can be

controlled. One could also argue that without inflammation most disease would not even exist. Take a look at this list of diseases and their relationship to inflammation:

Disease	Mechanism
Allergy	4 Immune Mediated Types + Sensitivities, all of which cause inflammation
Alzheimer's	Chronic inflammation destroys brain cells
Anemia	Inflammatory cytokines attack erythropoietin production
Ankylosing Spondylitis	Inflammatory cytokines induce autoimmune reactions against joint surfaces
Asthma	Inflammatory cytokines induce autoimmune reactions against airway lining
Arthritis	Inflammatory cytokines destroy joint cartilage
Autism	Inflammatory cytokines induce autoimmune reactions in the brain arresting right hemisphere development
Carpal Tunnel Syndrome	Chronic inflammation causes excessive muscle tension shortening tendons in the forearm and wrist compressing nerves
Celiac	Chronic immune mediated inflammation damages intestinal lining
Crohn's Disease	Chronic immune mediated inflammation damages intestinal lining
Congestive Heart Failure	Chronic inflammation contributes to heart muscle wasting
Eczema	Chronic inflammation of the gut and liver with poor detoxification and often antibodies against Transglutaminase-3
Fibrosis	Inflammatory cytokines attack traumatized tissue
Fibromyalgia	Inflamed connective tissue often food allergy related and exacerbated by secondary nutritional and neurological imbalances
Gall Bladder Disease	Inflammation of the bile duct due to excess HDL cholesterol plugging, produced in response to gut inflammation
GERD	Inflammation of the esophagus and digestive tract nearly always food sensitivity and pH driven
Guillain-Barre	Autoimmune attack of the nervous system often triggered by autoimmune response to external stressors such as vaccinations
Hashimoto's Thyroiditis	Autoimmune reaction originating in the gut triggered by antibodies against thyroid enzymes and proteins
Heart Attack	Chronic inflammation contributes to coronary atherosclerosis
Kidney Failure	Inflammatory cytokines restrict circulation and damage nephrons and tubules in the kidneys
Lupus	Inflammatory cytokines induce an autoimmune attack against connective tissue

Disease	Mechanism
Multiple Sclerosis	Inflammatory cytokines induce autoimmune reactions against the myelin
Neuropathy	Inflammatory cytokines induce autoimmune reactions against myelin and vascular connective tissues which irritate nerves
Pancreatitis	Inflammatory cytokines induce pancreatic cell injury
Psoriasis	Chronic inflammation of the gut and liver with poor detoxification
Polymyalgia Rheumatica	Inflammatory cytokines induce autoimmune reactions against muscles and connective tissue
Rheumatoid Arthritis	Inflammatory cytokines induce autoimmune reactions against joints
Scleroderma	Inflammatory cytokines induce an autoimmune attack against connective tissue
Stroke	Chronis inflammation promote thromboembolic events
Surgical Complications	Inflammatory cytokines (OFTEN PRE-DATING the surgery) slow or prevent healing

Imagine presenting to your primary care manager (PCM) with any of the above mentioned symptoms or issues (because you know full-well that you have, at some point or another). How would they broach the issue, how would they treat it? Maybe they'd prescribe a new and improved "allergy medication" to calm your "over-active" immune system, or a non-steroidal anti-inflammatory to keep your inexplicable chronic pain somewhat manageable, or even a new prescription laxative that's way better than anything available over-the-counter. After all, they did just have a fabulous "drug rep dinner" at a local eatery the other night. Who knows, maybe that drug rep taught them something they weren't already privy to in medical school. It's not as though there's a "federally mandated incentive program that uses a combination of incentive payments and payment adjustments to encourage electronic prescribing by eligible professionals." Wait, what? Yes, it's called the eRx Incentive Program. Google it.

Apropos of newly developed drugs to "treat" anything, I came across the website of one online that was most educational where the disorder of "allergic asthma" is concerned. From the site of a new subcutaneous injection for allergic asthma:

> You may not be surprised to hear that about 25 million people in the U.S. have asthma. But did you know that about 60% of those people have allergic asthma? For those whose asthma is moderate to severe and uncontrolled, getting the right diagnosis can be hard. This is because people with allergic asthma don't always realize their asthma is triggered by allergens. They simply think they have asthma and allergies.

The symptoms of asthma and allergic asthma are the same. [Italics are mine]
Asthma is a chronic condition with inflammation and narrowing of the airways, as well as tightening of the muscles around the airways. This can lead to wheezing, shortness of breath, chest tightness, and coughing. Allergic asthma is a type of asthma. So, if you have allergic asthma, you may experience these symptoms. With allergic asthma, it's the triggers that are different. All asthma attacks and symptoms are triggered by something. In the case of allergic asthma, these symptoms are brought on by exposure to allergens in the air, including pet dander, dust mites, and cockroaches.

How do triggers impact allergic asthma?

If you have allergic asthma, allergens like pet dander, dust mites, and cockroaches can trigger your asthma symptoms and attacks.

• When an allergen enters your body, your immune system identifies it as something harmful

• Your immune system responds by releasing a substance called immunoglobulin E (or IgE).

• IgE plays a key role in your allergic asthma. It works by binding to allergens, which causes the release of chemicals that can lead to inflammation (swelling) in and around the lungs. This can trigger an asthma attack.

People with allergic asthma may have higher levels of IgE because of the way their immune system reacts to allergens. For some, blocking IgE has been shown to be a helpful part of their allergic asthma treatment plan. If you think you may have allergic asthma, ask your doctor about how much IgE is in your body. [So they can prescribe you a drug to help you ignore the fact that the food you're eating is most likely the strongest trigger of IgE.]

Can you believe that nowhere on the site of XOLAIR® (omalizumab), manufactured by Novartis Pharmaceuticals Corporation, is the subject of a food allergy brought up as a possible trigger to allergic asthma? Even though the immune system responds with the same substance, IgE, when it encounters a protein like casein or gluten? Totally rhetorical: has your primary care manager ever mentioned the fact that there most likely is a nutritional root to all of those problems, and crazier yet, insisted that if your symptoms are to be eliminated, your consumption of dairy or any other food, for that matter, containing digestively-questionable proteins, and inflammation inducing compounds, must also cease? If your PCM is a naturopath, homeopath, chiropractic or holistically-practicing medical or osteopathic physician, then your answer might be, Of course they have! Good on you, by the way, if your circumstances have allowed you to be fortunate enough to be able to select any of those professionals to be your guide in maintaining optimal physical, mental, and emotional wellness.

Unfortunately, if you're like the majority of the population of the United States and Canada forced into allopathic care, you may want to rethink your plan for staying healthy "with the help of your doctor". Allopathy is the system of "medicine" that aims to deal with disease by using drugs or surgery, methods which themselves produce additional effects that are different from or aggravating of those of the disease being treated. This just so happens to be the system used by most *conventional* medical doctors, and doctors of osteopathy, DOs, (don't assume that *all* DOs practice holistic or functional medicine- they don't!) Simply because allopaths are the only ones that accept insurance, is not a good enough reason to subject yourself to their practice. It may be time for you to start investing in your wellness by paying for true healing "as you go", instead of allowing your ailments and disorders to be subsidized by monthly insurance premiums and co-pays.

This chapter was meant to be about how cow's milk is intended for baby cows. It has explored many, but definitely not all the problems that can arise if humans consume cow's milk. It was about giving you all the information you need to quit dairy cold turkey, today. Connect the dots about how an American dietary staple has wreaked, and continues to wreak absolute havoc on so many lives. The last straw is an example of why we must keep cow's milk, in every way shape or form, out of the bodies of infants who don't have access to human breastmilk, to avoid the other potential problems that result when we attempt to replace the original.

When we have to add individual synthetic vitamins and minerals to cow's milk to make it remotely (but not really) acceptable to feed human infants with, we run the risk of setting ourselves up for failure. Commercial infant formula is an embarrassment. The soy versions, the dairy versions, even the organic versions, are all an insult. We can't sincerely believe that a product whose ingredients list begins with "corn syrup solids", and ends with vitamin and mineral isolates, synthetically-derived in a laboratory, could actually be a solid foundation on which to continue the development of a biologically sound human being. About a year ago, I came across some very depressing information in a post on the website www.greenmedinfo.com, in the article, *Why Is Pesticide Used as an Ingredient in Infant Formula?*

> Why is cupric sulfate -- a known herbicide, fungicide and pesticide -- being used in infant formula? And why is it displayed proudly on product labels as a presumably nutritious ingredient?
>
> Used to kill fungus, aquatic plants and roots of plants, parasitic infections in aquarium fish and snails, as well as algae and bacteria such as Escherichia coli, cupric sulfate hardly sounds fit for human consumption, much less for infants.
>
> Indeed, infants are all too often looked at as "miniature adults" from the perspective of toxicological risk assessments, rather than what they are: disproportionately (if not exponentially) more susceptible to the adverse effects of environmental exposures. Instead of reducing or altogether eliminating avoidable infant chemical exposures (the precautionary principle), the chemical industry- friendly focus is always on determining "an acceptable level of harm" – as if there were such a thing!
>
> It boggles the imagination how cupric sulfate ended up in infant formula, as well as scores of other consumer health products, such as Centrum and One-A-Day vitamins? After all, it is classified, according to the Dangerous Substance Directive (one of the main European Union laws concerning chemical safety), as "Harmful (Xn), Irritant (Xi) and Dangerous for the environment (N)."
>
> Moreover, the U.S. Environmental Protection Agency (EPA) requires that the warning signal "DANGER" appear on the labels of all copper sulfate end-products containing 99% active ingredient in crystalline form.

The anger that had been festering in me quickly turned into a relentless determination to glean as much information about the blue substance I remember using in the chemistry lab, and to expose the facts as quickly as possible. I researched the data for days, even visiting the local mega-grocery-mart and examining every container of formula on the shelves (over 20 varieties), to verify that indeed, cupric sulfate was an ingredient in all of them. What I discovered only added to my fury. The actual amount of copper in every suggested serving varied from 70 mcg to 80 mcg.

Consider that an infant is fed at least every 4 hours and that according to the government agency, the National Institutes of Health (NIH), the daily recommended allowances of copper are as follows:

- for infants 0-6 months is 200 mcg
- for infants 7-12 months, 220 mcg
- for children 1-3 years, 340 mcg
- for children 4-8 years, 440 mcg
- for children 9-13 years, 700 mcg
- adolescents 14-18 years, 890 mcg

That would mean that between the ages of 0-6 months, a formula-fed infant who drinks 6 bottles of 5 fluid ounces, is taking in between 420 and 480 mcg of copper, daily. And that's a conservative estimate, because they do go through growth spurts! That's more than twice what the NIH recommends for a child that age, and even more than the recommended daily allowance for a 7 year old! Turning our attention to the risks associated with too much copper in the diet, we find: nausea, vomiting, diarrhea and even kidney damage, anemia and death. According to an article on Dr. Joseph Mercola's site, www.Mercola.com, about the whether or not your multivitamin should contain copper, we see some alarming symptoms related to getting too much copper:

> ...copper can cause other health problems in addition to mental decline. If you consume too much copper, you may have abdominal pain, cramps, nausea, diarrhea, vomiting and liver damage. Elevated copper levels have also been linked to conditions including: schizophrenia, hypertension, stuttering, fatigue, headaches, muscle and joint pain, autism, childhood hyperactivity, depression, insomnia, senility, premenstrual syndrome.

Now, clearly PMS is not a symptom you're going to find in a 6 month old, but fatigue, headaches, muscle and joint pain, depression, insomnia? How else would you describe colic?

I created a flyer with the information and even advertised it in the newsletter of the local wives club on our base, hoping to inform as many people as I could. Not one individual contacted me to ask if the information was legitamate or to express concern. I felt like my sole responsibility from that moment on was to put an end to the needless suffering of every infant who's ever had the misfortune of being fed what Dr. Robert Mendelsohn, renowned pediatrician and author, referred to as "the granddaddy of all junk food". I'm not sure how many people I actually reached with those sophomoric efforts, but at this point, bound and with an ISBN, the secret's out.

The pesticide in question, *copper II or cupric sulfate,* indeed has an abundance of warnings listed on its Material Safety Data Sheet (MSDS). The shocking part was what I would find on a subdomain of cornell.edu: EXTOXNET, Extension Toxicology Network, described as "A Pesticide Information Project of Cooperative Extension Offices of Cornell University, Michigan State University, Oregon State University, and University of California at Davis. Major support and funding was provided by the USDA/Extension Service/National Agricultural Pesticide Impact Assessment Program". So, here it is, here's what a government-funded, academically-based authority has to say about an ingredient found in every commercial infant formula on the market in the United States (yes, even the organic ones!):

TRADE OR OTHER NAMES:
Basic copper sulfate: BSC Copper Fungicide; Bordeaux Mixture is a combination of hydrated lime and copper sulfate.

REGULATORY STATUS:
Copper sulfate is classified as a general use material by the U.S. Environmental Protection Agency (EPA). The warning signal "DANGER" must appear on the labels of all copper sulfate end-products containing 99% active ingredient in crystalline form.

INTRODUCTION:
Copper sulfate is a fungicide used to control bacterial and fungal diseases of fruit, vegetable, nut and field crops. Some of the diseases that are controlled by this fungicide include mildew, leaf spots, blights and apple scab. It is used in combination with lime and water as a protective fungicide, referred to as Bordeaux mixture, for leaf application and seed treatment. It is also used as an algaecide, an herbicide in irrigation and municipal water treatment systems, and as a molluscicide, a material used to repel and kill slugs and snails. Copper sulfate is a naturally-occurring inorganic salt and copper is an essential trace element in plant

and animal nutrition. It is available in the following formulations: dusts, wettable powders, and fluid concentrates.

TOXICOLOGICAL EFFECTS:

ACUTE TOXICITY
Copper is one of 26 essential trace elements occurring naturally in plant and animal tissue. The usual routes by which humans receive toxic exposure to copper sulfate are through skin or eye contact, as well as by inhalation of powders and dusts. Copper sulfate is a strong irritant.

Copper sulfate is only moderately toxic upon acute oral exposure. There have been reports of human suicide resulting from the ingestion of gram quantities of this material. The lowest dose of copper sulfate that has been toxic when ingested by humans is 11 mg/kg. Ingestion of copper sulfate is often not toxic because vomiting is automatically triggered by its irritating effect on the gastrointestinal tract. Symptoms are severe, however, if copper sulfate is retained in the stomach, as in the unconscious victim. Some of the signs of poisoning which occurred after 1-12 grams of copper sulfate was swallowed include a metallic taste in the mouth, burning pain in the chest and abdomen, intense nausea, vomiting, diarrhea, headache, sweating, shock, discontinued urination leading to yellowing of the skin. Injury to the brain, liver, kidneys and stomach and intestinal linings may also occur in copper sulfate poisoning.

Copper sulfate can be corrosive to the skin and eyes. It is readily absorbed through the skin and can produce a burning pain, along with the same severe symptoms of poisoning from ingestion. Skin contact may result in itching or eczema. It is considered a skin sensitizer and can cause allergic reactions in some individuals. Eye contact with this material can cause: conjunctivitis, inflammation of the eyelid lining, excess fluid buildup in the eyelid; cornea tissue deterioration due to breaks, or ulceration, in the eye's mucous membrane; and clouding of the cornea.

The amount of copper sulfate that is lethal to one-half (50%) of experimental animals fed the material is referred to as its acute oral lethal dose fifty, or LD50. The LD50 for copper sulfate is 30 mg/kg in rats. Ingestion by animals of three ounces of a 1% solution of copper sulfate will produce extreme inflammation of the gastrointestinal tract, with symptoms of abdominal pain, vomiting, and diarrhea.

When copper sulfate is given intravenously, or injected into the vein, as little as 2 mg/kg copper sulfate is lethal to guinea pigs; and 4 mg/kg is lethal to rabbits.

CHRONIC EFFECTS

Vineyard sprayers experienced liver disease after 3 to 15 years of exposure to copper sulfate solution in Bordeaux mixture. Long-term effects are more likely in individuals with Wilson's disease, a condition which causes excessive absorption and storage of copper. Chronic exposure to low levels of copper can lead to anemia. *The biological or chemical manner by which excessive doses of copper sulfate work is not well understood.* [Italics are mine.]

The growth of rats was retarded when 25 mg/kg of copper sulfate was included in their diets. 200 mg/kg caused starvation and death. Sheep with access to salt licks that contained five to nine percent copper sulfate showed signs of absence of appetite (anorexia), anemia, and degenerative changes, followed by death within one or two days of exposure. This material caused a significant increase in the death rates in mice that were exposed to an air level equivalent to human inhalation exposures.

The EPA limit for copper sulfate in drinking water is 1 ppm. This limit has been set to prevent a disagreeable taste from copper in drinking water, as well as to provide adequate protection from toxicity.

REPRODUCTIVE EFFECTS:

Developing embryos were resorbed in pregnant hamsters given copper salts intravenously on the eighth day of gestation. Testicular atrophy increased in birds as they were fed larger amounts of copper sulfate. Sperm production was also interrupted to varying degrees. Reproduction and fertility was affected in pregnant rats given this material on the third day of pregnancy. EPA does not require data on the reproductive effects of copper sulfate in mammals.

TERATOGENIC EFFECTS:
Heart disease occurred in the surviving offspring of pregnant hamsters given intravenous copper salts on the eighth day of gestation. EPA does not require data on the teratogenic effects of copper sulfate.

MUTAGENIC EFFECTS:
At 400 and 1,000 ppm, copper sulfate caused mutations in two types of micro- organisms. Data on the potential mutagenic effects of this material is not required by the EPA.

CARCINOGENIC EFFECTS:
Ten mg/kg of copper sulfate caused endocrine tumors in chickens given the material parenterally, that is, outside of the gastrointestinal tract through an intravenous or intramuscular injection. EPA does not require this data for copper sulfate.

ORGAN TOXICITY:
Examinations of copper sulfate-poisoned animals showed signs of acute toxicity in the spleen, liver and kidneys. Injury may also occur to the brain, liver, kidneys and gastrointestinal tract in response to overexposure to this material.

FATE IN ANIMALS AND HUMANS:
Absorption of copper sulfate into the blood occurs primarily under the acidic conditions of the stomach; the mucous membrane lining of the intestines acts to some extent as a barrier to absorption of ingested copper. After ingestion, more than 99% of copper is excreted in the feces. Copper is an essential trace element that is strongly bio-accumulated. It is stored primarily in the liver, brain, heart, kidney and muscles. About one-third of all the copper in the body is contained in the liver and brain. Another third is contained in the muscles. The remaining third is dispersed in other tissues.

So after read all this, I couldn't help but be taken back to the sadness and guilt I felt when I ended up having to decide what I would feed my first-born daughter, after my milk had dried up when she was almost 6 months old. Up until that time, I had been pumping my milk for her because of nursing difficulties when she was born. Every symptom she exhibited when I started her on formula was on the list of acute toxico-logical symptoms listed above, so the same evening I came across the article on greenmedinfo.com, I looked up the documented symptoms of infant reflux and landed on the website of a trusted authority in allopathic care, the Mayo Clinic.

According to Mayo Clinic Staff, the causes of infant reflux are as follows:

Infant reflux is related to a number of factors, often in combination with one another. In infants, the ring of muscle between the esophagus and the stomach- the lower esophageal sphincter (LES)- is not yet fully mature, allowing stomach contents to flow backward. Eventually, the LES will open only when baby swallows and will remain tightly closed the rest of the time, keeping stomach contents where they belong.

Babies are lying flat most of the time, which makes reflux more likely. Moreover, their diet is completely liquid, also favoring infant reflux. Sometimes air bubbles in the stomach may push liquids backward. In other cases, your baby may simply drink too much, too fast. Although infant reflux most often occurs after a feeding, it can happen anytime your baby coughs, cries or strains. In a small number of cases, the symptoms of infant reflux are caused by something else. Among the possibilities:

• Allergic gastroenteritis is an intolerance to something in food, usually a protein in cow's milk.

• Gastroesophageal reflux disease (GERD) is a more severe condition where the reflux is acidic enough to actually irritate and damage the lining of the esophagus.

• Eosinophilic esophagitis is a condition where a particular type of white blood cell (eosinophil) builds up and injures the lining of the esophagus.

• Obstruction is a blockage or narrowing in the esophagus (esophageal stricture) or between the stomach and small intestine (pyloric stenosis)."

Hey, Mayo Clinic Staff, did you know there's a fungicide in infant formula masquerading as a mineral supplement, in a dose that the NIH would consider overabundant, and whose acute toxicological effects mimic those of infant reflux and GERD? When a baby experiences "frequent spitting up or vomiting, irritability when feeding, or refusing food because of a burning pain in the chest and abdomen, intense nausea, vomiting, diarrhea, headache, sweating", how could we dismiss that as something they'll probably just "outgrow"? Whether formula manufacturers are using copper (II) cupric sulfate as a mold inhibitor or as a source for the trace mineral copper, they're exposing babies to a toxic, "corrosive...fungicidal...skin sensitizer... the biological or chemical manner by which excessive doses work is not well understood". That should make you mad, not indifferent.

Remember that "Copper sulfate is only moderately toxic upon acute oral exposure..." and that "ingestion of copper sulfate is often not toxic because vomiting is automatically triggered by its irritating effect on the gastrointestinal tract," except when it's crammed down the throat of a helpless infant every four hours. And now the even more heart-breaking fact: "Symptoms are severe, however, if copper sulfate is retained in the stomach, as in the unconscious victim." Or a baby put down for a nap after feeding. There's nothing gentle or soothing about that.

So, at the end of day, what's a parent to do if their hand is forced into feeding their baby something other than breastmilk? Before I answer that I want to stress the importance of mother's milk from the very beginning. And in order for a mother to be able, physically, to nurse her newborn, we have to actually go back before she even conceives. Yes, that far back. A woman with truly healthy eating habits, who isn't starving her body of saturated fat, cholesterol, organic superfoods like green leafy veggies, herbs, spices, berries, and eggs, is going to be a better host to the new life she's building inside of her. A woman who isn't taxing her immune system and thyroid by eating inflammatory foods like grains and pasteurized dairy, unfermented soy, and damaged oils, will have an enjoyable pregnancy. She will not develop pre-eclampsia or gestational diabetes, excessive swelling throughout her body or high blood pressure. She will be able to labor and birth her baby much easier than if she had gained 40, 50 and even 60 pounds in 4 to 6 months. And I say that because usually pregnancy weight gain doesn't begin until close to the end of the first trimester.

Natural labor, unaided by synthetic hormones introduced into the woman's body leads to the natural progression of the reproductive cycle, and after labor, lactation is the next step in the woman's reproductive cycle. The reproductive cycle actually starts with ovulation, hopefully leading to fertilization, next is conception, followed by gestation, labor, and finally lactation. So nursing is necessary for the well-being of the mother as much as it is for the newborn. If something along that journey goes awry and the nursing relationship must be cut short or cannot begin, you can make your own baby formula using a combination of goat milk and coconut milk. You can add whole food supplements to it along with probiotics, coconut and olive oil, essential fatty acids, as well, and you can prevent the needless suffering that can result from the consumption of commercial formula. Please don't take this subject lightly, and please share this with anyone you know who is either about to have a baby and is still debating whether or not to nurse, or someone whose hand has already been forced to feed their infant formula.

Censored Nutritional Gem #5: Cow's Milk is For Calves

Suggested Reading:

Whitewash: The Disturbing Truth About Cow's Milk and Your Health, Joseph Keon PhD

Pottenger's Cats: A Study in Nutrition, Francis M. Pottenger, Jr., MD

Take Control of Your Health, Joseph Mercola, DO

Why Do I Still Have Thyroid Symptoms? When My Lab Tests Are Normal, Datis Kharrazian, DHSc, DC, MS

Brain Receptor Methodologies Part B Amino Acids. Peptides. Psychoactive Drugs, A collection of neurobiological research, Edited by Paul J. Marangos, Iain C. Campbell, Robert M. Cohen

Survival in The 21st Century, Viktoras H. Kulvinskas, MS

Suggested Reading for Optimal Reproductive Cycle Health:

Trust Your Body, Trust Your Baby, Henci Goer

Birth Without Violence, Frederick Laboyer, MD

The Womanly Art of Breastfeeding, Diane Wiessinger, Diana West and Teresa Pitman, published by La Leche League International
Raising a Vaccine Free Child, Wendy Lydall

Spiritual Midwifery, Ina May Gaskin

Herbs and Helps in Pregnancy, Katherine Tarr

The last word on [bovine] casein goes to...

Vaccines containing casein, bovine extract, soy peptones, lactose, and egg proteins. All of which pose a risk of antibody production against more than just childhood diseases. The following pages are modified from *The Vaccine Excipient & Media Summary*, available on the CDC website. For a PDF of the original file, Google "Vaccine Excipient List".

The Vaccine Excipient & Media Summary
Excipients Included in U.S. Vaccines, by Vaccine
This table includes not only vaccine ingredients (e.g., adjuvants and preservatives), but also substances used during the manufacturing process, including vaccine-production media, that are removed from the final product and present only in trace quantities. In addition to the substances listed, most vaccines contain Sodium Chloride (table salt).
Last Updated September 2013
All reasonable efforts have been made to ensure the accuracy of this information, but manufacturers may change product contents before that information is reflected here.
If in doubt, check the manufacturer's package insert.

Adenovirus, Source: Manufacturer's P.I. Dated March, 2011
sucrose, D-mannose, D-fructose, dextrose, potassium phosphate, plasdone C, anhydrous lactose, micro crystalline cellulose, polacrilin potassium, magnesium stearate, cellulose acetate phthalate, alcohol, acetone, castor oil, FD&C Yellow #6 aluminum lake dye, human serum albumin, fetal bovine serum, sodium bicarbonate, human-diploid fibroblast cell cultures (WI-38), Dulbecco's Modified Eagle's Medium, monosodium glutamate
Anthrax (Biothrax), Source: Manufacturer's P.I. Dated May 2012
aluminum hydroxide, benzethonium chloride, formaldehyde, amino acids, vitamins, inorganic salts and sugars
BCG (Tice), Source: Manufacturer's P.I. Dated February 2009
glycerin, asparagine, citric acid, potassium phosphate, magnesium sulfate, Iron ammonium citrate, lactose
DT (Sanofi), Source: Manufacturer's P.I. Dated December 2005
aluminum potassium sulfate, peptone, bovine extract, formaldehyde, thimerosal (trace), modified Mueller and Miller medium, ammonium sulfate

DTaP (Daptacel), Source: Manufacturer's P.I. Dated July 2012

aluminum phosphate, formaldehyde, glutaraldehyde, 2-Phenoxyethanol, Stainer-Scholte medium, modified Mueller's growth medium, modified Mueller-Miller casamino acid medium (without beef heart infusion), dimethyl 1-beta-cyclodextrin, ammonium sulfate

DTaP (Infanrix), Source: Manufacturer's P.I. Dated July 2012

formaldehyde, glutaraldehyde, aluminum hydroxide, polysorbate 80, Fenton medium (containing bovine extract), modified Latham medium (derived from bovine casein), modified Stainer-Scholte liquid medium

DTaP-IPV (Kinrix), Source: Manufacturer's P.I. Dated July 2012

formaldehyde, glutaraldehyde, aluminum hydroxide, Vero (monkey kidney) cells, calf serum, lactalbumin hydrolysate, polysorbate 80, neomycin sulfate, polymyxin B, Fenton medium (containing bovine extract), modified Latham medium (derived from bovine casein), modified Stainer-Scholte liquid medium

DTaP-IPV/Hib (Pentacel), Source: Manufacturer's P.I. Dated July 2012

aluminum phosphate, polysorbate 80, formaldehyde, gutaraldehyde, bovine serum albumin, 2-phenoxethanol, neomycin, polymyxin B sulfate, Mueller's Growth Medium, Mueller-Miller casamino acid medium (without beef heart infusion), Stainer-Scholte medium (modified by the addition of casamino acids and dimethyl-beta-cyclodextrin), MRC-5 (human diploid) cells, CMRL 1969 medium (supplemented with calf serum), ammonium sulfate, and medium 199

DTaP-HepB-IPV (Pediarix), Source: Manufacturer's P.I. Dated August 2012

formaldehyde, gluteraldehyde, aluminum hydroxide, aluminum phosphate, lactalbumin hydrolysate, polysorbate 80, neomycin sulfate, polymyxin B, yeast protein, calf serum, Fenton medium (containing bovine extract), modified Latham medium (derived from bovine casein), modified Stainer-Scholte liquid medium, Vero (monkey kidney) cells

Hib (ActHIB), Source: Manufacturer's P.I. Dated November 2012

ammonium sulfate, formalin, sucrose, Modified Mueller and Miller medium

Hib (Hiberix), Source: Manufacturer's P.I. Dated March 2012

formaldehyde, lactose, semi-synthetic medium

Hib (PedvaxHIB), Source: Manufacturer's P.I. Dated December 2010

aluminum hydroxphosphate sulfate, ethanol, enzymes, phenol, detergent, complex fermentation medium

Hib/Hep B (Comvax), Source: Manufacturer's P.I. Dated December 2010
yeast (vaccine contains no detectable yeast DNA), nicotinamide adenine dinucleotide, hemin chloride, soy peptone, dextrose, mineral salts, amino acids, formaldehyde, potassium aluminum sulfate, amorphous aluminum hydroxyphosphate sulfate, sodium borate, phenol, ethanol, enzymes, detergent

Hib/Mening. CY (MenHibrix), Source: Manufacturer's P.I. Dated 2012
tris (trometamol)-HCl, sucrose, formaldehyde, synthetic medium, semi-synthetic medium

Hep A (Havrix), Source: Manufacturer's P.I. Dated June 2013
aluminum hydroxide, amino acid supplement, polysorbate 20, formalin, neomycin sulfate, MRC-5 cellular proteins

Hep A (Vaqta), Source: Manufacturer's P.I. Dated November 2012
amorphous aluminum hydroxyphosphate sulfate, bovine albumin, formaldehyde, neomycin, sodium borate, MRC-5 (human diploid) cells

Hep B (Engerix-B), Source: Manufacturer's P.I. Dated July 2012
aluminum hydroxide, yeast protein, phosphate buffers

Hep B (Recombivax), Source: Manufacturer's P.I. Dated July 2011
yeast protein, soy peptone, dextrose, amino acids, mineral salts, potassium aluminum sulfate, amorphous aluminum hydroxyphosphate sulfate, formaldehyde, phosphate buffer

Hep A/Hep B (Twinrix), Source: Manufacturer's P.I. Dated August 2012
formalin, yeast protein, aluminum phosphate, aluminum hydroxide, amino acids, phosphate buffer, polysorbate 20, neomycin sulfate, MRC-5 human diploid cells

Human Papillomavirus (HPV) (Cerverix), Source: Manufacturer's P.I. Dated Aug 2012
vitamins, amino acids, lipids, mineral salts, aluminum hydroxide, sodium dihydrogen phosphate dehydrate, 3-O-desacyl-4' Monophosphoryl lipid A, insect cell, bacterial, and viral protein.

Human Papillomavirus (HPV) (Gardasil), Source: Manufacturer's P.I. Dated March 2013
yeast protein, vitamins, amino acids, mineral salts, carbohydrates, amorphous aluminum hydroxyphosphate sulfate, L-histidine, polysorbate 80, sodium borate

Influenza (Afluria), Source: Manufacturer's P.I. Dated April 2013
beta-propiolactone, thimerosol (multi-dose vials only), monobasic sodium phosphate, dibasic sodium phosphate, monobasic potassium phosphate, potassium chloride, calcium chloride, sodium taurodeoxycholate, neomycin sulfate, polymyxin B, egg protein, sucrose
Influenza (Agriflu), Source: Manufacturer's P.I. Dated June 2012
egg proteins, formaldehyde, polysorbate 80, cetyltrimethylammonium bromide, neomycin sulfate, kanamycin
Influenza (Fluarix), Source: Manufacturer's P.I. Dated May 2013
octoxynol-10 (Triton X-100), α-tocopheryl hydrogen succinate, polysorbate 80 (Tween 80), hydrocortisone, gentamicin sulfate, ovalbumin, formaldehyde, sodium deoxycholate, sucrose, phosphate buffer
Influenza (Flublok), Source: Manufacturer's P.I. Dated December 2012
monobasic sodium phosphate, dibasic sodium phosphate, polysorbate 20, baculovirus and host cell proteins, baculovirus and cellular DNA, Triton X-100, lipids, vitamins, amino acids, mineral salts
Influenza (Flucelvax), Source: Manufacturer's P.I. Dated October 2012
Madin Darby Canine Kidney (MDCK) cell protein, MDCK cell DNA, polysorbate 80, cetyltrimethlyammonium bromide, β-propiolactone, phosphate buffer
Influenza (Fluvirin), Source: Manufacturer's P.I. Dated January 2012
nonylphenol ethoxylate, thimerosal (multidose vial–trace only in prefilled syringe), polymyxin, neomycin, beta-propiolactone, egg proteins, phosphate buffer
Influenza (Flulaval), Source: Manufacturer's P.I. Dated February 2013
thimerosal, formaldehyde, sodium deoxycholate, egg proteins
Influenza (Fluzone: Std, High-Dose, & Intradermal), Source: Manufacturer's P.I. Dated Apr 2013
formaldehyde, octylphenol ethoxylate (Triton X-100), gelatin (standard trivalent formulation only), thimerosal (multi-dose vial only), egg protein, phosphate buffers, sucrose
Influenza (FluMist), Source: Manufacturer's P.I. Dated July 2013
ethylene diamine tetraacetic acid (EDTA), monosodium glutamate, hydrolyzed porcine gelatin, arginine, sucrose, dibasic potassium phosphate, monobasic potassium phosphate, gentamicin sulfate, egg protein
Japanese Encephalitis (Ixiaro), Source: Manufacturer's P.I. Dated May 2013

aluminum hydroxide, Vero cells, protamine sulfate, formaldehyde, bovine serum albumin, sodium metabisulphite, sucrose

Meningococcal (MPSV4-Menomune), Source: Manufacturer's P.I. Dated October 2012
thimerosal (multi-dose vial only), lactose, Mueller Hinton casein agar, Watson Scherp media, detergent, alcohol

MMR (MMR-II), Source: Manufacturer's P.I. Dated December 2010
Medium 199, Minimum Essential Medium, phosphate, recombinant human albumin, neomycin, sorbitol, hydrolyzed gelatin, chick embryo cell culture, WI-38 human diploid lung fibroblasts

MMRV (ProQuad), Source: Manufacturer's P.I. Dated August 2011
sucrose, hydrolyzed gelatin, sorbitol, monosodium L-glutamate, sodium phosphate dibasic, human albumin, sodium bicarbonate, potassium phosphate monobasic, potassium chloride, potassium phosphate dibasic, neomycin, bovine calf serum, chick embryo cell culture, WI-38 human diploid lung fibroblasts, MRC-5 cells

Pneumococcal (PCV13 – Prevnar 13), Source: Manufacturer's P.I. Dated January 2013
casamino acids, yeast, ammonium sulfate, Polysorbate 80, succinate buffer, aluminum phosphate, soy peptone broth

Pneumococcal (PPSV-23 – Pneumovax), Source: Manufacturer's P.I. Dated October 2011
phenol.

Polio (IPV – Ipol), Source: Manufacturer's P.I. Dated December 2005
2-phenoxyethanol, formaldehyde, neomycin, streptomycin, polymyxin B, monkey kidney cells, Eagle MEM modified medium, calf serum protein, Medium 199

Rabies (Imovax), Source: Manufacturer's P.I. Dated December 2005
Human albumin, neomycin sulfate, phenol red indicator, MRC-5 human diploid cells, beta-propriolactone

Rabies (RabAvert), Source: Manufacturer's P.I. Dated March 2012
β-propiolactone, potassium glutamate, chicken protein, ovalbuminegg protein, neomycin, chlortetracycline, amphotericin B, human serum albumin, polygeline (processed bovine 14 gelatin), sodium EDTA, bovine serum

Rotavirus (RotaTeq), Source: Manufacturer's P.I. Dated June 2013
sucrose, sodium citrate, sodium phosphate monobasic monohydrate, sodium hydroxide, polysorbate 80, cell culture media, fetal bovine serum, vero cells [DNA from porcine circoviruses (PCV) 1 and 2 has been detected in RotaTeq. PCV-1 and PCV-2 are not known to cause disease in humans.]

Rotavirus (Rotarix), Source: Manufacturer's P.I. Dated September 2012
amino acids, dextran, sorbitol, sucrose, calcium carbonate, xanthan, Dulbecco's Modified Eagle Medium (DMEM) [Porcine circovirus type 1 (PCV-1) is present in Rotarix. PCV-1 is not known to cause disease in humans.]

Smallpox (Vaccinia – ACAM2000), Source: Manufacturer's P.I. Dated September 2009
human serum albumin, mannitol, neomycin, glycerin, polymyxin B, phenol, Vero cells, HEPES

Td (Decavac), Source: Manufacturer's P.I. Dated March 2011
aluminum potassium sulfate, peptone, formaldehyde, thimerosal, bovine muscle tissue (US sourced), Mueller and Miller medium, ammonium sulfate

Td (Tenivac), Source: Manufacturer's P.I. Dated December 2010
aluminum phosphate, formaldehyde, modified Mueller-Miller casamino acid medium without beef heart infusion, ammonium sulfate

Td (Mass Biologics), Source: Manufacturer's P.I. Dated February 2011
aluminum phosphate, formaldehyde, thimerosal (trace), ammonium phosphate, modified Mueller's media (containing bovine extracts)

Tdap (Adacel), Source: Manufacturer's P.I. Dated April 2013
aluminum phosphate, formaldehyde, glutaraldehyde, 2-phenoxyethanol, ammonium sulfate, Stainer-Scholte medium, dimethyl-beta-cyclodextrin, modified Mueller's growth medium, Mueller-Miller casamino acid medium (without beef heart infusion)

Tdap (Boostrix), Source: Manufacturer's P.I. Dated February 2013
formaldehyde, glutaraldehyde, aluminum hydroxide, polysorbate 80 (Tween 80), Latham medium derived from bovine casein, Fenton medium containing a bovine extract, Stainer-Scholte liquid medium

Typhoid (inactivated – Typhim Vi), Source: Manufacturer's P.I. Dated December 2005
hexadecyltrimethylammonium bromide, phenol, polydimethylsiloxane, disodium phosphate, monosodium phosphate, semi-synthetic medium

Typhoid (oral – Ty21a), Source: Manufacturer's P.I. Dated August 2006
yeast extract, casein, dextrose, galactose, sucrose, ascorbic acid, amino acids, lactose, magnesium stearate
Varicella (Varivax), Source: Manufacturer's P.I. Dated December 2012
sucrose, phosphate, glutamate, gelatin, monosodium L-glutamate, sodium phosphate dibasic, potassium phosphate monobasic, potassium chloride, sodium phosphate monobasic, potassium chloride, EDTA, residual components of MRC-5 cells including DNA and protein, neomycin, fetal bovine serum, human diploid cell cultures (WI-38), embryonic guinea pig cell cultures, human embryonic lung cultures
Yellow Fever (YF-Vax), Source: Manufacturer's P.I. Dated January 2010
sorbitol, gelatin, egg protein
Zoster (Shingles – Zostavax), Source: Manufacturer's P.I. Dated June 2011
sucrose, hydrolyzed porcine gelatin, monosodium L-glutamate, sodium phosphate dibasic, potassium phosphate monobasic, neomycin, potassium chloride, residual components of MRC-5 cells including DNA and protein, bovine calf serum

A table listing vaccine excipients and media by excipient can be found in: Grabenstein JD. ImmunoFacts: Vaccines and Immunologic Drugs – 2013 (38th revision). St Louis, MO: Wolters Kluwer Health, 2012.

Notes

6
Unfermented Soy is Unfit
(For human consumption.)

Soy, your doctor tells you it's good for your heart. You hear about it being the solution to preventing world hunger and how it allows vegans to have their soysages and soycon, tofurkey and motor oil all from the same plant. After all, what other plant is so versatile? It's a vegetable, it's a grain, it's the bun, burger, and the cheese, and it has industrial applications! You can douse it with herbicides, and it won't die (only 90% of the varieties grown in the US can claim that honorable distinction though). We hear all these things about it as though they were sales clinchers. But we don't realize that the insidiousness of this plant across all categories of products we consume in the place of REAL food, has facilitated some huge problems- for all humans- men, women, and children alike.

As Dr. Kaayla Daniel PhD sees it, the stuff has a "dark side". And very soon, you may begin to agree wholeheartedly. Soy is a legume, first and foremost, just like a peanut. I think we'd scratch our heads at the idea of a peanut being referred to as a vegetable or a grain, the way soy is, but because of the massive cash crop status soy enjoys in this country, it seems to be a little "above the law" (starring Steven Soygal), yet soy has actually never even been granted GRAS status by the FDA. GRAS stands for Generally Regarded As Safe, basically for any human consumption. When something is granted GRAS status, it means that there is no age limitation or other consumption restriction on it as a food. Children, pregnant and nursing moms, the elderly, it's generally regarded as safe for all. But soy has not enjoyed that privilege, yet it's revered as though it's the nectar of the Gods. Visit Dr. Daniel's website, www.NaughtyNutritionist.com, and pick up her book, *The Whole Soy Story*, heavily referenced with research not funded by Monsanto (creators of the Round-up Ready Soybean), or the Demonic Soy Cult, I mean the United Soybean Board.

The bit of truth that is associated with the health claims about soy is actually referring to traditionally fermented soy foods like miso, natto, tempeh, tamari- all used in Asia as condiments, not primary sources of food or substitutes for animal protein. The media may try to make us believe that Asian cultures owe their longevity to consumption of *unfermented* soy, but as Dr. Daniel explains, there is indeed a dark side to America's favorite health food. The following are soy derivatives and ingredients you may find on anything in the grocery store that comes premade or processed:

• Soybean oil- actually labelled vegetable oil if you can imagine. Why? To deceive folks, that's why. It sounds much healthier to say you're using oil extracted from vegetables than from SOY. Can you name a few *vegetables* that are rich enough in oils to actually be sources of them, because I can't.

• Soy flour- If you've ever seen a package of soy flour with the words "whole grain" on it, you have definitely witnessed semantics at their best. I don't think you'll come across a food with so many personalities, one moment it's a vegetable, the next it's a grain. Whatever the unsuspecting public may have been tricked into thinking is the next healthy thing for them to consume- that's what soy will dress up as for Halloween.

• Soy lecithin- a cheap emulsifier used in the candy-making industry, also found in salad dressing, cake mix, teabags! It is collected from the sludge remaining after soybeans are pressed for their oil. It is loaded with residues of all of the herbicides, pesticides, and fertilizers applied to the crop. A note about lecithin- a little goes a long way, and what I mean by that is that it only takes a tiny amount to trigger a big reaction in someone that is sensitive enough.

• Soy Milk- also something to avoid- opt for coconut milk, or water!

• Soy protein Isolate- You're going to find this "anti-food" in low quality: protein powders, meal replacement shakes, snack bars, and other *froods* (that's short for Frankenfoods), and the reason I'm referring to them in that less than flattering way is because unfermented soy protein is extremely difficult for humans to digest. And remember that incompletely broken down protein can and will trigger immune-mediated activity and subsequently inflammation.

If you have protein supplements or bars or treats in the pantry and there are soy ingredients in them, please realize that 90% of soy crops in the U.S. come from genetically modified seeds, Roundup Ready. Those products in your cupboard are about the lowest quality you can find. Unfermented soy is not a superfood, it's toxic.

The soy industry has manipulated and continues to manipulate both the media and the FDA to allow soy to carry the health claim of reducing heart disease and cholesterol. About five years ago, they even tried to secure the claim of reducing the risk of cancer. Dr. Daniel was able to effectively prevent that claim from being approved, but if it had been approved, consumption of the problematic legume would likely have doubled to more than $8 billion in annual U.S. sales. Clearly that's a motivating factor for the marketing department at the United Soybean Board.

If you want a website littered with lies upon lies, visit www.SoyConnection.com and if you decide to take the trash strewn on that site as gospel, get ready for a plethora of health issues from gas and bloating, to hormone dysfunction and endocrine disruptions, and possibly even cancer. Yes, I said cancer, namely thyroid, but don't rule out breast cancer and ovarian or uterine.

I strongly encourage you to pick up Dr. Daniel's book, *The Whole Soy Story,* flip through it, go to the back 50 pages full of references, and see if you can take her advice with a grain of salt, because I'm certain if you are consuming anything from commercially bottled salad dressing to bread and vegetable oil, you're eating a whole lot more soy than you think. You can also visit the website of the Weston A. Price Foundation, at www.WestonAPrice.org and search the word "soy". From the brochure "Soy Alert!" published by the Weston A. Price Foundation for Wise Traditions in Food, Farming, and the Healing Arts, the myths and truths about soy (reprinted with permission):

> Myth: Use of soy as a food dates back many thousands of years.
>
> *Truth: Soy was first used as a food during the late Chou dynasty (1134-246 BC), only after the Chinese learned to ferment soy beans to make foods like tempeh, natto and tamari.*
>
> Myth: Asians consume large amounts of soy foods.
>
> *Truth: Average consumption of soy foods in Japan and China is 10 grams (about 2 teaspoons) per day. Asians consume soy foods in small amounts as a condiment, and not as a replacement for animal foods.*
>
> Myth: Modern soy foods confer the same health benefits as traditionally fermented soy foods.
>
> *Truth: Most modern soy foods are not fermented to neutralize toxins in soybeans, and are processed in a way that denatures proteins and increases levels of carcinogens.*
>
> Myth: Soy foods provide complete protein.
>
> *Truth: Like all legumes, soy beans are deficient in sulfur-containing*

amino acids methionine and cystine. In addition, modern processing denatures fragile lysine.

Myth: Fermented soy foods can provide vitamin B12 in vegetarian diets.

Truth: The compound that resembles vitamin B12 in soy cannot be used by the human body; in fact, soy foods cause the body to require more B12

Myth: Soy formula is safe for infants.

Truth: Soy foods contain trypsin inhibitors that inhibit protein digestion and affect pancreatic function. In test animals, diets high in trypsin inhibitors led to stunted growth and pancreatic disorders. Soy foods increase the body's requirement for vitamin D, needed for strong bones and normal growth. Phytic acid in soy foods results in reduced bioavailabilty of iron and zinc which are required for the health and development of the brain and nervous system. Soy also lacks cholesterol, likewise essential for the development of the brain and nervous system. Megadoses of phytoestrogens in soy formula have been implicated in the current trend toward increasingly premature sexual development in girls and delayed or retarded sexual development in boys.

Myth: Soy foods can prevent osteoporosis.

Truth: Soy foods can cause deficiencies in calcium and vitamin D, both needed for healthy bones. Calcium from bone broths and vitamin D from seafood, lard and organ meats prevent osteoporosis in Asian countries—not soy foods.

Myth: Modern soy foods protect against many types of cancer.

Truth: A British government report concluded that there is little evidence that soy foods protect against breast cancer or any other forms of cancer. In fact, soy foods may result in an increased risk of cancer.

Myth: Soy foods protect against heart disease.

Truth: In some people, consumption of soy foods will lower cholesterol, but there is no evidence that lowering cholesterol with soy protein improves one's risk of having heart disease.

Myth: Soy estrogens (isoflavones) are good for you.

Truth: Soy isoflavones are phyto-endocrine disrupters. At dietary levels, they can prevent ovulation and stimulate the growth of cancer cells. Eating as little as 30 grams (about 4 tablespoons) of soy per day can result in hypothyroidism with symptoms of lethargy, constipation, weight gain and fatigue.

Myth: Soy foods are safe and beneficial for women to use in their postmenopausal years.

Truth: Soy foods can stimulate the growth of estrogen-dependent tumors and cause thyroid problems. Low thyroid function is associated with difficulties in menopause.

Myth: Phytoestrogens in soy foods can enhance mental ability.

Truth: A recent study found that women with the highest levels of estrogen in their blood had the lowest levels of cognitive function; In Japanese Americans tofu consumption in mid-life is associated with the occurrence of Alzheimer's disease in later life.

Myth: Soy isoflavones and soy protein isolate have GRAS (Generally Recognized as Safe) status.

Truth: Archer Daniels Midland (ADM) recently withdrew its application to the FDA for GRAS status for soy isoflavones following an outpouring of protest from the scientific community. The FDA never approved GRAS status for soy protein isolate because of concern regarding the presence of toxins and carcinogens in processed soy.

Myth: Soy foods are good for your sex life.

Truth: Numerous animal studies show that soy foods cause infertility in animals. Soy consumption enhances hair growth in middle-aged men, indicating lowered testosterone levels. Japanese housewives feed tofu to their husbands frequently when they want to reduce his virility.

Myth: Soy beans are good for the environment.

Truth: Most soy beans grown in the US are genetically engineered to allow farmers to use large amounts of herbicides. Think Monsanto's Roundup Ready strain of soybeans that resist application of said herbicide and still grow and survive without issue.

Myth: Soy beans are good for developing nations.

Truth: In third world countries, soybeans replace traditional crops and transfer the value-added of processing from the local population to multinational corporations.

Soy Dangers Summarized

• High levels of phytic acid in soy reduce assimilation of calcium, magnesium, copper, iron and zinc. Phytic acid in soy is not neutralized by ordinary preparation methods such as soaking, sprouting and long, slow cooking. High phytate diets have caused growth problems in children.

• Trypsin inhibitors in soy interfere with protein digestion and may cause pancreatic disorders. In test animals soy containing trypsin inhibitors caused stunted growth.

• Soy phytoestrogens disrupt endocrine function and have the potential to cause infertility and to promote breast cancer in adult women.

• Soy phytoestrogens are potent antithyroid agents that cause hypothyroidism and may cause thyroid cancer. In infants, consumption of soy formula has been linked to autoimmune thyroid disease.

• Vitamin B12 analogs in soy are not absorbed and actually increase the body's requirement for B12. [Pernicious anemia is a deficiency in B12]

• Soy foods increase the body's requirement for vitamin D.

• Fragile proteins are denatured during high temperature processing to make soy protein isolate and textured vegetable protein.

• Processing of soy protein results in the formation of toxic lysinoalanine and highly carcinogenic nitrosamines.

• Free glutamic acid or MSG, a potent neurotoxin, is formed during soy food processing and additional amounts are added to many soy foods.

• Soy foods contain high levels of aluminum which is toxic to the nervous system and the kidneys.

Censored Nutritional Gem #6: Unfermented Soy is Unfit (For human consumption.)

Suggested Reading:

The Whole Soy Story: The Dark Side of America's Favorite Health Food, Kaayla T. Daniel, PhD

Take Control of Your Health, Joseph Mercola, DO

Food Allergy Guide to Soy: How to Eat Safely and Well Soy-Free, Bill Bowling

Excitotoxins: The Taste That Kills, Russell L. Blaylock, MD

Seeds of Deception: Exposing Industry and Government Lies About the Safety of the Genetically Engineered Foods You're Eating, Jeffrey M. Smith

The last word...
(From Dr. Christiane Northrup's website www.DrNorthrup.com)

Christiane Northrup, M.D., is a visionary pioneer and the world's leading authority in the field of women's health and wellness. Dr. Northrup is a leading proponent of medicine that acknowledges the unity of mind, body, emotions, and spirit. Internationally known for her empowering approach to women's health and wellness, Dr. Northrup teaches women how to thrive at every stage of life.

Estrogen Dominance: What You Need To Know

The conventional medical mindset is that menopause is an estrogen deficiency disease resulting from ovarian failure. Women have been led to believe that at the slightest symptoms, they should run out and get estrogen replacement. While estrogen levels will decrease during menopause, the truth is, estrogen levels do not fall appreciably until after a woman's last period. In fact, far more women suffer from the effects of "estrogen dominance" during the transition—that is, they have too much estrogen relative to progesterone. And some women can suffer from the symptoms of estrogen dominance for 10 to 15 years, beginning as early as age 35.

Listen To Your Body

The symptoms listed below, as well as many others, often arise when estrogen overstimulates both the brain and body. All of these symptoms are exacerbated by stress of all kinds. Many women in their thirties and early forties find that they experience moderate to severe symptoms of estrogen dominance as they approach perimenopause.

- Decreased sex drive
- Irregular or otherwise abnormal menstrual periods
- Bloating (water retention)
- Breast swelling and tenderness
- Fibrocystic breasts
- Headaches (especially premenstrually)
- Mood swings (most often irritability and depression)
- Weight and/or fat gain (particularly around the abdomen and hips)
- Cold hands and feet (a symptom of thyroid dysfunction)
- Hair loss
- Thyroid dysfunction

• Sluggish metabolism
• Foggy thinking, memory loss
• Fatigue
• Trouble sleeping/insomnia
• PMS

Estrogen dominance has also been linked to allergies, autoimmune disorders, breast cancer, uterine cancer, infertility, ovarian cysts, and increased blood clotting, and is also associated with acceleration of the aging process.

What Causes This

When a woman's menstrual cycle is normal, estrogen is the dominant hormone for the first two weeks leading up to ovulation. Estrogen is balanced by progesterone during the last two weeks. As a woman enters perimenopause and begins to experience anovulatory cycles (that is, cycles where no ovulation occurs), estrogen can often go unopposed, causing symptoms. Skipping ovulation is, however, only one potential factor in estrogen dominance. In industrialized countries such as the United States, there can be many other causes, including:

• Excess body fat (greater than 28%)
• Too much stress, resulting in excess amounts of cortisol, insulin, and norepinephrine, which can lead to adrenal exhaustion and can also adversely affect overall hormonal balance
• A low-fiber diet with excess refined carbohydrates and deficient in nutrients and high quality fats
• Impaired immune function
• Environmental agents

Spiritual and Holistic Options

Here's what you can do to decrease estrogen dominance: Increase nutrients in the diet; take a high potency multivitamin/mineral combination [we should hope Dr. Northrup also meant to add "bioavailable" to the description of that supplement], as well as:

1. Follow a hormone-balancing diet: Eat lots of fresh fruits and vegetables, adequate protein, and moderate amounts of healthy fat. Remember to get enough fiber. Estrogen is excreted by the bowel; if stool remains in the bowel, estrogen is reabsorbed.

2. Lose excess body fat and get regular exercise—especially strength training.

3. Detoxify your liver: Traditional Chinese Medicine explains that menopausal symptoms are caused by blocked liver and kidney chi. This makes sense. The liver acts as a filter, helping us screen out the harmful effects of toxins from our environment and the products we put in our bodies. When the liver has to work hard to eliminate toxins such as alcohol, drugs, caffeine, or environmental agents, the liver's capacity to cleanse the blood of estrogen is compromised.

4. Decrease stress: Learn how to say no to excessive demands on your time. Remember, perimenopause is a time to reinvent yourself. This means investing time and energy in yourself, not everyone else.

Notes

7

Save the Olive Oil for Salads
(Don't cook with it.)

Why can't I cook with olive oil? We talked about the structure of unsaturated fatty acids in chapter 1 and how those substances are not stable in the presence of heat and oxygen. According to Udo Erasmus, PhD, "when extra virgin olive oil is fried, it is extensively damaged. It should not be used for frying, but should be added to foods after they come off the heat." *But it says that it's safe for medium heat right there on the bottle!* It's wrong. Take the word of a PhD (Udo Erasmus) with graduate studies in genetics and biochemistry, who has devoted the last almost twenty years of his professional life to researching fats and oils and their role in the human body, over the marketing claims of an oil manufacturer trying to make millions of dollars by ensuring his product has as widespread a use as possible. Be smart about the information you use to make daily choices and when you find consistency across your sources, and all of those sources don't have the financial backing of multi-billion dollar chemical and frankenfood companies, go with them.

When you heat pourable oils, like olive and even grapeseed oil, you damage them, even more than they may already be due to what they had to go through during the manufacturing process. But heating them definitely turns them into something toxic (with inflammatory potential) to the body. Does that mean that we should avoid oils altogether since they have to be treated so carefully? Absolutely not. Our bodies require both saturated and unsaturated fatty acids obtained from our diets, in order to function properly and for all body systems to have at their disposal the raw materials required to synthesize necessary life chemicals. We simply have to be aware that oils, since they are composed primarily of unsaturated fatty acids, have to be treated with respect.

The long and short of it is that by documented chemical structure, certain bonds are very susceptible to alteration and disruption and those happen to also be the bonds in oils. Oils are liquid at room temperature, that's how you can tell them apart from fats- which are solid at room temperature. When you do require fat for cooking and baking, choose unrefined coconut oil and organic palm shortening, and follow the "low and slow" rule. Don't exceed low-medium heat on the stove top, and try not to bake at over 350 degrees Fahrenheit because all fats, oils and proteins can be damaged when exposed to high temperatures. How easy was that?

Censored Nutritional Gem #7: Save the Olive Oil for Salads

8
Fat, Friendly Flora, and Lacto-Fermentation Facilitate Flushing
(Way more than fiber alone.)

How many times a day should you go Number 2? Some of us would say once, while others would pause uncomfortably to remember just how many days it's actually been since their last round of elimination. I'm going to try to give you the ideal explanation with as few puns and plays on words as possible. How many times you should have a bowel movement is going to depend loosely on how many times a day you eat. If you only eat once a day, are you going to be making three separate trips to the bathroom between sun up and sun down? Probably not. Conversely, just because you eat six times a day, doesn't mean you'll be eliminating that many times either. How efficient your bowels are at cleaning themselves out is really going to depend on what they're processing. Give them lots of meat and refined carbohydrates, with nary a salad or vegetable to speak of and you're going to be lucky to visit the WC once a week, if that.

If you're eating three meals a day, you should eliminate at least twice anywhere from 9 to 24 hours later, provided the meals you consumed were of quality nutrition. Did you know the number one reason Americans present to their primary care manager is for constipation? Without doing a thorough inventory but giving you an average, I'd say the shelf space devoted to laxatives is considerably more than that devoted to olive oil. We are the Constipation Nation. If there's any doubt, just walk through your local mega mart and look at the distention of people's midsections. They're not going to the bathroom. They're not able to go to the bathroom, even though they're getting 6 to 12 servings of whole grains a day. They're holding it all in, not willingly mind you, and it's making them miserable, and sick.

So, is fiber the answer? Is that why people aren't able to empty their bowels efficiently enough to prevent putrefaction of our intestines? Fiber is definitely an important aspect of our diet where regularity is concerned but that's not the only thing that will clean out your system and make sure you're not distended and backed up. I think a huge misconception in the United States and Canada is that fiber is the be-all and end-all in maintaining regularity, but that's simply not the case. The typical mindset is also to get your fiber from whole grains, since they present with such an "abundance" of it. Eat 6 to 12 servings of grains a day, no or low fat, no lacto-fermented food, a gram of protein for every pound you weigh and take in the amount of water we're notorious for consuming and I guarantee you, you'll stop yourself up faster than you can say "megacolon". So you say, well of course you'll get constipated doing that, you're not eating any fruits or veggies. Does America eat enough fruits and veggies, America? Could we fathom that all we need to do to improve our regularity is add the recommended 5 servings of fruits and veggies a day to our diets? Ketchup will count as one serving; a little bag of mechanically cut up, smoothed out, and bleached carrots could be the second. The third could be a cup of iceberg lettuce drowned in ranch dressing, and the fourth and fifth, a double serving of creamed corn. Do all those count? Apparently not because those are the fruits and veggies we're eating and we're still full of it. And corn is not a vegetable, it's a grain!

You're going to get more fiber from dark green leafy veggies, grapefruit, strawberries, beans and lentils than you're going to get from that whole wheat bread you're toasting. And if you are getting your fiber from veggies and fruits, in addition to fiber, you're also going to get enzymes, water, and phytochemicals that are all going to help more than just your digestive system work efficiently. So yes, eat lots of beans, and fresh, organic veggies and fruits, and you'll be providing your digestive system the highest quality fiber to give it the upper hand in preventing putrefaction.

From the book, *Plant Fiber in Foods*, by James W. Anderson, "A high fiber diet can help lower cholesterol, control blood sugar (soluble fiber), and prevent constipation (insoluble). Aim for 25-35 grams (g) of total fiber each day, or 6-8 grams per meal, and 3-4 grams per snack, choosing foods from all the categories listed… Increase your fiber intake gradually, over 2 or 3 weeks, so your system can adapt to the added bulk without discomfort. Drink plenty of fluids, at least 6-8 cups of caffeine-free liquid daily." By reviewing the table below, you can see that simply eating 2 cups of a 4-bean veggie chili containing a combination of pinto beans, navy beans, black beans and light red kidney beans will yield a total fiber intake of 26.6 grams for a total of 4 servings.

Legumes (cooked)	Serving Size	Total Fiber	Soluble	Insoluble
Black beans	½ cup	6.1	2.4	3.7
Black-eyed peas	½ cup	4.7	0.5	4.2
Chick peas, dried	½ cup	4.3	1.3	3.0
Kidney beans, light red	½ cup	7.9	2.0	5.9
Lentils	½ cup	5.2	0.6	4.6
Lima beans	½ cup	4.3	1.1	3.2
Navy beans	½ cup	6.5	2.2	4.3
Pinto beans	½ cup	6.1	1.4	4.7

Adapted from Nutrition Services, Harvard University Health Services

Vegetables (cooked)	Serving	Total fiber	Soluble	Insoluble
Asparagus	½ cup	2.8	1.7	1.1
Beets, flesh only	½ cup	1.8	0.8	1.0
Broccoli	½ cup	2.4	1.2	1.2
Brussels sprouts	½ cup	3.8	2.0	1.8
Carrots, sliced	½ cup	2.0	1.1	0.9
Cauliflower	½ cup	1.0	0.4	0.6
Green beans, canned	½ cup	2.0	0.5	1.5
Kale	½ cup	2.5	0.7	1.8
Okra, frozen	½ cup	4.1	1.0	3.1
Peas, green, frozen	½ cup	4.3	1.3	3.0
Potato, sweet, flesh	½ cup	4.0	1.8	2.2
Potato, russet, baked	1 med	4.7	1.2	3.5
Spinach	½ cup	1.6	0.5	1.1
Tomato sauce	½ cup	1.7	0.8	0.9
Turnip	½ cup	4.8	1.7	3.1
Raw Vegetables				
Avocado, sliced	½ cup	5.0	2.0	3.0
Cabbage, red	1 cup	1.5	0.6	0.9
Carrots, fresh	1, 7½ in.	2.3	1.1	1.2
Celery, fresh, diced	1 cup	1.7	0.7	1.0
Cucumber, fresh	1 cup	0.5	0.2	0.3
Lettuce, iceberg	1 cup	0.5	0.1	0.4
Mushrooms, fresh	1 cup	0.8	0.1	0.7
Onion, fresh, chopped	½ cup	1.7	0.9	0.8
Green pepper, diced	1 cup	1.7	0.7	1.0
Tomato, fresh	1 medium	1.0	0.1	0.9

Adapted from Nutrition Services, Harvard University Health Services

Using the table above how many servings of vegetables would it take to bring you into compliance with at least 25 grams of fiber in one day? Try the 9 below for total fiber of 25.2 grams.

- 1 cup cooked broccoli (2 servings): Total fiber 4.8 g
- 2 cups spinach salad (4 servings): Total fiber 6.4 g
- 1 cup avocado (2 servings): Total fiber 10.0 g
- 1 medium baked potato (1 serving): Total fiber 4.7 g

Fruits	Serving	Total fiber	Soluble	Insoluble
Apple, red, fresh w/skin	1 small	2.8	1.0	1.8
Applesauce, canned	½ cup	2.0	0.7	1.3
Apricots, dried	7 halves	2.0	1.1	0.9
Apricots, fresh w/skin	4	3.5	1.8	1.7
Banana, fresh	½ small	1.1	0.3	0.8
Blueberries, fresh	¾ cup	1.4	0.3	1.1
Cherries, black, fresh	12 large	1.3	0.6	0.7
Figs, dried	1 ½	3.0	1.4	1.6
Grapefruit, fresh	½ medium	1.6	1.1	0.5
Grapes, fresh w/skin	15 small	0.5	0.2	0.3
Kiwifruit, flesh	1 large	1.7	0.7	1.0
Mango, flesh only	½ small	2.9	1.7	1.2
Melon, cantaloupe	1 cup cubed	1.1	0.3	0.8
Orange, fresh	1 small	2.9	1.8	1.1
Peach, fresh, w/skin	1 medium	2.0	1.0	1.0
Pear, fresh, w/skin	½ large	2.9	1.1	1.8
Plum, red, fresh	2 medium	2.4	1.1	1.3
Prunes, dried	3 medium	1.7	1.0	0.7
Raisins, dried	2 tbsp	0.4	0.2	0.2
Raspberries, fresh	1 cup	3.3	0.9	2.4
Strawberries, fresh	1 ¼ cup	2.8	1.1	1.7
Watermelon	1 ¼ cup cubed	0.6	0.4	0.2

Adapted from Nutrition Services, Harvard University Health Services

When it comes to fruits, you really need to keep in mind that even *fructose*, fruit sugar, is sugar, and that keeping your intake of *any sugar* at around 25 grams per day is truly optimal. One cup of strawberries contains only 7 grams of fructose, where 1 medium apple contains 19 grams. Limit your fruit consumption to 2 servings per day, or opt for berries as your fruit servings, many of which are powerful super foods (low caloric content with exceptionally high micronutrient content).

How many servings would it take to get the minimum recommended grams of fiber from the list of whole grain foods, if you didn't want to eat boxed breakfast cereal? The following examples would give you a total fiber intake of 25.1 grams from 11.5 servings of the number one recommended media source of fiber.

- 2 slices whole wheat bread (2 servings): Total fiber 3.0 g
- 1/3 cup dry oatmeal (1 serving): Total fiber 2.7 g
- 1 bran muffin (1 serving, recipe for 12 calls for 1 cup of bran): Total fiber 2.0g
- 2 slices rye bread (2 servings): Total fiber 3.6g
- 2 cups whole wheat spaghetti (4 servings): Total fiber 10.8
- 4 1/2 cups popcorn (1.5 serving): Total fiber 3.0 g

Pasta, Rice, Grains	Serving	Total Fiber	Soluble	Insoluble
Popcorn, popped	3 cups	2.0	0.1	1.9
Rice, white	½ cup	0.8	trace	0.8
Spaghetti, white	½ cup	0.9	0.4	0.5
Spaghetti, whole wheat	½ cup	2.7	0.6	2.1
Wheat bran	½ cup	12.3	1.0	11.3
Wheat germ	3 tbsp	3.9	0.7	3.2
Breads and Crackers				
Pumpernickel	1 slice	2.7	1.2	1.5
Rye	1 slice	1.8	0.8	1.0
White	1 slice	0.6	0.3	0.3
Whole wheat	1 slice	1.5	0.3	1.2
Cereals				
All Bran	1/3 cup	8.6	1.4	7.2
Benefit	¾ cup	5.0	2.8	2.2
Cheerios	1 ¼ cup	2.5	1.2	1.3
Corn flakes	1 cup	0.5	0.1	0.4
Cream of wheat, regular	2 ½ tbsp	1.1	0.4	0.7
Fiber One	½ cup	11.9	0.8	11.1
Grapenuts	¼ cup	2.8	0.8	2.0
Oat bran, cooked	¾ cup	4.0	2.2	1.8
Oatmeal, dry	1/3 cup	2.7	1.4	1.3
Puffed Wheat	1 cup	1.0	0.5	0.5
Raisin Bran	¾ cup	5.3	0.9	4.4
Rice Krispies	1 cup	0.3	0.1	0.2
Shredded Wheat	1 cup	5.2	0.7	4.5
Special K	1 cup	0.9	0.2	0.7

Adapted from Nutrition Services, Harvard University Health Services

So you can easily tell that getting your minimum recommended fiber intake from whole grain breads and pastas can only happen if you're consuming close to the maximum number of servings. Grains have considerably less regularity-promoting insoluble fiber than most fruits and vegetables, and simply can't even measure up to the amounts in beans and lentils. The only real way for whole grains to compete (barely) with the fiber content of beans is to be consumed through breakfast cereals, and even then, cup for cup, beans outrank. Listen carefully to those radio and TV ads that promote fiber intake through whole grains, and feel free to lose all faith in the credibility of the source, because now you know better.

Fiber aside, did you know you could add so much more power to peristalsis with a little help from friendly flora? Probiotics are the friendly microorganisms that break down everything the digestive process didn't get a chance to so that it can pass through that colon without beginning to decompose anaerobically (putrefaction!). Nowadays, a supplement may be the best option for most of us. A healthy colon should contain 2 to 3 pounds of friendly flora or beneficial bacteria, and that's kind of a misnomer I just realized because flora refers to plant life and bacteria are not considered plants, so maybe they'd be more aptly named friendly *fauna,* but I digress.

Consider the fact that the body doesn't produce the probiotics residing in the gut, they must be introduced through our food. In an article on his website, www.Mercola.com, Dr. Mercola recently wrote:

> Your gastrointestinal tract houses some 100 trillion bacteria—about two to three pounds worth. In all, the bacteria outnumber your body's cells by about 10 to 1.

> Your intestinal bacteria are part of your immune system, and researchers are discovering that microbes of all kinds play instrumental roles in countless areas of your health. For example, beneficial bacteria, also known as probiotics, have been shown to:

> • Modulate your immune response and reduce inflammation
> • Produce vitamins, absorb minerals, and eliminate toxins
> • Control asthma and reduce risk of allergies
> • Benefit your mood and mental health
> • Boost weight loss

> Beneficial bacteria also control the growth of disease-causing bacteria by competing for nutrition and attachment sites in your colon. This is

of immense importance, as pathogenic bacteria and other less beneficial microbes can wreak havoc with your health if they gain the upper hand. It can also affect your weight.

When it comes to diet, you want to eat mostly whole, fresh, unadulterated foods, taking pains to avoid sugars and processed/pasteurized and genetically engineered foods of all kinds. Add to that a healthy amount of traditionally fermented foods each day and you're off to a good start. Examples of healthy fermented foods include:

- Sauerkraut, pickles [traditionally fermented, not the vinegar added variety], and other fermented vegetables
- Fermented dairy products, such as yoghurt and kefir made from raw, (unpasteurized) dairy
- Miso
- Tempeh
- Olives

A strong case can be made for eating organic to protect your gut flora as agricultural chemicals take a heavy toll on beneficial microbes—both in the soil in which the food is grown, and in your body. Glyphosate (Roundup), used in particularly hefty amounts on genetically engineered crops, appears to be among the worst of the most widely used chemicals in food production. As for general lifestyle advice, you'll want to avoid well-known culprits that kill beneficial bacteria, such as:

- Antibiotics (also note that most store-bought beef typically comes from cattle raised with antibiotics. To avoid getting a dose of antibiotics in every piece of meat you eat, make sure your meat is grass-fed and finished)
- Chlorinated water
- Antibacterial soap
- Pollution

If your doctor has ever suggested you take a spoonful of mineral oil to help get your bowels moving again, I, personally, would fire them. Mineral oil is no more meant for human consumption than petroleum jelly. Why do they suggest it? According to www.WebMD.com:

... it is known as a lubricant laxative. It works by keeping water in the stool and intestines. This helps to soften the stool and also makes it easier for stool to pass through the intestines." There are of course possible side effects, "this medication should not be used in older adults, children younger than 6 years, or in people who are bedridden…

Because this drug can interfere with the absorption of certain vitamins (fat-soluble vitamins including A, D, E, K), take this medication on an empty stomach… This product may decrease the absorption of other medications you may be taking. Take this product at least 2 hours from your other medications… It may take 6 to 8 hours before this medication causes a bowel movement. Tell your doctor if your condition persists or worsens, or if bleeding from the rectum occurs.

That's just lovely. But we can see that it has indeed been documented that *oil* is an intestinal lubricant that helps keep water in the stool and intestines, while also softening the stool which makes it easier to pass through said intestines. Now, why couldn't they have suggested you take a spoonful of coconut oil, or olive oil, to do the exact same thing, without the worry of interference of absorption of the fat soluble vitamins? Good question. The fantastic thing to recognize is that the right fats, high quality fats and oils like coconut oil, and cold-pressed extra virgin olive oil, keep your colon well-lubricated so that everything *does* slide through without delay. In addition, as Gem # 1 clearly explains, it does so much more than that! People on low fat diets can attest to this, if you're not loading up on the leafy greens and water, you get constipated. Let's stop underestimating the role fat plays when it comes to efficient elimination, and also embrace the idea that whole grains come with a lot more baggage than just bulk fiber.

Censored Nutritional Gem #8:
Fat, Friendly Flora, and Lacto-Fermentation Facilitate Flushing
(Way more than fiber alone.)

The last word on lacto-fermentation goes to...

Dr. Stephan Guyenet, an obesity researcher and neurobiologist, enjoys "synthesizing and communicating science for a general audience" on his blog, wholehealthsource.blogspot.com. And for that we are most grateful! According to Dr. Guyenet:

> ...most if not all dairy-eating cultures ferment their milk... [whether it's] kefir from Caucasia, laban from the Middle East, dahi from India, creme fraiche from Western Europe, piima from Finland, mursik from Kenya... these cultures knew cultured milk was delicious and nutritious. It is the process by which "friendly" microorganisms, called probiotics, "consume" the proteins and carbohydrates present in foods and basically pre-digest those macromolecules for us, thereby easing the burden on our own digestive systems. Long before the times of pasteurization and modern refrigeration, the only way we had to preserve and store foods for later use was by lacto-fermenting them. Many of the world's oldest cultures actually eat a traditionally fermented food with every meal.

9
A Good Egg is a Raw Egg

Don't raw eggs give you salmonella? Dr. Mercola is going to come to our rescue on this issue once again:

Salmonella infections are usually present only in traditionally raised commercial hens. If you are purchasing your eggs from healthy chickens this infection risk are obtaining high quality, cage-free, organically fed, chicken eggs as recommended above, the risk virtually disappears. But before you eat eggs - raw or not - you should thoroughly examine them for signs of infection:

• Always check the freshness of the egg right before you consume the yolk.

• If you are uncertain about the freshness of an egg, don't eat it- that's one of the best safeguards against salmonella infection.

• If there is a crack in the shell, don't eat it. You can easily check for this by immersing the egg in a pan of cool, salted water. If the egg emits a tiny stream of bubbles, don't consume it as the shell is porous/contains a hole.

• If you are getting your eggs fresh from a farmer it is best to not refrigerate them. This is the way most of the world stores their eggs; they do not refrigerate them. To properly judge the freshness of an egg, its contents need to be at room temperature. Eggs that are stored in the fridge and opened immediately after taking them out will seem fresher than they actually are. Eggs that you want to check the freshness of should be kept outside the fridge for at least an hour prior to opening them.

• First, check all the eggs by rolling them across a flat surface. Only consume them if they roll wobbly.

• Open the egg. If the egg white is watery instead of gel-like, don't consume the egg. If the egg yolk is not convex and firm, don't consume the egg. If the egg yolk easily bursts, don't consume the egg.

• After opening the egg you can put it up to your nose and smell it. If it smells foul you will certainly not want to consume it. The traditional nutritional dogma states that raw egg whites contain a glycoprotein called avidin that is very effective at binding biotin, one of the B vitamins. The concern is that this can lead to a biotin deficiency.

The simple solution was to cook the egg whites as this completely deactivates the avidin. The problem is that it also completely deactivates nearly every other protein in the egg white. While you will still obtain nutritional benefits from consuming cooked egg whites, from a nutritional perspective it would seem far better to consume them uncooked.

The basic composition of the egg more than compensated for this. It contains tons of biotin in the egg yolk. Egg yolks have one of the highest concentrations of biotin found in nature. So it is likely that you will not have a biotin deficiency if you consume the whole raw egg, yolk and white. It is also clear, however, that if you only consume raw egg whites, you are nearly guaranteed to develop a biotin deficiency unless you take a biotin supplement."

It has also been revealed that the soy-rich feed commercial laying hens are fed deposits residues of soy protein in the egg itself. For people sensitive enough to soy, especially those suffering from eczema, this confounds the issue of elimination attempts since eggs now become a potential source of a well-known allergen. Tropical Traditions, a family-owned company with the website of the same name, offers a bountiful assortment of coconut products, grass-finshed meats, as well as pastured eggs from laying hens fed the company's own soy-free *CocoFeed*. Brian Shilhavy, CEO of Tropical Traditions, along with his wife, Marianita, a Certified Nutritionist/Dietician in the Philippines, also run and edit the company's sister site www.HealthImpactNews.com. Their free e-Newsletter, *Health Impact News Daily*, provides subscribers "the latest news regarding issues that impact your health you may find difficult to find in other media sources".

From the website www.HealthImpactNews.com, some interesting conclusions have been drawn from pro-soy research being conducted at Ohio State University:

Professor M. Monica Giusti, a poultry biologist of The Ohio State University, is one of the few people who has done research on soy isoflavones appearing in commercial egg yolks. She has designed lab tests to detect soy isoflavones. In 2009 one of her students published a master's thesis on the transfer of the soy protein into egg yolks and chicken tissue: *Quantification of Soy Isoflavones in Commercial Eggs and Their Transfer from Poultry Feed into Eggs and Tissues.* The results of the study as stated in the abstract:

> Isoflavones are potent phytoestrogens found in soy-beans. Soybean meal constitutes a main ingredient of poultry feed and isoflavones may transfer into eggs and tissues. Our objective was to determine the transfer and accumulation of isoflavones from the feed into hen eggs and tissues, making them isoflavone sources in the human diet. Isoflavone content of commercial eggs with different claims were analyzed by HPLC-MS after hydrolysis. All commercial samples contained soy isoflavones and the metabolite equol. Then, 48 laying hens were fed soy-free, regular (25% soybean meal) or isoflavone rich diet. Isoflavones were found in experimental eggs and tissues. Enhancement of the diet with 500 mg isoflavones/100g feed result-ed on egg yolks containing 1000µg isoflavones/100g while livers, kidneys, hearts and muscles contained 7162 µg/100g, 3355 µg/100g, 272 µg/100g and 97 µg/100g , respectively. The results showed that diet can be altered to modulate isoflavone content in hen eggs and tissues.

The author of the study has a pro-soy view of soy protein, so the study was designed to encourage more soy protein to be transferred to egg yolks and poultry tissue. The parameters of the study included comparing chickens fed a soy-free feed, and at the time Tropical Traditions' soy-free Cocofeed was the only feed available for them to use. Since they started with laying hens that had been raised on a soy-based diet, they conducted periodic tests to determine how long it took the soy-protein to not show up in egg yolks after starting on the soy-free Cocofeed. No trace of the soy isoflavone was found after 10 days following the conversion to the soy-free Cocofeed. So if you think you are allergic to eggs, it could be that you are actually allergic to soy protein, which is present in virtually all commercial eggs, including organic ones.

Not sure how much clearer this point could be made- you're eating what your food ate. If your food ate yellow food coloring to dress up the poor excuse for a yolk it's forced to produce, you're eating yellow food coloring too. If your food was pumped full of tranquilizers to prevent it from pecking out the eyes of its roommates, you're going to get a steady dose of tranquilizers too. According to Ruth Harrison's book, *Animal Machines: The New Factory Farming Industry,* at the time of first publishing in 1964, only 20 percent of laying hen flocks in England and Wales were on range, while the rest had gone indoors. The hens may have been denied green pastures and the sun's rays, but their food could now be easily adjusted to control the chemical composition of the egg. "One could change the chemical composition of an egg by putting certain substances in the diet but it did not necessarily pay to do so. One could feed to produce eggs with higher vitamin A and D, for instance, but the producer would not get any more money for a super-vitaminised product." More still from *Animal Machines:*

> Increased egg production brings headaches as far as egg quality is concerned. Poor shells, pale yolks, watery whites, all prove a problem. For poor shells and thin shells improvement can be made with additions to the diet, while emulation of the golden yolked free range egg can be got by feeding dried grass or, if that proves too expensive, by feeding a yellow dye to the bird. In Australia, producers receive a premium for golden yolks, and this is beginning to operate in some packing stations here [England 1964]. The housewife, curious creature that she is, feels the egg she used to know had more quality than its pale yolked successor. She sticks to this idea stubbornly, against all assurances to the contrary, and is willing to pay more for her free range eggs, so the free range egg must be simulated as far as possible. The bird can only co-operate in this endeavor as far as she is able. 'Severe de-beaking can lead to poor shell quality by restricting the birds' ability to eat calcium grit' comments a report in *Farming Express,* 31st January 1963.

Stubborn housewife that I am, I have to throw in here how much we love raising our own laying hens. They're so easy to care for and we control the extra food they get beyond green grass, bugs, grubs and worms, by ordering organic soy-free feed from www.CountrysideOrganics.com, based in Fishersville, Virginia. We order about 500 pounds of feed, three times a year, and take the utmost pleasure in knowing what our little betties are eating. It's so gratifying to go out to your own backyard and bring in this full meal-deal, freshly laid and ready to nourish you. So, eat your eggs raw and enjoy the fact that if you don't damage the proteins by cooking, the majority of which are actually in the yolk (sorry bodybuilders!), it is the yardstick by which the quality of all protein we consume is measured against. Don't forget, the cholesterol is contained in the yolk and cooking will oxidize it, consequently rendering it an acid-forming, inflammatory substance for the immune system to deal with. But if you leave it unsullied, the body can actually use it to *reduce* inflammation throughout the body, as well as make you happy.

Censored Nutritional Gem #9: A Good Egg is a Raw Egg
(Pastured and soy-free.)

Suggested Reading:

Take Control of Your Health, Joseph Mercola, DO

Animal Machines, Ruth Harrison

The Whole Soy Story, Kaayla T. Daniel, PhD

Dr. Mercola's Total Health Program, Joseph Mercola, DO

Diet for a Small Planet, Frances Moore Lappé

10
Ideal Body Weight is a Result of Nourished Cells
(You're not fat, you're inflamed.)

There are so many times I see posts in my social media news streams about someone becoming a "health coach" with one company or another that promises weight loss above all, and better health as a result (when it should actually be the other way around). Yes, the various programs incorporate some healthy lifestyle pointers, like "loving yourself" and doing some form of exercise that you enjoy, every day. Those same people will accompany their posts with before and after pictures of themselves (most still sporting visibly noticeable signs of inflammation either in their faces and/or all over their bodies), and how they feel the "best" they've ever felt in their "entire" lives. I immediately seek out the product or supplement credited with their "transformation" and go right to the ingredients label (aka, the jugular). It is in those details that you will deem the worthiness of two things: their products for your consumption, and their consumption of your heard-earned money in exchange for their products.

When a dietary supplement, weight loss product, meal replacement shake or bar is full of synthetic vitamins and minerals, artificial sweeteners, flavors, and preservatives, damaged oils, hydrogenated oils, and allergenic proteins, health and wellness are going to be an unattainable goal. If people do happen to lose weight while consuming the product it's usually because of calorie restriction, and the simultaneous removal of junk foods, refined carbohydrates, and liquid calories (sweet tea, soft drinks, fruit juices, etc.) from their diets, along with the increase of consumption of fresh vegetables and fruits. They would have most likely lost more weight had they simply done every one of the activities in the last sentence, minus consuming the product in question! It is the betterment of the diet through the removal of foods that are known to be inflammation producing and the increase in consumption of anti-inflammatory foods that yields true health and wellness, on a cellular level, and consequently, the automatic optimization of body weight.

Perhaps the bombardment of our minds via certain media sources on the subject of food additives, like artificial sweeteners, colors, and preservatives, has desensitized us to the hazards their consumption presents, accepting their presence in food products almost as readily as we accept "growing old". Perhaps we're so sick of hearing about "lactose intolerance" and "gluten sensitivity" that we've become allergic to the mere utterance of the words. If that's the case, then the degenerative state of our mental, emotional, and physical health, as a population, leaves little to be justified. In addition to artificial ingredients, all too often a review of the ingredients label will reveal the presence of at least 3 of the 8 "Most Allergenic Foods". According to the FDA , the governmental authority charged with "Protecting and Promoting your Health", and for your deciphering pleasure, some "FoodFacts" about food allergies:

> Each year, millions of Americans have allergic reactions to food. Although most food allergies cause relatively mild and minor symptoms, some food allergies can cause severe reactions, and may even be life-threatening. There is no cure for food allergies. Strict avoidance of food allergens, and early recognition and management of allergic reactions to food, are important measures to prevent serious health consequences.

What Are Major Food Allergens?

While more than 160 foods can cause allergic reactions in people with food allergies, the law identifies the eight most common allergenic foods. These foods account for 90 percent of food allergic reactions, and are the food sources from which many other ingredients are derived.

The eight foods identified by the law are:

- Cow's Milk
- Eggs
- Fish (e.g., bass, flounder, cod)
- Crustacean shellfish (e.g. crab, lobster, shrimp)
- Tree nuts (e.g., almonds, walnuts, pecans)
- Peanuts
- Wheat
- Soybeans

These eight foods, and any ingredient that contains protein derived from one or more of them, are designated as "major food allergens" by FALCPA.

I don't think that we've written off the hazards of what is offered up on grocers' shelves and through direct marketing companies (trying to convince people they're

"Creating Health, Hope and Happiness"), but I have to believe that people sincerely don't realize the toxic potential of the convenience they're ingesting. Conveniences like soups, and meal-like alternatives that all you have to do is add hot water to and ta-da!, something resembling fresh, garden-plucked wholesomeness (only the label reads like anything but) provide a false sense of security that the individual is eating healthfully. But due to the very nature of the lack of naturally-present nutritive value in the ingredients, the "meal" is fortified with synthetic vitamins and mineral isolates, which the cells scoff at, and which also contribute to acidifying the body of most sympathetic nervous system dominant individuals (those of the chronically stressed variety).

Medifast®, a company that originally only sold their dehydrated soups, desserts, snack bars, and various other "foods" meant for "healthy weight loss" directly to physicians to "dispense", now also enlists the networking talents of enterprising individuals to market the following products. The ingredients in italics are controversial at best, if not downright hazardous. See if you can guess what's what (answers on page 133):

> 1. *Soy protein isolate*, dehydrated beef, tomato powder, *modified potato starch*, chicory root extract (inulin), dehydrated potatoes, dehydrated carrots, *yeast extract,* dehydrated green beans, dehydrated cabbage, beef stock, dehydrated tomato, *canola oil, hydrolyzed soy, corn and wheat gluten protein,* xanthan gum, dehydrated celery, dehydrated minced onion, spices, *salt, natural flavors, soy lecithin, autolyzed yeast extract, dl-methionine*, garlic powder, vegetable stock (carrot, onion, celery).

> 2. *Textured soy protein concentrate, soy protein isolate, parboiled long grain white rice, wild rice*, carrots*, *natural chicken flavor*, peas*, chicory root extract (inulin), cooked chicken*, shitake mushrooms*, *yeast extract, canola oil,* xanthan gum, celery*, salt, onion powder, minced onion*, *soy lecithin, natural flavor, autolyzed yeast, l-cysteine hydrochloride*, black pepper, garlic powder, parsley*. *dehydrated

> 3. Dehydrated potato flakes, *milk protein concentrate,* gum acacia, *skim milk, calcium caseinate, whey protein isolate, dried egg whites, salt, natural flavors, dried sour cream (cultured cream, nonfat milk),* potato starch, dehydrated chive flakes, *yeast extract, soy lecithin,* onion powder, cellulose gum, *whey, autolyzed yeast extract, dry buttermilk, torula yeast*, xanthan gum, tapioca dextrin, *carrageenan, sunflower oil.*

All of the items above are fortified with the following blend of vitamins and minerals, and of special note, provide either 20 or 25% of your RDA of copper from copper sulfate, which if you recall from chapter 4, is the fungicide also used in commercial infant formula:

> Vitamins and Minerals: Calcium phosphate, calcium carbonate, magnesium oxide, ascorbic acid, ferric orthophosphate, vitamin E acetate, niacinamide, zinc oxide, calcium pantothenate, manganese sulfate, *copper sulfate,* pyridoxine hydrochloride, riboflavin, thiamin mononitrate, vitamin A palmitate, chromium chloride, folic acid, sodium molybdate, biotin, potassium iodide, sodium selenite, vitamin K1, vitamin D3, vitamin B12.

Breakfast, dessert, and snack options are equally questionable:

> 4. *Rolled oats, soy protein isolate, oat fiber, brown sugar, soy lecithin, salt, acesulfame potassium, dl-methionine, natural and artificial flavors, sucrose, caramel color, molasses, sulfiting agents.*

> 5. *Soy protein isolate, polydextrose, soluble corn fiber, glycerine, whey protein isolate, sugar, peanut flour, milk protein isolate,* water, *fructose, peanuts,* inulin, fractionated palm kernel oil, unsweetened chocolate, natural flavors, *cocoa (processed with alkali), soy lecithin, salt, whey, nonfat dry milk, cocoa butter, sucralose.*

> 6. *Soy protein isolate,* tapioca starch, *corn flour,* pea fiber, *soybean oil, whey, dextrin, cheddar cheese (cultured milk, salt, enzymes), salt, maltodextrin,* onion powder, chili pepper, garlic powder, *buttermilk solids,* spice, *torula yeast, natural flavor, lactic acid,* jalapeno pepper, *yeast extract, paprika extract (flavor and color),* turmeric extractives (spice and color), potato starch, *corn starch,* guar gum.

> 7. *Soy protein isolate, fructose, dextrin, cocoa (processed with alkali), whey protein concentrate, modified food starch,* chicory root extract (inulin), *soy lecithin, salt,* cellulose gum, natural and a*rtificial flavor, acesulfame potassium, corn syrup,* xanthan gum, *carrageenan, caramel color.*

> 8. *Calcium caseinate, sugar, fructose, sunflower oil,* chicory root extract (inulin), *dextrin, maltodextrin, whey protein concentrate,* instant coffee, cellulose gum, dried egg whites, *sodium casein-*

ate, xanthan gum, *acesulfame potassium, mono and diglycerides,* natural and *artificial flavors, carrageenan, soy lecithin, caramel color.*

9. *Soy protein isolate, whey protein concentrate*, dried blueberries, *rice flour, oat fiber, resistant corn starch,* dried apples, dried egg whites, *sunflower oil, maltodextrin*, natural and *artificial flavors*, baking powder (sodium acid pyrophosphate, sodium bicarbonate, *corn starch,* and calcium phosphate), xanthan gum, *soy lecithin, sugar, sodium caseinate, acesulfame potassium, citric acid, mono and diglycerides, sucralose*, lemon juice concentrate, molasses, *caramel color, salt.*

Loaded with allergens like indigestible protein from soy and cow's milk, artificial flavors, colors and bulking agents to give a "thick and creamy" impression of what would otherwise be unpalatable, time-crunched consumers are deceived into believing meal replacement shakes provide "balanced nutrition" :

10. *Isolated soy protein, whey protein concentrate, whey protein isolate*, glycerin, *corn syrup*, maltitol, chocolate coating (*whey protein concentrate*, palm kernel oil, maltitol, cocoa powder, *sugar, soy lecithin [an emulsifier], vanillin [an artificial flavor]*), water, *soy fiber, maltodextrin, peanut flour,* coconut oil, inulin, ascorbic acid, beta carotene, biotin, calcium pantothenate, tricalcium phosphate, ferric orthophosphate, folic acid, magnesium phosphate, niacin, magnesium and calcium phosphates, pyridoxine hydrochloride, riboflavin, thiamine hydrochloride, palmitate, cyanocobalamin, cholecalciferol, tocopheryl acetate, guar gum, natural and *artificial flavor.*

11. *Whey protein concentrate, calcium caseinate, milk protein isolate,* L-glutamine, L-lysine, L-leucine, L-isoleucine, L-valine, crystalline fructose, dicalcium phosphate, potassium citrate, potassium chloride, magnesium oxide, ascorbic acid, choline bitartrate, ferrous fumarate, inositol, vitamin E acetate, zinc oxide, niacinamide, vitamin A palmitate, copper gluconate, calcium pantothenate, manganese sulfate, chromium citrate, riboflavin, pyridoxine hydrochloride, selenomethionine, thiamine hydrochloride, biotin, folic acid, phytonadione, cholecalciferol, sodium molybdate, potassium iodide (iodine), cyanocobalamin, maltodextrin, gum arabic, natural and *artificial flavors,* guar gum, beet root extract (for color), xanthan gum, medium-chain triglycerides, citric acid, malic acid, oat fiber, cellulose powder, citrus pectin, *soy lecithin, sucralose,* bromelain, papain.

12. *Soy protein isolate, fructose,* cellulose powder, *corn bran, artificial French vanilla flavor,* guar gum, potassium chloride, calcium phosphate, *calcium caseinate, casein, rice fiber, soy lecithin, canola oil,* medium chain triglycerides, *carrageenan, dl-methionine,* inulin, magnesium oxide, silicone dioxide, licorice flavor, natural vanilla flavor, ginger root powder, psyllium husk powder, citrus pectin, proteases derived from Apsergillus niger and Aspergillus oryzae (both from Aminogen®), honey powder, ascorbic acid, *dl-alpha tocopheryl acetate,* papaya fruit powder, blueberry powder, pomegranate powder, biotin, niacinamide, beta carotene, ferrous fumarate, zinc oxide, copper gluconate, calcium d-pantothenate, bromelain, cyanocobalamin, folic acid, cholecalciferol, pyroxidine hydrochloride, thiamine mononitrate, riboflavin, chromium chloride, sodium molybdate and sodium selenite.

13. *Soy protein isolate,* digestive resistant maltodextrin (from Fibersol™), *whey protein hydrolysate, whey protein concentrate,* dicalcium phosphate, *sunflower oil,* natural and *artificial flavor,* medium chain triglycerides, maltodextrin, gum arabic, xanthan gum, *sodium caseinate,* dimagnesium phosphate, magnesium oxide, *soy lecithin, mono and diglycerides,* patented protease (from Aminogen), dipotassium phosphate, *sucralose,* ascorbic acid, vitamin E acetate, chromium amino acid chelate, molybdenum amino acid chelate, selenium amino acid chelate, biotin, vitamin A palmitate, niacinaminde, potassium iodide, zinc oxide, copper gluconate, calcium pantothenate, cyanocobalamin, manganese sulfate, cholecalciferol, pyridoxine hydrochloride, thiamin E mononitrate, riboflavin, phytomenadione, and folic acid.

14. Proprietary Blend of 2,231 mg: *Soy lecithin (97% phosphatides), soy protein isolate,* Spirulina pacifica, apple fiber, barley grass, eleuthero root extract, *brown rice flour,* alfalfa leaf, *barley malt,* beet juice powder, royal jelly, Bacillus coagulans (LactoSpore™), acerola, chlorella, milk thistle seed, astragalus root extract, green tea leaf extract, Ginko biloba leaf extract, dulse, bilberry extract, and aloe vera gel. Proprietary Blend of 330 mg: Broccoli, black walnut leaf powder, blackberry fruit, blueberry fruit, corn silk stylus, cranberry, dandelion leaf, goldenseal herb (aerial parts), kale, lemon grass, marshmallow root, meadowsweet herb (aerial parts), oat straw (aerial parts), papaya leaf, parsley, pau d'arco bark, plantain leaf, red raspberry leaf, rose hips, rosemary leaf, slippery elm bark, spinach, strawberry fruit, tomato, turmeric root, watercress, white willow bark, and okra.

In the interest of making an honest living on their own terms by "owning their own business while helping others", well-meaning, albeit inadequately-versed individuals promote products that can quite possibly do more harm than good. They don't realize that the ingredients in the products they're not only selling, but also consuming, are of questionable origin, and potentially problematic for an increasing number of people. If you rely on processed foods that are "ready-to-go" from freezer to microwave, or from box to plate, it's time to gut your pantry of products that could not only be contributing to hidden food allergies, but could also be increasing your risk of endocrine and reproductive system dysfunction, and eventually cancer (refer to chapter 6 for information on the dangers of unfermented soy, and realize that all of the aforementioned products contain numerous unfermented soy additives as ingredients). I urge you to beware of the following ingredients, and if there *are* products in your kitchen and gym bag with said ingredients, throw them out!

Ingredients with allergic and adverse reaction potential:

All soy and derivatives including but not limited to:
- Soy protein isolate (isolated soy protein)
- Soybean oil (often labeled as vegetable oil)
- Soy lecithin
- Soy flour
- Soy milk
- Textured soy protein (concentrate)
- Soy fiber

All milk ingredients including but not limited to:
- Milk protein concentrate
- Whey protein concentrate
- Casein
- Calcium caseinate
- Sodium caseinate
- Whey protein hydrolysate

All unfermented grains, including corn, rice, and oats, are hidden sources of gluten:
- Corn bran
- Corn syrup
- Corn starch
- Rice bran
- Rice syrup

- Rice flour
- Barley malt extract

All Artificial sweeteners:
- Acesulfame potassium
- Sucralose (also the active ingredient in Splenda®)
- Aspartame
- Saccharin
- Neotame
- Advantame

Artificial colors and preservatives including but not limited to:
- Caramel color
- FD&C Blue No. 1, Brilliant Blue
- FD&C Blue No. 2, Indigotine
- FD&C Green No. 3, Fast Green
- FD&C Red No. 3, Erythrosine
- FD&C Red No. 40, Allure Red
- FD&C Yellow No. 5, Tartrazine
- FD&C Yellow No. 6, Sunset Yellow
- Sodium benzoate
- Sodium metabisulfite

As more and more awareness is raised about the importance of getting our vitamins and minerals from actual food sources, such as vegetables, fruits, herbs, and spices, there are thousands of products being introduced that attempt to meet the demands of consumers who are attempting to take control of their health and remedy occasional inadequacies in their daily diets. These consumers have done their research and realize the best way to nourish their bodies is through the consumption of high quality organic vegetables, fruits, and general clean eating, but due to hectic schedules and limited time, also realize they have to supplement in one way or another.

Hundreds of manufacturers are clamoring to gain market share in an industry that in 2012 produced $32 billion in revenue with nutritional supplements alone. That leaves consumers in the typical "buyer beware" position to ensure their hard-earned dollars stretch as far as possible on quality supplements. We know our cells are starving, but lab-synthesized multivitamins are not going to fool them. The question of supplements is a dicey one because we really must get our nutrition from whole food. And I believe we have yet to patent a version of a naturally occurring vitamin, mineral, bioflavenoid, or any biochemical substance that remotely resembles the quality of the original.

We also know our diets are deficient in the amounts of nutrients we need to function optimally, because the way we live today makes our body a glutton for cellular nutrition. And I use the word glutton because we really are so stressed out, and so sleep-deprived, and cholesterol deprived, that we go through nutrients extraordinarily faster than someone living on a tropical island with nothing to do but get off their hammock during their afternoon nap because a fleeting downpour is approaching. We demand super-charged output from our system and it will only oblige if it has the basic tools to run efficiently and repair itself at will.

At the same time, our soils are depleted and shoddily "renovated" with fertilizers, and the produce we buy has either been doused with pesticides, fungicides, and herbicides, or is often cost-prohibitive for many who would like to opt for the organic versions of what is seasonally available. The bottom line is that if it's not at least our part-time job (10 to 15 hours a week), it can be challenging to get enough of the right foods in our diets on a daily basis. We've actually known this for quite some time. Otherwise, we wouldn't have created food "enrichment" and "fortification", or that multivitamin. Even if you eat "healthy", your body can be deficient. You must get that "insurance policy" from whole food supplementation, not from a lab-synthesized, pressed-sawdust horse pill.

So you should absolutely supplement, not replace a meal with a food-like imposter. What are the most important factors to be included? In chapter 8, *Fat, Friendly Flora and Lacto-Fermentation Facilitate Flushing*, we discussed that a quality probiotic supplement and some sort of traditionally fermented food, both on a daily basis, can do wonders for digestion, and even affect other aspects of your health in a beneficial manner. The next most important supplement is going to be a broad spectrum enzyme supplement, containing both digestive enzymes such as amylase, protease, and lipase, which will assist with the digestion of starches, proteins, and fats, respectively.

There are therapeutic enzyme formulas that contain pancreatic enzymes as well as proteolytic enzymes like nattokinase or an extract thereof. Nattokinase is a fibrinolytic enzyme found in the traditionally fermented soy cheese eaten in Japan called natto. Nattokinase has been shown to digest not only fibrin (the tough protein found in blood clots both inside the body and in scabs on the outside), but also other plasmin substrates. Basically, they have the ability to break up blood clots that may be floating through your arteries ready to wreak havoc if they get to a narrow enough space where they stop traffic. If you're curious to learn more, check out the academic version of Google at scholar.google.com and simply type in "nattokinase". You'll find numerous scholarly papers dating back to 1993 about this alternative to pharmaceutical blood thinners.

What else should you be supplementing with? A quality mineral supplement, in the perfect ratio between cofactors for maximum absorption into the cells and bones.   One that will provide the essential support our metabolic processes require to stay on top of balancing pH, facilitating normal muscle contraction and relaxation, and so much more. One with maximum bioavailability, as opposed to being deposited on the artery walls the way calcium can be found in arterial plaque; on the bones as is the case with bone spurs; or in the kidneys as stones). Himalayan pink salt is a wonderful source of over 80 trace minerals, and should be used liberally in all your cooking and baking endeavors.

Remember that the body is not capable of producing its own minerals; it must get them from our diet. Examples of minerals are zinc, magnesium, calcium, selenium, iron, manganese, chromium, iodine, and a host of others required only in trace amounts (but if we're deficient in them, we open the door for dysfunction). And if you noticed, I did put magnesium before calcium because in order to properly absorb calcium, the body not only requires that magnesium is present simultaneously, along with vitamin D, but that it's also in a higher quantity than calcium, actually about a 2:1 ratio.

Then there's something simply called a "whole food supplement". These are supplements where the only ingredients are real vegetables and fruits. It is of paramount importance to look at the supplement you're thinking of taking and if it contains foods that you have ready-access to like green peppers, garlic, celery, onions, carrots, beans, grapefruit, apples, strawberries, etc, just increase your daily intake of those foods. I'm not going to take a garlic supplement if I can just add it to the hummus I make twice a week, and where I also happen to be getting protein and fiber from the garbanzo beans, freshly squeezed lemon juice, and essential fatty acids from the tahini the recipe calls for. Be prudent in your supplementing, get what you can from real food, and what you don't have access to, in whole food supplement form.

So the must-haves in your supplement arsenal are going to be: probiotics, enzymes, a whole food supplement, and a high quality absorbable mineral complex. If you're going to choose the individual supplement route, I recommend Dr. Mercola's brand available on his site, www.Mercola.com, or even comparing his with another great brand, Garden of Life. The only downside to taking all of those in pill form is the potential handful of 10 to 15 capsules a day that you'll have to down either before breakfast or throughout the day. For years I used to take numerous natural supplements including probiotics, green food caplets, vitamin C, effervescent magnesium powder, beta glucans, and raw organic prenatal capsules (entirely from whole foods). I felt pretty good with that regimen since, once I started working outside the home, I wasn't able to regularly juice organic leafy greens four times a week like I used to. I wanted to make doubly sure that I was getting enough nutrients via high quality supplements. How great would it have been if someone had came up with a way to put all of that stuff in one container? Oh, wait. They did.

If you want a foundational whole food supplement, which also happens to be fermented for maximum bio-availability while also containing a hefty dose of organic superfoods and cultured minerals that we seem to deplete of at a higher rate, then Akea Fermented Superfoods and Probiotics (distributed by Asantae) could quite frankly be the most bulletproof whole food supplement available on the market today. It's definitely one that your entire family can safely consume and benefit from. With over 30 organic superfoods from the world's Longevity Hot Spots, including Okinawa; Symi, Greece; Sardinia, Italy; Nicoya, Costa Rica, and also a proprietary blend of the better-known powerful superfoods like cacao, noni, chlorella and spirulina, Akea gives you that cornucopia of cell-centric nutrition your cells are starving for.

Longevity Hot Spots are places around the world where people live considerably longer than we do, with a fraction of the degenerative diseases that plague the modern world including cancer, heart disease, and diabetes. Okinawans have a 300 percent greater chance of reaching the age of 100 than we do! They not only live longer-they live *better*, and I'm sure we can all agree that when we talk about life, tied for first with quantity is quality.

Since those organic superfoods are also fermented, you have the best opportunity to make sure all of the micronutrients in those foods are going to make it to your cells (and not just pass on through to the potty). A customized blend of the minerals magnesium, zinc, selenium, calcium, manganese, chromium, molybdenum, iodine, and potassium, which are in the perfect ratio required for optimal assimilation, are also added to the superfoods before the fermentation process rendering them cultured, and thus adding to their bioavailability even more. Roughage is great and all, but in those leaves of spinach, kale and romaine lettuce that your teeth failed to grind up completely and that your digestive enzymes were deficient in breaking down that plant fiber, there are still viable nutrients that the body could have benefitted from.

Only juicing or blending can extract the most juice and increase the surface area of those leafy greens enough to make sure you're getting every last microgram of phytochemicals. Fermentation uses friendly microorganisms (probiotics!) to also pre-digest macronutrients like proteins and carbohydrates, into forms we can easily process, as well as making the micronutrients such as vitamins and minerals more bioavailable.

After the fermentation process, Akea is fortified with not only digestive enzymes but also, Nattozimes®, formulated to provide a blend of proteases which have been shown to break down standard fibrin substrates in a manner similar to nattokinase. According to the National Enzyme Company, manufacturer of Nattozimes, "In vitro research has shown that the proteases used in Nattozimes possess fibrinolytic activity. Nattozimes proteases support healthy protein metabolism, both within the digestive tract and systemically." Right before Akea is packaged for distribution, they add ten strains of live probiotics which replenish the ones we've decimated by drinking chlorinated water and dosing up with antibiotics when we get a runny nose. Akea truly is all food, no synthetics, no fillers or stimulants or diuretics.

It's not a meal replacement or a protein shake so you have to make sure you're actually eating food with macronutrients as well. Macronutrients are proteins, fats and carbohydrates and we cannot live without the first two because they're largely what our bodies are made of. And carbohydrates, believe it or not, on their own, may only provide the body with *energy*, but they are carriers for what is essential for life and that is the plethora of micronutrients found in plants, veggies, herbs, spices, and fruits. And all those foods we just mentioned are comprised mostly of water and carbohydrates, so when you eat them, consider those carbs the transporters of vitamins, minerals, antioxidants, bioflavonoids, and enzymes. These are the nutrients that we require to thrive, and live vibrant, quality lives. My daily dose of Akea (22 grams) gives me the ORAC value of 5 organic fruits and vegetables, the oa t beta glucans of 8 bowls of oatmeal, the live probiotics of 6 servings of yogurt, and the resveratrol of 28 glasses of wine. All of that packs a heck of a nutritional punch that allows you to navigate life at break-neck speed (slow down though!), without so much as a hint of windburn, all while providing a quantity of nutrition that opens the door for therapeutic benefit.

Censored Nutritional Gem #10:
Ideal Body Weight is a Result of Nourished Cells
(You're not fat, you're inflamed and undernourished.)

Mystery Meals:

1. Vegetable Beef Soup from Medifast®, Inc., All Rights Reserved
2. Wild Rice and Chicken Flavored Soup from Medifast®, Inc.
3. Mashed Potatoes from Medifast®, Inc.
Vitamins and Minerals content from Medifast®, Inc.
4. Maple and Brown Sugar Oatmeal from Medifast®, Inc.
5. Peanut Butter Chocolate Chip Chewy Bar from Medifast®, Inc.
6. Chili Nacho Cheese Puffs from Medifast®, Inc.
7. Dutch Chocolate Smoothie from Medifast®, Inc.
8. Coffee Soft Serve from Medifast®, Inc.
9. Blueberry Muffin Soft Bake from Medifast®, Inc.
10. AdvoBar® Meal , AdvoBar® is a registered trademark AdvoCare International, L.P., Plano Texas
11. AdvoBar®Meal Replacement Shake
12. Formula 1 Healthy Meal Nutritional Shake is a registered trademark of Herbalife® International of America
Aminogen® is a registered trademark of Triarco Industries, Inc.
13. ViSalus® Vi-Shape®Nutritional Shake Mix,
Vi-Shape®and ViSalus® are registered trademarks of Blyth, Inc., Delaware
LactoSpore® is registered trademark of Sabinsa Corporation, New Jersey
14. Greens® by It Works!®, registered trademarks of It Works! Global, Bradenton, Florida

11
Spuds Are Spectacular

How did potatoes get such a bad reputation in popular "nutrition"? How could a food loaded with fiber, usable protein, vitamins and minerals, be as ostracized from our diets as much as potatoes have? Do I need to tell you the story about cholesterol and saturated fat again? If you thought all they were filled with was bad carbs and weight-gain potential, all I am saying is give potatoes a chance. I was able to give up wheat products, pasta, rice, and oatmeal because I knew I would have my potatoes to hug and kiss. My favorite meal growing up was my mother's pan-fried potatoes and I could have eaten them every day, twice a day, had she been willing to make them. They're not grains. They're not useless and if you prepare and consume them correctly, they're pretty wicked awesome.

So then, why the debate? I honestly think when we realized how void of nutrients typical "white processed food" was, like white sugar, white flour, polished white rice, we just kind of kept firing away at anything else that was white, to include potatoes (although why we kept cow's milk I'm not quite sure). But think about it: potatoes are not refined, they're rich in complex carbohydrates, they have more net usable protein than a piece of string cheese, and when it comes to mineral content, including magnesium, phosphorus, potassium, zinc, B vitamins and vitamin C, potatoes have it all. From a book originally published in 1905, Practical Dietetics With Special Reference To Diet In Disease, Dr. William Gilman Thompson puts the perfection of potatoes into perspective:

> The potato ranks first in importance among the class of tubers which serve man for food, both on account of its easy cultivation in a great variety of soils and on account of its digestibility when properly cooked. As an exclusive article of diet the potatoes too largely composed of starch to be of much nutritive value, and enormous quantities have to be eaten (several pounds a day) in order to supply enough nitrogen for the energy of the body.

> The potato, however, has less starch than rice, peas, or lentils. It also has less woody fibre than most underground vegetables. In Ireland this vegetable constitutes a greater proportion of the daily food than in almost any other country, and in periods of famine has been known to form four fifths of the entire food for a time, but of late years it has been largely

supplemented by the cultivation of Indian corn and other products. The flavour and quality of the potato is influenced very much by the soil and climate in which it grows, a sandy soil being best. König gives the percentage composition of the potato as water, 75.77; nitrogenous materials, 1.79 (others give 2.10); fat, 1.60; starch, 20.56; cellulose, 0.75-; ash, 0.97. It is thus seen to contain about one fourth solid matter. The potato becomes a much more strengthening food when eaten, as it usually is, with meat gravy, fat, or butter and salt. Potato juice has a faintly acid reaction, and its vegetable acids are mainly combined with salts of potassium, but also with sodium and calcium. It also contains traces of iron, phosphoric and sulphuric acids, chlorine, silica, and magnesia.

Owing to the large proportion - from 12 to 24 per cent - of nearly pure starch which is found in the potato, it is very extensively used in this country and elsewhere for the manufacture of laundry starch. Old potatoes, and those which have been long kept, show some alteration in the quantity of their starch, and a part is converted into sugar and gum. Potato starch, as compared with other starches, is thoroughly digestible, but much depends upon the cooking. The starchy granules are tough and absorb water from the acid juices which surround them and from water added in cooking, and when properly prepared the potato becomes soft and mealy. When this is not the case, however, it remains hard and soggy, and is thoroughly indigestible.

The following statement in regard to the potato is made in a recent report of the British Commissioners of Prisons:

> "Within and surrounding the cells is a fluid or juice the albuminous constituents of which are coagulated during the process of cooking. The watery part of this juice is absorbed by the starch granules, which swell up and distend the cells in which they are contained, so that they no longer adhere together, and the result is the loose flocculent mass which is described as a floury or mealy potato. Unless the potato be properly cooked, the fluid referred to is only partially absorbed, the cells do not become sufficiently distended and separated, and the potato is then described as 'waxy' and 'dense.' In this condition it is not digested, and consequently does not

furnish to the system the antiscorbutic principle in which
resides its chief value as an article of diet".

When potatoes are cooked in water, it is desirable not to remove their skins, for the latter prevent to a great extent the passage of the salts out into the fluid. The fact that potatoes will not decay if kept dry for a length of time makes them very useful vegetables upon sea voyages, when their antiscorbutic properties are especially serviceable. Potatoes are more digestible when cooked by baking in their skins than by any other process. They then become mealy and their starch is digested with comparative ease by invalids. They are also quite digestible if steamed, or if boiled and mashed through a colander.

So as it turns out, potatoes have a fantastic NPU or *net protein utilization* of 60 on that scale which ranges from 1 to 100. NPU, not to be confused with NPR, is a combination of a protein's *biological value*, as well as its *digestibility*. Biological value is the percentage of absorbed protein that your body actually uses, and digestibility is indicative of how much protein is broken down or digested and then absorbed into the body through the digestive system. But the journey doesn't end there. Once it's absorbed from the digestive system, it has to make its way to the cells and to various other locations in the body where hormones are going to be synthesized and enzymes manufactured, etc. and that's where biological value takes over. So a food's NPU is actually comprised of both those factors: biological value and digestibility.

From Frances Moore Lappe's book Diet for a Small Planet:

The NPU of a food is largely determined by how closely the essential amino acids in its protein match the body's one utilizable pattern... The proteins which our bodies are made of are comprised of varying combinations of 22 different amino acids. 8 of these amino acids cannot be synthesized by the body; they must be obtained from food sources. These 8 amino acids are tryptophan, leucine, isoleucine, valine, threonine, methionine and cysteine, and histadine. Our bodies need all of the essential amino acids simultaneously in order to carry out protein synthesis. We live, heal, and die by protein synthesis!

So not only do these 8 essential amino acids have to be present at the same time, but they also need to be present in the correct proportion so they can be properly absorbed. So that's basically what the one utilizable pattern is- the presence of all 8 essential amino acids in the correct proportion, all at the same time [an NPU of 100].

The NPU of egg protein is 94, it actually most nearly matches the body's one utilizable pattern, so it is used as the model for measuring amino acids patterns in other foods. The NPU of Swiss cheese is less than 70; kidney beans have an NPU of 38; soybean flour disgraces at 16, and chicken breast is just under 65. All of that just to tell you potatoes are great sources of usable protein! One very important thing to mention is that conventionally grown potatoes consistently test high in pesticide residues, so the organic version is going to be worth every penny. Google "produce dirty dozen list" to find out which vegetables and fruits are best purchased organic, and which conventionally-grown ones are somewhat innocuous.

Let's turn our attention to the use of potatoes for something else you may have been in the dark about. Being happy. About seven years ago, when we were living in the Eastern Panhandle of West Virginia, I had heard of a book called *Potatoes not Prozac.* I chuckled at the clever title but since I had never been on Prozac or thought I needed to be, it just stuck in my mind as a book for "depressed people trying to get off their meds". It was while doing the research for *SatFatRox* that I finally bought the book, *Potatoes not Prozac*, by Dr. Kathleen DesMaisons, a PhD who specializes in combining medical and holistic approaches to treating alcoholism, drug addiction, depression, and compulsive behavior, and flipped eagerly through it to find the specific reference to potatoes.

Imagine my serendipity when I came across the chapter where she grants us carte blanche of eating a potato every night before bedtime, but exactly three hours after eating dinner. Remember what I said earlier about being able to give up all the pasta and bread in the world for being able to eat my potatoes? Turns out, there's a reason for that. I'm sugar sensitive (always have been, just thought my "sweet tooth" was cute as opposed to debilitating). Over the past year, twice weekly, after we bake our 3-day supply of potatoes in the evening, I usually find myself eating one- right before I go to bed. I add a tablespoon of coconut oil, pink salt, and sometimes some hot sauce, but never once thought I was intuitively heeding my body's request. Your instructions for being happier, from *Potatoes not Prozac:*

> Every night, just before bed, have a potato with its skin. Ideally (for biochemical reasons), have it three hours after dinner. This may sound too simple to be part of your healing, but eating the potato will help your body raise your serotonin level and make you feel more confident, competent, creative, and optimistic...

> You can eat your potato baked, mashed, roasted, cut into oven fries, or grated into hash browns. Just make sure you cook the potato and eat

the skin. You can top it with anything you like except foods that contain protein. (If you eat protein along with the potato at bedtime, it will interfere with your serotonin-making process.)

If you find you're having wild dreams on the nights you have your potato, this is a clue that you have very low serotonin. Eating the nightly potato is giving you a bigger hit of serotonin than you're ready for. You need the serotonin, but it is better to go more slowly. Ease into it and let your brain catch up…Your body is talking to you. Listen.

Who would have ever thought that a potato could be prescribed to increase serotonin levels? Is it any wonder we're so down and depressed? Our tools to produce our feel good brain chemicals have been demonized and wrongly-implicated in a destroying our health. But don't worry, there's nothing a little antidepressant can't fix! Serotonin is a neurotransmitter (brain chemical) that promotes relaxation and makes us feel hopeful and optimistic, reflective and thoughtful, able to concentrate, with more creativity and better focus. Serotonin also influences your self-control, impulse control, and your ability to plan ahead. Your body makes serotonin from the essential amino acid tryptophan, but just eating food high in tryptophan is not going to ensure that you're making enough serotonin. Dr. DesMaisons goes on to explain exactly how potatoes work their magic:

Tryptophan comes from the protein you're eating during the day. But having tryptophan available for making serotonin requires more than simply eating foods that contain it. After you eat protein, your body breaks it down into its different amino acids. These amino acids travel to the brain in your bloodstream. They cannot immediately enter your brain cells, however, because there is a blood-brain barrier that controls what gets into your brain at any given time.

Tryptophan swims up to the blood-brain barrier with all the other amino acids. But it can't get in right away. There are far fewer tryptophan molecules than other amino acid molecules. It is outnumbered and loses out in the competition to cross the barrier. Think of tryptophan as a runt who gets left behind in the shuffle. This means that even if you eat protein with high levels of tryptophan, that alone won't do the trick. The runt needs help.

Your body has a special way to help the runt get across the blood-brain barrier. When the body releases insulin, the insulin seeks out amino acids to use for building muscle. But insulin isn't interested in the runt. It only wants the big guys. So it carries off the other amino acids to other parts of the body where muscle can be found, leaving little tryptophan behind to hop across the blood-brain barrier and be put to use making serotonin. And more serotonin makes you feels better…

Since all carbohydrates raise your level of insulin, it is complex carbs like those in potatoes that will give you a slow and gradual insulin response, not a blood sugar spike. Potatoes also have a high level of potassium, which is known as a cofactor for insulin, and gives the potato a potent effect. Also contributing to the pros list of potatoes is the fact that they seem to provide an emotional comfort factor as well. The "satiety index" assigns a value to how full certain foods make people feel after eating them. In a study by S. Holt et al., referenced by Dr. DesMaisons in her book, the satiety index of potatoes, 323, was more than double its closest competitors, whole-grain bread and popcorn, at values of 157, and 154, respectively. So basically, "eating potatoes is not only satisfying; it actually changes your brain chemistry."

After all is said and done, it should come as no surprise that potatoes will always be a part of my repertoire as long as they're organic, and baked or boiled in their skins. We pre-bake our organic russets and store them in the fridge in a sealed container until we're ready to eat them (they'll last about 4 days). After slicing them up in bite-size pieces, gently pan-warm them on low/medium heat in coconut oil and season them with pink salt and herbs and spices: Country Fried Potatoes! If you're making mashed potatoes, choose organic red potatoes, boil them whole, with their skins on, making sure you don't overcook them.

These were a huge staple when I was growing up and my mom always peeled them and cut them up into cubes to boil them. Turns out you wash all that wonderful mineral content down the drain. Make sure you tend them as they simmer, turn them over once in the water so they cook quicker but don't overcook them, if they begin to split, again, you run the risk of leaking nutrients out into our cooking water. Looks like spuds are back on the menu boys!

Censored Nutritional Gem #11: Spuds are Spectacular

Suggested Reading:

Potatoes not Prozac, Kathleen DesMaisons, PhD, Addictive Nutrition

Diet for a Small Planet, Frances Moore Lappé

Notes

12
The Right Salt is Pink Salt

To salt or not to salt? That, my friends, is the question. We overlook the importance of salting the foods we cook because of the terrible wrap the very word "salt" has received over the past hundred years for causing high blood pressure, water retention, and weight gain, destroying your kidneys, etc. The human body needs only as little as 500 milligrams of sodium per day and that can be obtained from 1/4 teaspoon or just under 1000 mg of Himalayan Pink Salt, but it needs a bunch of other trace minerals every day as well. Trace minerals which you're not going to find anywhere near the sources of our daily "salt" intake.

The USDA recommends no more than 2,500 milligrams of sodium per day (which clearly is already five times more than what the body requires but that seems to be a detail lost on that governing body). The average American takes in more than 5,000 milligrams a day. We're talking about *one* mineral. Where are we getting all of that from? Go to your pantry and start reading some ingredient labels: sodium benzoate, sodium caseinate, sodium aluminosilicate, sodium aluminum phosphate, sodium nitrite, sodium nitrate, monosodium glutamate. Good grief! Did you know that a chicken sandwich from a certain Southern-bred chicken sandwich fast food joint contains over 1300 milligrams of sodium? Not of "salt", of sodium. All sourced from the sodium-based chemicals I just listed. Now, we need sodium ions for conducting nerve impulses and maintaining the resting membrane potential of a neuron along with many other functions to keep our bodies running optimally but, 1300 milligrams of sodium alone in one sandwich? That's just criminal.

The refining process of table salt, aka sodium chloride removes 82 of the 84 naturally occurring minerals, while having chemicals added to prevent it from absorbing moisture, so it can flow freely from the salt shaker. It is then bleached similar to the process used to whiten refined sugar and flour. Dr. Esterban Genao, a Florida pediatrician stated in an interview, "I am convinced that the refining of salt, the refining of sugar, and of oils, is going to be shown to be responsible for a great majority of our physical problems." What's so wrong with table salt? As George Malkmus, founder of Hallelujah Acres, www.HAcres.com, explains:

1. Mineral Depletion

Table salt leads to a poorly functioning immune system along with the initiation and acceleration of chronic illness. It depletes calcium, potassium, and magnesium and is directly related to cardiovascular disease. The ingestion of large amounts leads to mineral deficiency. [You're craving salt because you're mineral deficient, and salty is what the tongue associates with sources of minerals. Only you're not giving the body what it thinks it's going to get.]

2. Acid Formation

Due to its lack of buffering minerals, it becomes an acidifying substance within the body, and joins the other acidifying substances found in the "World's Diet." All animal products (both flesh and dairy), all refined sugars, and refined flour are acidifying, making it difficult for the body to maintain its alkalinity. [That's where the "acid meadow" comes in and starts eating away at your happiness.]

3. Fluid Imbalance

Table salt is toxic to the body and responsible for upsetting the fluid balance, debilitating the circulatory system (that would include the heart), and aggravating a number of salt pathologies.

One ounce (28 grams) of ingested table salt will cause the body to retain 3 quarts of water (6 pounds of excess bodily fluids), in an attempt to dilute this extremely toxic substance. That's basically a week's worth of salt consumption for the average American. And if you factor in how dehydrated we are 6 pounds is on the light side. So what do you do? Well, for one thing, you stop eating anything that comes in a box, sealed bag, can, or pouch, manufactured on an assembly line that has added sodium. You then begin adding Himalayan Pink Salt, also known as Himalayan Crystal Salt, to your own food prep at home. It's a superfood in its own right. It balances the body's fluid levels, and some sources say it can even help the body to eliminate stored refined salt deposits and kidney stones. Interestingly enough, the etiology of the word salvation comes from the Latin word for salt, *sal.*

From www.HimalayanCrystalSalt.com, the website of the Original Himalayan Crystal Salt®, some historical facts about salt:

Just what is salt?

As common as salt is to our tables, we have come to accept its presence in our lives as ordinary. But in the not-too-distant past, wars were fought over its possession and civilizations rose and fell in pursuit of what came to be called "white gold." In times past, common rock salt was given to the common people and the highly valued crystal salt, like Original Himalayan Crystal Salt®, was reserved for royalty. Primitive man had no concerns about salt. He got his daily requirement of salt from consuming the blood of the animals he ate. We know that blood consists of mostly salt and a full complement of minerals. In this way, early civilizations received the benefits of salt and its included mineral nutrients.

As humans became civilized and moved towards agriculture and the domestication of animals, the demand for salt increased. Besides being valued as a seasoning, we discovered the ability of salt to preserve food. This freed us from our dependency on seasonal availability of food as we could now preserve our food. This opened the possibility for traveling and carrying our food with us.

Paid in salt? It happened…

But salt was always difficult to come by and it became a highly valued item of trade. So valued in fact, that it served as a monetary exchange. The early Romans controlled the price of salt and would increase the price to fund their wars then reduce the price so as to make salt available to the common citizen. In fact, Roman soldiers were paid in salt.

The word salary comes from the Latin world salarium, which means payment in salt. Sal is Latin for salt. This is also the time when the phrase "worth ones salt" originated. The Romans actually built roads specifically for making the transportation of salt more convenient. One such road, the Via Salaria, led from Rome to the Adriatic sea, where salt was produced by evaporating sea water, a common method still used today.

Early America: Salt and War…

There are stories surrounding salt throughout American history. Salt is thought to be a major factor in the outcome of many wars fought on American soil. During the Revolutionary War, the British used Americans who were loyal to the British crown to intercept the rebels' salt supply. This action destroyed the rebels' ability to preserve food.

During the War of 1812, soldiers in the field received salt brine as payment because the government was too poor to pay them with money. Prior to Lewis and Clark's expedition to the West, President Jefferson referred in his address to Congress about a mountain of salt believed to lie near the Missouri River, which would have been of enormous value if the two pioneers could verify the story.

Censored Nutritional Gem #12 The Right Salt is Pink Salt.

Notes

13
Artificial Sweeteners Kill
(Brain cells at least.)

Whatever the rationale, whatever the logic- nothing can justify the destructive potential of artificial stimulation of the brain's pleasure centers. This is certainly the case with artificial sweeteners; they are lab-created drugs meant to fool the brain into thinking something sweet has been placed in the mouth. Regardless of their lack of calories, they actually trigger appetite, and fat storage, and bio-accumulation. They are not an acceptable replacement for caloric sweeteners (notice I didn't say natural because nowhere in nature will you find a mound of white sugar piled high and ready to snort, I mean bake with.) And I say that because they are addictive. Anything that stimulates the pleasure centers of the brain, the areas that process feelings of euphoria, comfort, and well-being, are referred to as pleasure centers. You might ask, so what's wrong with a little artificial stimulation? It's deadly. You're exciting the brain cells (neurons) so much so that they die remarkably before their time.

If you're trying to lose weight by cutting out sugar from sodas and replacing them with diet ones, you may be doing more harm than you think. According to a review by scientists from the University of Pretoria and the University of Limpopo, consumption of the artificial sweetener aspartame may inhibit the ability of enzymes in your brain to function normally. The review found that high doses of the sweetener may lead to neurodegeneration. It has also previously been found that it can also cause neurological and behavioral disturbances in sensitive individuals. Specifically, the review found a number of direct and indirect changes that occur in your brain as a result of high consumption levels of aspartame, including disturbing:

- The metabolism of amino acids
- Protein structure and metabolism
- The integrity of nucleic acids
- Neuronal function
- Endocrine balances

Further, the breakdown of aspartame into aspartic acid, phenylalanine (an excitatory amino acid) and methanol (aka wood alcohol), causes nerves to fire excessively, which can lead to depolarization or even death of the affected neurons. Chronic illnesses which may be caused by long-term exposure to excitatory amino acid damage include:

- Multiple sclerosis, Parkinson's disease and Alzheimer's disease
- Memory and hearing loss
- Hormonal problems
- Epilepsy
- Brain Lesions
- Neuroendocrine disorders

With methanol further being broken down by the body into formic acid (what fire ants inject into a bite) and formaldehyde (a deadly neurotoxin), the U.S. Environmental Protection Agency states that methanol "is considered a cumulative poison due to the low rate of excretion once it is absorbed, with both aforementioned metabolites being toxic." They recommend a limit of consumption of 7.8 mg/day, but a one-liter aspartame-sweetened beverage contains about 56 mg of methanol. The symptoms of methanol poisoning are numerous and varied and can include:

- Vision problems
- Headaches, ear buzzing, dizziness
- Nausea and gastrointestinal disturbances
- Weakness, numbness and shooting pains in your extremities
- Behavioral disturbances
- Memory lapses

Aside from the damage it can do to your brain, aspartame has been linked to an increase risk of cancer. One well-controlled, peer-reviewed, seven-year study even found that as little as 20 milligrams of aspartame per day can cause cancer in humans; one 12-ounce diet soda contains about 180 milligrams of aspartame. So before you reach for that quart of diet soda at the gas station or even give it to your kids thinking it's better than all that sugar- think again. You may just be jumping from the frying pan into a blazing inferno.

Artificial sweeteners and other artificial flavoring aids such as sodium nitrate and sodium nitrite found copiously in luncheon meats and hotdogs are called excitotoxins because they do just that- excite the brain to toxic levels. They're also so concentrated that they wreak havoc on the digestive system, well-known to cause bloating, gas, diarrhea, or constipation. We know how harmful sugar is, otherwise we wouldn't have tried for over a hundred years to find its "innocuous" replacement.

Below is a list of the artificial sweeteners currently on the market, as well as hiding in foods such as commercially prepared salad dressings, mayonnaise, and electrolyte-balancing beverages meant for dehydrated children (Pedialyte® Bubble Gum Flavor ingredients: Water, Dextrose. Less than 2% of the Following: Citric Acid, Potassium Citrate, Salt, Sodium Citrate, Artificial Flavor, Sucralose, Acesulfame Potassium, Zinc Gluconate, and Red 40.):

• Aspartame

• Acesulfame potassium or acesulfame-K, K being the symbol for potassium in the periodic table of elements: composed of carbon, nitrogen, oxygen, hydrogen, sulfur, and potassium- all elements found in fertilizer. An FDA report from 1994 admits "Methylene chloride, a carcinogenic chemical, is a potential impurity in acesulfame-K resulting from its use as a solvent in the initial manufacturing step of the sweetener."

• Sucralose, the active ingredient in Splenda, quite simply put, is a chlorinated molecule of sugar. Don't forget that chlorine is poisonous. Sucralose has about as much business being associated with the natural "goodness" of sugar as crack has with the innocuousness of baking soda. Not to mention that the first 2 ingredients in Splenda are dextrose and maltodextrin, corn-derived sugars. How the manufacturer of Splenda managed to get that one past the FDA is beyond many, but telling the public that something that so clearly contains sugar is safe for people trying to avoid sugar borders on criminal. Sucralose may not have a glycemic index or calories, but there's more to Splenda than just sucralose. If you see sucralose as an ingredient in a product you've been indulging in, discard that product immediately. Its chemical formula is closer to that of the pesticide DDT than to the addictive drug sugar.

• Saccharine- a derivative of coal tar (you may as well start smoking). We should not be eating things derived from petrochemicals, or coal, or tar, regardless if they've been added, removed, added, and removed, added yet again, sure to be removed after a significantly higher number of birth defects have been associated with their consumption(?), from Proposition 65.

- Neotame- that's a new spin on the same poisonous pony- if a lab or pharmaceutical company is behind it, it's not food. And if it's not food, don't put it in your mouth.

- Advantame- The manufacturer behind this most recent formula to trick the brain into thinking it's tasting sweetness   reports that advantame is 100 times sweeter than aspartame, and at least as many times more safe.

There are acceptable low-calorie or even no-calorie sweeteners out there that are not toxic; my personal favorite, stevia extract. The stevia plant is also known as the sweetleaf plant, and a version of it happens to grow very well here in North Carolina. It has also been used for thousands of years in South America; the Japanese had been sweetening their Diet Coke with it since the seventies. In a nutshell, it is the extract of a plant, containing naturally-occurring substances called steviocides, which are upwards of 300 times sweeter than sugar, but with no caloric value and no effect on blood-glucose levels. Its extremely concentrated nature will require it to have been *diluted,* so to speak, with either erythritol (a sugar alcohol derived from fruit with no caloric value) if it is in powdered form; or with purified water as the carrier in liquid form (usually naturally preserved with grapefruit seed extract). It will come with a dropper and you can literally sweeten a full glass of fluid with as few as 4 to 6 drops.

Censored Nutritional Gem #13: Artificial Sweeteners Kill (Brain cells at least.)

Suggested Reading:

Sweet Deception: How Splenda and the FDA May Be Hazardous to Your Health, Drs. Joseph Mercola DO and Kendra Degen Pearsall, ND

Excitotoxins: The Taste That Kills, Russell Blaylock, MD

Sugar Blues, William Dufty

14
Your Body Hates Chlorinated Water

How much water is enough water? This is going to be a quick one when we're talking about quantity. The rule of thumb is 8 ounces per waking hour. So, consider that you stop drinking about 2 hours before you lie down at night because you want to avoid trips to the bathroom in the middle of the night, and that you've stayed hydrated throughout the day, and that you should avoid drinking water with your meals because it dilutes the acids in your stomach that are imperative for proper digestion, that would leave an individual that rises at 6 am and goes to bed by 10 pm, consuming 10 to 12, 8-ounce glasses of water per day. That's barring any strenuous exercise or being outside in high temperature situations, like digging trenches in the middle of July. I guess a second part to that question should be, is bottled water the best or will tap water suffice? We'll get that shortly but first, from another hero among men, Dr. William Gilman Thompson on "The Classes Of Foods. Part I Water" :

> It is estimated that water composes about 70 per cent of the entire body weight, and it is an almost universal solvent. Its importance to the system, therefore, cannot be overrated. The elasticity or pliability of muscles, cartilages, and tendons, and even of bones, is in great part due to the water which these tissues contain. As Solis-Cohen says, "the cells of the body are aquatic in their habits." The amount of water required by a healthy man in twenty-four hours is, on the average, between 65 and 70 ounces, besides about 20 ounces taken in as an ingredient of solid food, thus making a total of 85 to 90 ounces. The elimination of this water is divided as follows: 28 per cent through the skin, 20 per cent through the lungs, 50 per cent through the urine, 2 per cent through other secretions and the feces. This is, of course, a very general computation, for there is constant variation in the activity of different organs.

> A large proportion of the water is taken in the form of beverages composed chiefly of it, and by many persons they are substituted for plain water altogether. In some countries light wines, beer, and other fermented drinks wholly replace drinking water. This may be due to habit and custom, or to necessity from lack of pure natural water, but in all cases the quantity of water required to maintain the functions of the body in healthful activity remains the same, whether it be drunk

pure or in beverages, or taken with succulent fruits and vegetables, or in koumiss, etc.

One of the most universal dietetic failings is neglect to take enough water into the system.

The uses of water in the body may be summarised as follows:

1. It enters into the chemical composition of the tissues.
2. It forms the chief ingredient of all the fluids of the body and maintains their proper degree of dilution.
3. By moistening various surfaces of the body, such as the mucous and serous membranes, it prevents friction and the uncomfortable symptoms which might result from their drying.
4. It furnishes in the blood and lymph a fluid medium by which food may be taken to remote parts of the body and the waste matter removed, thus promoting rapid tissue changes.
5. It serves as a distributer of body heat.
6. It regulates the body temperature by the physical processes of absorption and evaporation.

All protoplasmic activity in cells ceases at once if they become dry. Elementary cells, such as the amoeba, cease to move, to digest, or to show any form of irritability or functional activity when dry, but if water be added to them their functions will be resumed, showing that they have been suspended and not necessarily destroyed.

The taking of much water into the stomach by its mechanical pressure excites peristalsis. One or two tumblerfuls of cold water taken into an empty stomach in the morning on rising favour evacuation of the bowels in this way. The water, moreover, is quickly absorbed and temporarily increases the fullness of the blood vessels. This promotes intestinal secretion and peristalsis. The increased activity of the lower bowel is explained in this way rather than by the idea that the water itself reaches the colon and washes out its contents.

This is something that we all need to be aware of and remedy the desensitization that has afflicted us. Pure, clean, drinking water is not something that the modern world should not have to obtain from a plastic bottle. But it doesn't end there. Merely bathing in chlorinated water can result in absorption of chlorine through the skin, and the hotter the water and longer the period of exposure, the greater the rate of absorption. According to the Wisconsin Department of Health Service website, "chlorine is a poisonous, greenish-yellow gas described as having a choking odor. It is a very corrosive, hazardous chemical… The proposed federal drinking water standard for chlorine is 4 parts per million (ppm). Many city water supplies are treated with chlorine to reduce the possible spread of bacterial disease. The system operators are required to maintain a detectable level of chlorine in the piping system. We suggest you stop drinking water that contains more than 4 ppm of chlorine on a regular basis." They go on to warn of the effects of short-term, high level exposures of breathing in chlorine gas:

- Immediately or shortly after exposure to 30 ppm or more of chlorine gas, a person may have chest pain, vomiting, coughing, difficulty breathing, or excess fluid in their lungs.

- Exposure to 430 ppm in air for 30 minutes will cause death.

- The health effects of breathing air that has less than 30 ppm of chlorine are the same as listed below for inhaling liquid bleach vapors.

- Liquid chlorine bleach and its vapors (at levels of 3-6 ppm in air) are irritating to eyes.

- At levels of 15 ppm in air people experience nose and throat irritation.

- Touching liquid chlorine bleach can cause skin irritation.

- Drinking levels over 4 ppm can cause throat and stomach irritation, nausea and vomiting.

So, is adding a poisonous, corrosive gas to our municipal water supplies the only way to reduce the risk of pathogenic factors and water borne illnesses? I found some great articles and resources online, one from the website that describes, "In 1908 the first addition of chlorine to a municipal water supply occurred in Jersey City, New Jersey, while at the same time near the Chicago Union Stockyards, chlorination transformed animal feed water from polluted to potable." Now, if you're drinking city water, as opposed to well water, chlorine is used to destroy pathogenic water-borne micro-organisms. Let it be known for a split second that chlorine is a poisonous gas and is deadly to *all* microorganisms, not just the pathogenic varieties, as well as humans, in just the right dose.

But it does more than just kill bacteria, it wreaks havoc on our cardiovascular system. As co-authors James B. Yoseph and Hannah Yoseph, MD, explain in their book, *How Statins Really Lower Cholesterol and Kill You One Cell at a Time:*

> Chlorine is a very strong oxidizer. It instantly reacts with water to form hypochlorous acid that kills microbes in seconds by oxidizing (destroying) their lipids. CVD plaques are full of oxidized cholesterol and dead mycoplasmas that normally circulate in arterial blood. White blood cells that ingest oxidized cholesterol in [an] attempt to clean up the mess are killed by apoptosis; these are called "foam cells".

> Arteries are our "pipes". Boiler engineers know that water must be completely chlorine-free before passing through metal pipes. If not, chlorine will oxidize (corrode) the inside of the pipes over years or decades- even stainless steel and titanium.

> If chlorine destroys the walls of metal pipes, what does it do to lipid-rich cell membranes that lines the walls of the arteries and the lipid-rich LDL cholesterol dissolved in the blood? If chlorine corrodes metal, what does it do to dissolved metals in the blood that are particularly important for normal heart and muscle function.

> Want to kill some marine life? Put them in a tank of chlorinated tap water and watch them slowly die. Chlorinated water is made safe for fish by adding enough vitamin C (a potent antioxidant) to neutralize the chlorine. While [they] bilk the public for billions of research dollars by blaming cholesterol for CVD, the verdict on chlorine was out long ago. Chlorinated water has been shown to:

> - Harden arteries (atherosclerosis)
> - Raise blood pressure (hypertension)
> - Enlarge the heart (cardiac atrophy)
> - Raise cholesterol (hypercholesterolemia)
> - Kill fish and other aquatic life

Consider the above explanation a possibility to account for a "three-fold increase in CVD since 1908 when chlorination of public water supplies and ingestion of phosphoric-acid containing sodas became increasingly popular…" Diverting your attention for a moment to a subject discussed earlier (sugar!), unfortunately, cardiovascular disease wasn't the only disease on the rise in America during that time. From an article written by Kevin Olsen, of Montclair State University, *Clear waters and a Green Gas: A History of Chlorine as a Swimming Pool Sanitizer in the United States*, the following excerpt gives us some interesting insight as "…the number of polio cases rose remarkably during the summer months…", [when children spent the bulk of their days at the community pool, splashing about and inadvertently ingesting some of that water?] Olsen further notes:

> Although the disease was first identified at the end of the 1800s, and the first serious outbreaks in the United States occurred at the time of WWI, polio was most common in the period between 1942 and 1953. The epidemic peaked in the summer of 1952 with 60,000 cases reported. Because polio outbreaks were most common in the summer months, anything associated with summer were suspect: flies, mosquitoes, strenuous exercise, eating ice cream and drinking cola.

It can take 4 to 21 days before symptoms appear and an infected person can pass the virus on to other people even before symptoms appear so a child could have been infected and still have been splashing about in a public pool for the first few days without feeling the slightest bit ill. Infection with polio happens when the virus enters the body through the mouth, it then multiplies in the throat and intestine, and spreads through the blood to the central nervous system.

What do ice cream and cola have in common? LOTS of sugar. Did you know that sugar is the most inflammatory substance we ingest as human beings? It depletes the immune systems and wreaks all sorts of havoc on all body systems. So here we are in the middle of the summer, swimming around in bath water, depleting our immune systems with a substance completely void of any nutrients that also happens to be more addictive than cocaine, but I digress. Ponder this passage from the same article for a moment:

> In March of 1903 Brown University began experiments with sterilizing pool water with chlorine. About the same time as the Lancet was publishing papers related to the bacterial contamination of swimming baths and means to sterilize them, including chlorination. A decade later (1913) the Lancet reported that chlorine levels of 0.5 to 1.0 ppm were sufficient for this purpose. By 1923 seven states had passed

regulations for the control of swimming pool sterilization and by 1946, announcements were made clearing the swimming pool as a potential source of the virus. [Since they had begun adding chlorine to every public and even private pool in existence.]

In January, 1946 The Journal of Pediatrics published a study on the means by which polio was transmitted. Although polio would continue to resist all prevention efforts of both laypersons and the medical community, a few useful facts did emerge. The authors concluded that there was no evidence that "water supplies, milk supplies, or swimming pools were means by which the disease was disseminated."

"Bullfeathers!", as my father would say. So you're swimming around in water that has bathed the rear ends of all the little kids in the neighborhood, and yes you're drinking the water, because you're a little kid and that's what it's there for! You're fresh off a break from drinking your Pepsi and slurping up the last of your scoop of ice cream loaded with immune-depleting substances and somehow can still find a way to deny the possibility of a connection there? That Journal of Pediatrics study seems like a bit of a *Diet-Heart Hypothesis* when you consider that over thirty years beforehand, the Lancet had reported that chlorination was sufficient enough a means to sterilize public pools. There are many other less toxic methods to sterilize our water supply.

In 1919, the Hotel Pennsylvania was advertising that its two swimming pools were "filtered clean, and then purified by violet rays. No Chlorine, no Chemicals." The hotel also offered "all electric treatments, baths, manicures, chiropody, and massage." Yet another instance, from the same article, where an alternative to chlorine was demonstrated to be superior involved W.A. Manheimer, Ph.D., the secretary of the American Association for Promoting Hygiene and Public Baths. In the early 1920s he conducted water purification experiments at the research laboratories of the New York State Department of Health. As a result of these experiments and subsequent field trials, Manheimer concluded that ozone was superior to chlorine for swimming pools. Chlorine was unsuited to waters with high concentrations of organic matter because of the odor problem. He went on to point out that since ozone is insoluble in water, there were no upper limits on the amounts that could be introduced. In 1934 a chemist named C. H. Brandes developed a method of introducing silver ions into a pool as a sterilizer, but the cost of treating pools by the electrolytic production of silver ions was considerably higher than that with chlorine.

Bottled water is a huge expense that is not only unnecessary but doesn't guarantee purity. It sits for months if not more in plastic bottles in all sorts of temperature extremes. We know these conditions compromise the integrity of the materials those bottles are made with and that runs the risk of actually releasing toxic chemicals into that water. The best thing you can do is have a whole-house water treatment system installed that removes the chlorine and other contaminants from your water before it even enters the pipes in your house. Understandably, that isn't going to be an option for everyone considering the upfront costs but if you are in a position to employ this method, find a reputable dealer in your area and get it done as soon as possible. The next best thing is to fix your drinking water with a reverse osmosis filtration system under your sink that will remove not only the chlorine, which decimates the probiotics in your gastrointestinal tract, but also heavy metals, fluoride, and other contaminants.

Why not distilled water? It's too pure. Think of it as "hungry water". According to the U.S. Environmental Protection Agency, "Distilled water, being essentially mineral-free, is very aggressive, in that it tends to dissolve substances with which it is in contact. Notably, carbon dioxide from the air is rapidly absorbed, making the water acidic and even more aggressive. Many metals are dissolved by distilled water." Because distilled water contains absolutely no trace minerals of any sort, it can upset the mineral balance in your body if you drink it too often or on a regular basis. Drinking clean, pure water is one of the keys to fantastic health. Next to cholesterol, it is the most necessary substance for human life (maybe clean air is a close second).

Signs of dehydration include muscle cramps, headache. The body tries to maintain cardiac output (the amount of blood that is pumped by the heart to the body); and if the amount of fluid in the intravascular space is decreased, the body tries to compensate for this decrease by increasing the heart rate and making blood vessels constrict to try to maintain blood pressure and blood flow to the vital organs of the body. The body shunts blood flow away from the skin to internal organs, for example, the brain, heart, lungs, kidneys, and intestines; causing the skin to feel cool and clammy. This coping mechanism begins to fail as the level of dehydration increases. With severe dehydration, confusion and weakness will occur as the brain and other body organs receive less blood.

The last massively important factor in optimal ousting of colon contents: water. If you're dehydrated, it will not bode well for any system in your body, but painfully so where the gut is concerned. How much *unchlorinated, unfluoridated* water? About a glass an hour, each hour you're awake!

Censored Nutritional Gem #14: Your Body Hates Chlorinated Water

Suggested Reading:

Alkalize or Die, Dr. Theodore A. Baroody

Your Body's Many Cries for Water, F. Batmanghelidj, MD

The Healthy Home: Simple Truths to Protect Your Family from Hidden Household Dangers, Dr. Myron Wentz and Dave Wentz, with Donna K. Wallace

How Statin Drugs Really Lower Cholesterol and Kill You One Cell at a Time, James B. Yoseph and Hannah Yoseph MD

Notes

15
Cook on Low, Cook it Slow
(Burnt food is toxic.)

Nothing says "America on a long weekend" louder and clearer than grill marks on a steak. Would it ever cross your mind that inside those tasty, seared markings lurk chemical compounds that are known carcinogens? Indeed they do, and we owe it all to something called the Maillard reaction. The Maillard (pronounced my-yard) reaction is a chemical reaction that occurs when heat is applied to something containing both amino acids (which remember are the tiny building blocks that proteins are made of) and reducing sugars, a few examples of which are glucose, fructose and lactose. The result is a complex mixture of molecules responsible for a range of odors and tastes. And the entire process is accelerated in an alkaline environment as when lye is used to darken pretzels. The specific type of amino acid present determines the resulting flavor and this entire process is the basis of the flavoring industry. So imagine for a second the taste of caramelized onions, or crème brûlée, or crispy fries. All of these different flavors are due chemical products formed during the Maillard reaction. Only one problem: the higher the temperature, the faster the reaction, meaning the browner something becomes, the greater the production of a "tasty" little agent called acrylamide.

Acrylamide is a chemical known as a *heterocyclic amine (HCA)*, or *heterocyclic aromatic amine (HAA)*. The problem is that acrylamide is also a known carcinogen (a substance that has been shown to produce cancer in laboratory tests). Acrylamide is not added to a food, it just happens to form naturally when anything that contains both proteins and sugars is heated past a certain temperature. It is also present in tobacco smoke, meanind that in addition to all the other toxic crud they're taking in, smokers are also exposed to particularly high levels of acrylamide. So, where and when are you going to find this substance that was added in 2011 to California's Propostion 65 list of chemicals?
- French fries,
- Potato and tortilla chips
- Coffee and roasted grain-based coffee substitutes
- Anything roasted or grilled with lovely dark brown or black char marks on it
- Canned black olives
- Roasted nuts
- Donuts
- Deep-fried foods
- Breakfast cereals, crackers, cookies, breads, and toast, all contain varying amounts of acrylamides

As German researcher Dr. Norbert U. Haase, explains, "acrylamide formation occurs in both industrial cooking and domestic preparation… [but] actual human exposure to acrylamide is highly variable because cooks and consumers have different preferences regarding discoloration and have developed individual preparation techniques to meet their specific requirements." That means the preparer of your meal has the power to increase the amount of cancer-causing substances in your food. That's sobering. Interestingly enough, when you boil or steam foods, you don't create acrylamide. We want some of the flavor that sautéing onions conveys or a little golden tone to a baked good we're making. So the key really is extreme caution with some things, moderation with others, and flat out avoidance with the flagrant. What do I mean by that? Don't allow *anything* you bake or cook in a pan to over-brown or burn. If it's burnt, throw it out. Avoid cooking on an open flame as your exposure to those heterocyclic amines increases considerably the more "well-done" your steak or chicken breast is cooked.

Mark G. Knize, Biosciences Directorate and researcher at the University of California, Lawrence Livermore National Laboratory, has written numerous academic articles on the effects of HAAs and their carcinogenic potential. In his piece, *Assessing Human Exposure to Heterocyclic Aromatic Amines,* he discusses the cumulative damage to our DNA that can result from a lifetime of consuming well-done meats:

> The hypothesis that HAA are involved in cancer etiology follows a logical mechanistic progression. HAA are present in some well-done meats, these meats are consumed over a lifetime, and the HAA are absorbed and metabolized to active intermediates that bind to DNA. It is these processes that can cause mutations leading to human cancer. The factors affecting the carcinogenic outcome are the exposure levels, possible susceptible periods during a human lifetime, the internal dose, the details of metabolic activation and detoxification, and repair of dam-aged macromolecules within the body's cells.

Yet another publication Knize co-authored involving the subject perfectly described by the study title, *Inhibition of fried meat-induced colorectal DNA damage and altered systemic genotoxicity in humans by crucifera, chlorophyllin, and yogurt,* suggests that the dietary intake of fermented foods, foods high in chlorophyll (dark green leafy vegetables), along with cruciferous vegetables like broccoli, have the potential to decrease DNA damage to the cells of the colon and rectum *that resulted from a high-temperature cooked meat diet.* The abstract of the study appears below:

Dietary exposures implicated as reducing or causing risk for colorectal cancer may reduce or cause DNA damage in colon tissue; however, no one has assessed this hypothesis directly in humans. Thus, we enrolled 16 healthy volunteers in a 4-week controlled feeding study where 8 subjects were randomly assigned to dietary regimens containing meat cooked at either low (100°C) or high temperature (250°C), each for 2 weeks in a crossover design. The other 8 subjects were randomly assigned to dietary regimens containing the high-temperature meat diet alone or in combination with 3 putative mutagen inhibitors: cruciferous vegetables, yogurt, and chlorophyllin tablets, also in a crossover design.

Subjects were nonsmokers, at least 18 years old, and not currently taking prescription drugs or antibiotics. We used the Salmonella assay to analyze the meat, urine, and feces for mutagenicity, and the comet assay to analyze rectal biopsies and peripheral blood lymphocytes for DNA damage. Low-temperature meat had undetectable levels of heterocyclic amines (HCAs) and was not mutagenic, whereas high-temperature meat had high HCA levels and was highly mutagenic. The high-temperature meat diet increased the mutagenicity of hydrolyzed urine and feces compared to the low-temperature meat diet. The mutagenicity of hydrolyzed urine was increased nearly twofold by the inhibitor diet, indicating that the inhibitors enhanced conjugation. Inhibitors decreased significantly the mutagenicity of un-hydrolyzed and hydrolyzed feces.

The diets did not alter the levels of DNA damage in non-target white blood cells, but the inhibitor diet decreased nearly twofold the DNA damage in target colorectal cells. To our knowledge, this is the first demonstration that dietary factors can reduce DNA damage in the target tissue of fried-meat associated carcinogenesis.

What does all this mean to you and your deep fryer, grill, smoker, spit, etc? It means the browner something gets, and the higher the temperature that it is cooked at, the higher the concentration of substances that can lead to colorectal DNA damage. Consider this a warning. Cook on low and slow down the process; and always use protective saturated fats as the barrier between your foods and heat. Keep in mind that although saturated fatty acids are much more stable in the presence of heat and oxygen than unsaturated fatty acids, they are by no means indestructible; they too can become damaged if you crank that burner or oven high enough. Those black marks are loaded with HAAs like acrylamide, as is anything that is deep-fried (including a turkey!), processed in an alkaline environment (canned black olives "Spanish-cured" in lye), or heavily processed like dehydrated soup mixes (see chapter 10 for examples of heavily processed dehydrated meal mixes to avoid like the plague). It also means that eating lacto-fermented food, leafy green and cruciferous vegetables has the potential to heal that poor colorectal DNA! And Mark G. Knize and his co-horts actually demonstrated this some time between 2005 and 2006! Interesting point, the study above was actually performed at the General Clinical Research Center (GCRC) of the University of North Carolina (Go Tar Heals!), with the involvement of the Laboratory of Molecular Carcinogenesis, National Institute of Environmental Health Sciences, National Institutes of Health, Department of Health and Human Services, at Research Triangle Park, North Carolina. If you'd like to review the study for yourself, visit www.ClinicalTrials.gov and enter the identifier, NCT00340743. Did I mention that according to the National Cancer Institute's website, www.Cancer.gov, based on 2008-2010 data, approximately 40.8 percent of men and women will be diagnosed with all cancer sites at some point during their lifetime? Coincidence? I think not.

Considering all of this information on the health-destructive potential of acrylamide, heterocyclic amines (HCA), and heterocyclic aromatic amines (HAA), one would think attempts to educate consumers clearly and concisely on how to reduce and even eliminate their intake would be vehemently publicized. Alas, industry attempts to diminish concerns and even discredit the abundant body of research devoted to the subject over the last 12 years are repulsively rampant.

The information for this chapter was obtained from both scholarly articles online and a book comprised of almost 500 pages of research studies from "authentic and highly regarded sources" around the world, on the subject in question. First published in 2006 by the Food Science, Technology, and Nutrition branch of Woodland Publishing Limited, in Cambridge, England, *Acrylamide and Other Hazardous Compounds in Heat-Treated Foods,* was edited by Kersten Skog, Professor in Food Chemistry at Lund University, Sweden; and Jan Alexander, Director for the Department for Food Toxicology at the Norwegian Institute of Public Health, and Professor in Environmental Medicine and Food Toxicology at the Norwegian University of Science and Technology.

Although the introduction to the publication includes the editors' acknowledgment that Maillard reaction products (acrylamide, HCAs and HAAs) are important for the sensory properties of heated and cooked foods such as color, flavor and aroma, they also warn that these compounds may not be beneficial, and may even be toxic to humans. I will take the findings of these academically accomplished individuals and the over 40 others just like them as gospel over the "opinions" of bought-and-sold charlatans like those appearing on a site much like the one doing damage-control for the soybean industry.

Shortly after the 2006 publication of *Acrylamide and Other Hazardous Compounds in Heat-Treated Foods,* a domain name and all of the possible suffixes associated with it were purchased to begin the propaganda against sound scientific findings on acrylamide. According to the WHOIS registry of active website domain names, on August 15th, 2007 a Corporation Service Company associated with approximately 21, 600 other domains registered the domain AcrylamideFacts.com, .net, .info, .biz, .us, and most unmeritedly AcrylamideFacts.org. Although the lines have been blurred in recent years about who is permitted to use one domain suffix over another (eg. only the U.S. Government is privy to the .gov suffix, and the .edu suffix can only be retained by educational institutions), the .org suffix was originally reserved for non-commercial organizations such as non-profits.

It seems the Grocery Manufacturers Association (GMA) joined the ranks of those non-profit organizations when it launched the site www.AcrylamideFacts.org and proceeded to forward www.AcrylamideFacts.com to the .org site. I wouldn't be surprised if in keeping with their ruthless attempts to undermine the efforts of Federally Funded Research and Development Centers (FFRDC), like the Lawrence Livermore National Laboratory, they would find a way to latch onto the .edu and .gov versions of AcrylamideFacts.

Paying a quick visit to either web address will land you on a page with a bountiful spread of all of the foods the research has proven to contain acrylamide, to include; french fries, canned black olives, grill-marked chicken breast, potato chips, pretzels, and even a cup of coffee (at least they're paying attention to what's being said about the wares they're peddling). I was having trouble deciding which aspect of the site's homepage was more unnerving, the photos, or the 3 rapidly-alternating quotes from two "experts", one on cancer and the other on nutrition:

> "Women should eat a balanced diet rich in fruit, vegetables, and fiber, and low in fat- that's the best dietary advice for reducing cancer risk."- Dr. Leslie Walker, Cancer Research U.K.

> "The evidence against acrylamide is based on high-dose animal studies or high-dose exposures in occupational studies- not on typical exposure in foods."- Ruth Kava, PhD, RD, Director of Nutrition, American Council on Science and Health

"Truth be told, there's just no evidence that acrylamide at the levels found in food presents either a toxic or carcinogenic hazard to people."- Ruth Kava, PhD, RD, Director of Nutrition, American Council on Science and Health

Honestly ladies? Do you kiss your children goodnight with those filthy lying mouths? Right after you've shared some pretzels and potato chips with them, I'm sure. A quick Google search on both of those "professionals" (trust me, I *am* holding back), will quickly demonstrate their partiality to the industry that sought their fundamentally worthless opinions to begin with. How else could one explain their willingness to trivialize a subject with such scientifically- demonstrated hazard potential?

If a visitor to the site isn't dissuaded from their information-gleaning efforts by the opinions of "Dr." Walker and Ruth Kava, and decides to peruse the site further, the "Home Cooking Tips" page will actually provide information that can be taken to heart, and that should be followed to the letter. That's a big "if" though because the site is also littered with efforts to trivialize the concerns of the world's leading researchers on the subject. When discussing what government authorities advise regarding dietary intake of acrylamide, they attempt to extinguish any consumer thoughts of reducing the consumption of junk food with cop-outs such as this:

> Although the formation of acrylamide in cooked foods is still being studied, a number of leading government food safety authorities around the world advise consumers to eat a healthy and balanced diet, rather than eliminate certain foods.
>
> For example, the U.S. Food and Drug Administration (FDA) recommends that the public eat a balanced diet, choosing a variety of foods that are low in trans fat and saturated fat, and rich in high-fiber grains, fruits, and vegetables.
>
> Similarly, the World Health Organization (WHO) reinforces general advice on healthy eating, including moderating consumption of fried and fatty foods. The WHO concludes that there is not enough evidence about the amounts of acrylamide in different types of food to recommend avoiding any particular food product.

As the GMA first introduces the consumer to acrylamide on their "educational" site, it's difficult to entertain their intentions as benevolent. While L.C. Maillard first recognized the formation of color through the interactions of amino acids and sugars in 1912, it wasn't until 1953 that Hodge would devise a schematic to provide the basis for our understanding of the reaction. Simply because humans have been facilitating the formation of acrylamide in foods "for as long as people have been baking, grilling, roasting, toasting, or frying foods", is not sufficient reason to dismiss the potential dangers of its overconsumption. From the GMA's site:

> *Acrylamide forms naturally in many plant-based, starch-rich foods when they are heated. Although acrylamide was first discovered to be present in food by the Swedish National Food Authority in 2002, we now know that acrylamide in foods is not new. Acrylamide has been present in the human diet for as long as people have been baking, grilling, roasting, toasting or frying foods.*

> *Acrylamide is present in many different foods regularly consumed around the world. For example, it is found in 40 percent of the calories consumed in the average American diet – in foods ranging literally from soup to nuts, and including baked and fried potatoes, cereals, coffee, crackers, olives, bread, asparagus, prune juice, dried fruit and many others. Acrylamide is produced by cooking foods, regardless of whether the food is made at home, in a restaurant or in a commercial setting. This widespread presence makes it highly unlikely that acrylamide can be completely eliminated from one's diet.*

> *While no health authority has recommended consumers change their eating behavior because of acrylamide, there are several practical methods to reduce acrylamide formation in many products. Food manufacturers and restaurants continue to explore and implement these solutions. Similarly, easy-to-follow advice is available for those consumers who want to reduce the formation of acrylamide while cooking at home.* [as opposed to those who are perfectly happy continuing to take in cancer-causing substances via 40 percent of the calories they consume.]

Try not to bake in an oven hotter than 350 degrees and don't take your stove-top burners past low-medium unless you're boiling water. And after you've reached a boil, you can conserve energy by puttin a lid on the pot and reducing the heat. Avoid well-done meats of any kind, and pan-sear as opposed to grilling on an open flame.

Censored Nutritional Gem #15 Cook on Low, Cook it Slow
(Burnt food is toxic.)

The last word on acrylamide and other cancer-causing chemicals goes to...

The State of California

Proposition 65 in Plain Language

Office of Environmental Health Hazard Assessment
California Environmental Protection Agency

What is Proposition 65?

In 1986, California voters approved an initiative to address their growing concerns about exposure to toxic chemicals. That initiative became the Safe Drinking Water and Toxic Enforcement Act of 1986, better known by its original name of Proposition 65. Proposition 65 requires the State to publish a list of chemicals known to cause cancer or birth defects or other reproductive harm. This list, which must be updated at least once a year, has grown to include over 800 chemicals since it was first published in 1987.

Proposition 65 requires businesses to notify Californians about significant amounts of chemicals in the products they purchase, in their homes or workplaces, or that are released into the environment. By providing this information, Proposition 65 enables Californians to make informed decisions about protecting themselves from exposure to these chemicals. Proposition 65 also prohibits California businesses from knowingly discharging significant amounts of listed chemicals into sources of drinking water.

The Office of Environmental Health Hazard Assessment (OEHHA) administers the Proposition 65 program. OEHHA, which is part of the California Environmental Protection Agency (Cal/EPA), also evaluates all currently available scientific information on substances considered for placement on the Proposition 65 list.

What types of chemicals are on the Proposition 65 list?

The list contains a wide range of naturally occurring and synthetic chemicals that are known to cause cancer or birth defects or other reproductive harm. These chemicals include additives or ingredients in pesticides, common household products, food, drugs, dyes, or solvents. Listed chemicals may also be used in manufacturing and construction, or they may be byproducts of chemical processes, such as motor vehicle exhaust.

How is a chemical added to the list?

There are four principal ways for a chemical to be added to the Proposition 65 list. A chemical can be listed if either of two independent committees of scientists and health professionals finds that the chemical has been clearly shown to cause cancer or birth defects or other reproductive harm. These two committees—the Carcinogen Identification Committee (CIC) and the Developmental and Reproductive Toxicant (DART) Identification Committee—are part of OEHHA's Science Advisory Board. The committee members are appointed by the Governor and are designated as the "State's Qualified Experts" for evaluating chemicals under Proposition 65. When determining whether a chemical should be placed on the list, the committees base their decisions on the most current scientific information available. OEHHA staff scientists compile all relevant scientific evidence on various chemicals for the committees to review. The committees also consider comments from the public before making their decisions.

A second way for a chemical to be listed is if an organization designated as an "authoritative body" by the CIC or DART Identification Committee has identified it as causing cancer or birth defects or other reproductive harm. The following organizations have been designated as authoritative bodies: the U.S. Environmental Protection Agency, U.S. Food and Drug Administration (U.S. FDA), National Institute for Occupational Safety and Health, National Toxicology Program, and International Agency for Research on Cancer.

A third way for a chemical to be listed is if an agency of the state or federal government requires that it be labeled or identified as causing cancer or birth defects or other reproductive harm. Most chemicals listed in this manner are prescription drugs that are required by the U.S. FDA to contain warnings relating to cancer or birth defects or other reproductive harm.

A fourth way requires the listing of chemicals meeting certain scientific criteria and identified in the California Labor Code as causing cancer or birth defects or other reproductive harm. This method established the initial chemical list following voter approval of Proposition 65 in 1986 and continues to be used as a basis for listing as appropriate.

What requirements does Proposition 65 place on companies doing business in California?

Businesses are required to provide a "clear and reasonable" warning before knowingly and intentionally exposing anyone to a listed chemical. This warning can be given by a variety of means, such as by labeling a consumer product, posting signs at the workplace, distributing notices at a rental housing complex, or publishing notices in a newspaper.

Once a chemical is listed, businesses have 12 months to comply with warning requirements.Proposition 65 also prohibits companies that do business within California from knowingly discharging listed chemicals into sources of drinking water. Once a chemical is listed, businesses have 20 months to comply with the discharge prohibition.

Businesses with less than 10 employees and government agencies are exempt from Proposition 65's warning requirements and prohibition on discharges into drinking water sources. Businesses are also exempt from the warning requirement and discharge prohibition if the exposures they cause are so low as to create no significant risk of cancer or birth defects or other reproductive harm. Health risks are explained in more detail below.

What does a warning mean?

If a warning is placed on a product label or posted or distributed at the workplace, a business, or in rental housing, the business issuing the warning is aware or believes that one or more listed chemicals is present. By law, a warning must be given for listed chemicals unless exposure is low enough to pose no significant risk of cancer or is significantly below levels observed to cause birth defects or other reproductive harm.

For chemicals that are listed as causing cancer, the "no significant risk level" is defined as the level of exposure that would result in not more than one excess case of cancer in 100,000 individuals exposed to the chemical over a 70-year lifetime. In other words, a person exposed to the chemical at the "no significant risk level" for 70 years would not have more than a "one in 100,000" chance of developing cancer as a result of that exposure.

For chemicals that are listed as causing birth defects or reproductive harm, the "no observable effect level" is determined by identifying the level of exposure that has been shown to not pose any harm to humans or laboratory animals. Proposition 65 then requires this "no observable effect level" to be divided by 1,000 in order to provide an ample margin of safety. Businesses subject to Proposition 65 are required to provide a warning if they cause exposures to chemicals listed as causing birth defects or reproductive harm that exceed 1/1000th of the "no observable effect level."

To further assist businesses, OEHHA develops numerical guidance levels, known as "safe harbor numbers" (described below) for determining whether a warning is necessary or whether discharges of a chemical into drinking water sources are prohibited. However, a business may choose to provide a warning simply based on its knowledge, or assumption, about the presence of a listed chemical without attempting to evaluate the levels of exposure. Because businesses do not file reports with OEHHA regarding what warnings they have issued and why, OEHHA is not able to provide further information about any particular warning. The business issuing the warning should be contacted for specific information, such as what chemicals are present, and at what levels, as well as how exposure to them may occur.

What are safe harbor levels?

As stated above, to guide businesses in determining whether a warning is necessary or whether discharges of a chemical into drinking water sources are prohibited, OEHHA has developed safe harbor levels. A business has "safe harbor" from Proposition 65 warning requirements or discharge prohibitions if exposure to a chemical occurs at or below these levels. These safe harbor levels consist of No Significant Risk Levels for chemicals listed as causing cancer and Maximum Allowable Dose Levels for chemicals listed as causing birth defects or other reproductive harm. OEHHA has established over 300 safe harbor levels to date and continues to develop more levels for listed chemicals.

What if there is no safe harbor level?

If there is no safe harbor level for a chemical, businesses that expose individuals to that chemical would be required to provide a Proposition 65 warning, unless the business can show that the anticipated exposure level will not pose a significant risk of cancer or reproductive harm. OEHHA has adopted regulations that provide guidance for calculating a level in the absence of a safe harbor level. Regulations are available at Article 7 and Article 8 of Title 27, California Code of Regulations. Determining anticipated levels of exposure to listed chemicals can be very complex. Although a business has the burden of proving a warning is not required, a business is discouraged from providing a warning that is not necessary and instead should consider consulting a qualified professional if it believes an exposure to a listed chemical may not require a Proposition 65 warning.

Who enforces Proposition 65?

The California Attorney General's Office enforces Proposition 65. Any district attorney or city attorney (for cities whose population exceeds 750,000) may also enforce Proposition 65. In addition, any individual acting in the public interest may enforce Proposition 65 by filing a lawsuit against a business alleged to be in violation of this law. Lawsuits have been filed by the Attorney General's Office, district attorneys, consumer advocacy groups, and private citizens and law firms. Penalties for violating Proposition 65 by failing to provide notices can be as high as $2,500 per violation per day.

How is Proposition 65 meeting its goal of reducing exposure to hazardous chemicals in California?

Since it was passed in 1986, Proposition 65 has provided Californians with information they can use to reduce their exposures to listed chemicals that may not have been adequately controlled under other State or federal laws. This law has also increased public awareness about the adverse effects of exposures to listed chemicals. For example, Proposition 65 has resulted in greater awareness of the dangers of alcoholic beverage consumption during pregnancy. Alcohol consumption warnings are perhaps the most visible health warnings issued as a result of Proposition 65.

Proposition 65's warning requirement has provided an incentive for manufacturers to remove listed chemicals from their products. For example, trichloroethylene, which causes cancer, is no longer used in most correction fluids; reformulated paint strippers do not contain the carcinogen methylene chloride; and toluene, which causes birth defects or other reproductive harm, has been removed from many nail care products. In addition, a Proposition 65 enforcement action prompted manufacturers to decrease the lead content in ceramic tableware and wineries to eliminate the use of lead-containing foil caps on wine bottles.

Proposition 65 has also succeeded in spurring significant reductions in California of air emissions of listed chemicals, such as ethylene oxide, hexavalent chromium, and chloroform.

Although Proposition 65 has benefited Californians, it has come at a cost for companies doing business in the state. They have incurred expenses to test products, develop alternatives to listed chemicals, reduce discharges, provide warnings, and otherwise comply with this law. Recognizing that compliance with Proposition 65 comes at a price, OEHHA is working to make the law's regulatory requirements as clear as possible and ensure that chemicals are listed in accordance with rigorous science in an open public process.

Where can I get more information on Proposition 65?

For general information on the Proposition 65 list of chemicals, you may contact OEHHA's Proposition 65 program at (916) 445-6900, or visit http://www.oehha.ca.gov/prop65.html . For enforcement information, contact the California Attorney General's Office at (510) 873-6321, or visit http://oag.ca.gov/prop65 .

Updated February 2013

Note: On the next page you will find an extremely truncated list of Proposition 65 Chemicals (full list is 23 pages), as I thought it of paramount importance to give you a glimpse into the potentially carcinogenic substances that are currently in use, either as prescription drugs, food additives, and even those whose years of lobbying to be removed actually paid off (artificial sweetener *saccharin*).

STATE OF CALIFORNIA
ENVIRONMENTAL PROTECTION AGENCY
OFFICE OF ENVIRONMENTAL HEALTH HAZARD ASSESSMENT
SAFE DRINKING WATER AND TOXIC ENFORCEMENT ACT OF 1986
CHEMICALS KNOWN TO THE STATE TO CAUSE CANCER OR REPRODUCTIVE
TOXICITY
JUNE 6, 2014

The Safe Drinking Water and Toxic Enforcement Act of 1986 requires that the Governor revise and republish at least once per year the list of chemicals known to the State to cause cancer or reproductive toxicity. The identification number indicated in the following list is the Chemical Abstracts Service (CAS) Registry Number. No CAS number is given when several substances are presented as a single listing. The date refers to the initial appearance of the chemical on the list. For easy reference, chemicals which are shown underlined are newly added. Chemicals or endpoints shown in strikeout were placed on the Proposition 65 list on the date noted, and have subsequently been removed.

Chemical	Type of Toxicity	CAS No.	Date Listed
Acrylamide	cancer	79-06-1	January 1, 1990
Acrylamide	developmental, male	79-06-1	Feb. 25, 2011
Saccharin, sodium	*cancer*	*128-44-9*	*January 1, 1988*
			Delisted January 17, 2003
Saccharin	*cancer*	*81-07-2*	*October 1, 1989*
			Delisted April 6, 2001
Sulfur dioxide	developmental	7446-09-5	July 29, 2011
Testosterone and its esters	cancer	58-22-0	April 1, 1988
Trichloroacetic acid	cancer	76-03-9	Sept. 13, 2013
D&C Orange No. 17	cancer	3468-63-1	July 1, 1990
D&C Red No. 8	cancer	2092-56-0	Oct. 1, 1990
D&C Red No. 9	cancer	5160-02-1	July 1, 1990
D&C Red No. 19	cancer	81-88-9	July 1, 1990
Citrus Red No. 2	cancer	6358-53-8	Oct. 1, 1989
Cocaine	developmental, female	50-36-2	July 1, 1989
Conjugated estrogens	developmental	---	April 1, 1990
Conjugated estrogens	cancer	---	Feb. 27, 1987
Clomiphene citrate	developmental	50-41-9	April 1, 1990
Clomiphene citrate	cancer	50-41-9	May 24, 2013
C.I. Disperse Yellow 3	cancer	2832-40-8	Feb. 8, 2013
Chloramphenicol sodium succinate	cancer	982-57-0	Sept. 27, 2013

Example Sources of the following Proposition 65 Chemicals:

• Acrylamide: canned soup, nuts, baked and fried potatoes, cereals, coffee, crackers, olives, bread, asparagus, prune juice, dried fruit.

> The proposed maximum allowable dose level (MADL) for acrylamide is 140 micrograms/day (μg/day). This value is based on the male reproductive effects of acrylamide as observed in the drinking water study in male rats by Tyl et al. (2000). The MADL is calculated based on a human male body weight of 70 kg (Title 27, California Code of Regulations, section 25803(b)

• Chloramphenicol sodium succinate: Intravenous (IV) antibiotic

• Clomiphene citrate: Prescription fertility (women) and low sperm count (for men) drug, Clomid

• Conjugated estrogens: Prescription menopause drug, Premarin (*pregnant mare urine*)

• Sulfur dioxide: Used to retain color of dried fruits, sun-dried tomaotes

• Testosterone and its esters: Prescription topical for males with low testosterone, AndroGel 1.62%

• Trichloroacetic acid: Used in cosmetics and chemical peels, and the treatment of genital warts

Afterthoughts on acrylamide and Proposition 65:

In December of 2002, hot on the heels of the report from the Swedish National Food Authority earlier that year identifying acrylamide as a potential carcinogen present in heat-treated foods (among others), *A Position Paper of the American Council on Science and Health*, by Joseph D. Rosen, Ph.D., Department of Food Science, at Rutgers University, was submitted to the California Office of Environmental Health Hazard Assessment (OEHHA), in a preemptive attempt to prevent the addition of acrylamide to the Proposition 65 list. The 17-page paper argues to diffuse concern of acrylamide's carciongenic potential by mockingly referring to other chemicals, at least one of which managed to buy its way off of the list (saccharin):

> So, is acrylamide formation in food really a cause for concern? Or will it turn out to be another one of those periodic food scares such as saccharin, aminotriazine in cranberries, cyclamates in diet soda, nitrosamines in bacon and luncheon meats, Red Dye #2 in processed foods...

Me thinks "The American Council on Science and Health" and the Grocery Manufacturers Association might go to drug rep dinners together on a weekly basis as the GMA continues to try and bully the California OEHHA into delisting acrylamide from Proposition 65.

Stand your ground Cali.

16
Excessive Protein Fertilizes the Acid Meadow
(One gram per pound of body weight at a time.)

Have you ever heard of an "acid meadow"? It's not what you're thinking. But if you allow this proverbial landscape to over-grow, advanced symptoms like Crohn's disease, lupus, cancer, and yes, schizophrenia can sprout and thrive. An acid meadow is what natural healers dub a body that has excess acid waste residues in its various tissues. The very nature of human life is acid-producing. Think about that; without breath in our lungs, we can't live. We exhale carbon dioxide, which happens to be the biggest source of acid in the body, as a result of inhaling "air" (which interestingly enough is comprised of approximately 78.09 percent nitrogen, 20.95 percent oxygen, 0.93 percent argon, and small amounts of other gases, including carbon dioxide).

We need oxygen to survive, and in order for plants to thrive and be able to produce it for us, they need our carbon dioxide to "breathe". How is carbon dioxide a source of acid? It binds to water in the blood and forms carbonic acid. Carbonic acid then dissociates into hydrogen (H+) ion and its buffer, bicarbonate (HCO_3-). The more hydrogen ions in a solution (hydrogen ion concentration), the lower its pH value is. Conversely, the more hydroxide (OH-) ions in a solution, the higher its pH value is. So, what's pH? Let's "squirrel" to a smidge of chemistry for that.

Potential hydrogen, abbreviated pH, is an important topic in physiology. It is the measure of acidity or alkalinity (basicity) of a solution. The pH scale ranges from 0, strongly acidic, to 14 strongly basic. Pure water has a pH of 7, symbolizing the measure of its neutrality: equal amounts of both hydrogen and hydroxide ions (H+ + OH- = H_2O). The hydrochloric acid in our stomachs (required for activation of the enzyme that digests protein), has a pH between 1 and 3; very *acidic*! On the other hand, sodium hypochlorite, better known as bleach, has a *basic* pH of 12; where drain cleaner is going to be considered *strongly basic* with a pH of 13. Note that I used the term basic as opposed to alkaline while referring to chemical solutions. When we discuss nutrition and body chemistry, I'm going to swap out basic for alkaline. The ideal pH of the blood should be very close to 7.4 (7.35 to 7.45), so slightly alkaline.

If the pH of the blood gets too low (too acidic) or too high (too alkaline), the structure of the proteins in your body can be affected and the proteins, denatured , a process that can affect their function. Unfortunately, it is much easier for the blood to become acidic (acidosis), rather than too alkaline (alkalosis). And when the blood does dip in pH, numerous symptoms and manifestations can emerge ranging from as inconvenient as acne, to as debilitating as arthritis, all the way to as deadly as cancer. Thank goodness you were not created in vain.

The body has exceptional systems in place to maintain homeostasis. We've discussed it before, but just for the record, homeostasis is that ideal state where variables are regulated so that internal conditions remain stable and relatively constant. Virtually every chemical reaction in the body requires some form of homeostatic control, especially the maintenance of optimal blood pH. Deviation from this value by more than a few tenths of a pH unit can be lethal, so your body is highly motivated to keep the blood pH as close to 7.4 as possible. Exhaling is a great way to eliminate acid from the body, and in order to exhale, you have to inhale, right? How many deep breaths have you taken today? Isn't that a novel idea- to increase the elimination of the most acid-forming factor from the body, you have the ability to consciously blow it out your nose and mouth. Keeping this in mind, you can see how not taking in enough oxygen (hypoventilation) allows for a buildup of carbon dioxide in the blood, which leads to respiratory acidosis. While on the flipside, hyperventilating, gives away too much carbon dioxide too quickly, thus producing respiratory alkalosis. Now, take a deep breath and blow it out with just a little more effort than you took it in. Do this a few times an hour, every waking hour. That's homeostasis in its simplest form.

Let it be known that the consumption, digestion, and subsequent processing, of certain foods greatly contributes to the formation of acid waste in the body. In the book *Alkalize or Die*, a definitive work about the subject, Dr. Theodore A. Baroody believes that, "acid wastes literally attack joints, tissues, muscles, organs, and glands, causing minor to major dysfunction. If they attack the joints, you might develop arthritis. If they attack the muscles, you could possibly end up with myofibrosis (aching muscles). If they attack the organs and glands, a myriad of illnesses and conditions could occur. The acid wastes set the stage for practically any and all opportunistic infections..." Let it also be known that when acid wastes are not eliminated when they should be (2 to 3 times per day!), they are reabsorbed from the colon into the liver, and put back into general circulation, where they will deposit in the tissues. So, considering the previous chapters you've read in this book on how inflammation has the potential to contribute to so many disorders and equally as much dysfunction, is the basis of disease acidosis or inflammation? The answer is both, as you're about to see how one begets the other.

Acid-forming foods are also known as mucus producers. How is mucus produced in the body? Thank goodness for glands- all sorts of them. The release of a chemical messenger of the immune system known as histamine, is responsible (among other actions), for triggering glandular secretions- mucus is a glandular secretion. Histamine is involved in regulating physiological function in the gut and also acts as a neurotransmitter. As part of an immune response to foreign pathogens (proteins!), histamine is produced by basophils and by mast cells found in nearby connective tissues to increase the permeability of the capillaries to white blood cells and some proteins. This allows the white blood cells to combat pathogens in the infected tissues. This also accounts for the runny nose and watering eyes you may experience as some type of airborne irritant has been inhaled.

Start bathing the tissues in an acidic medium and they become wounded, requiring the action of the immune system. The immune system then performs its duties via inflammatory reactions such as deployment of histamine. Excess mucus secretion reduces the respiratory system's ability to inhale and exhale, thereby reducing its ability to remove acid waste in the form of carbon dioxide. Now you're acidic. But wait, the plot thickens (as does the mucus because you're also perpetually dehydrated). The diet is depleted of nutrient-dense food so it lacks the ability to provide the body with raw materials to mediate toxicity. But it's also teeming with food-like imposters, tricking the immune system into thinking they're a target. So the immune system is now working triple-time to keep up. Only it can't- because the body's reserves from which it would fuel its efforts are non-existent. And now you have an autoimmune disorder, or two or three… Are you getting my clues?

As Dr. Baroody continues, "The ideal in dietary health is to eat as much fresh and raw food as possible." Since enzymes in raw food assist in its very digestion, taking in plenty of organic, colorful produce, like leafy green vegetables, tomatoes and berries, will assist the body in digesting other foods as well. It has been advised that if you do eat a considerable amount of cooked food (over 25 percent of your daily diet), that you supplement with digestive enzymes. The vast majority of individuals could replenish and sustain their body's alkaline reserves (elements the body uses to neutralize excess acidity), by taking in 80 percent of daily foods from those known to be alkaline-forming, and 20 percent of those from the acid-forming category. Animal protein, either from flesh or cow's milk, is one of the most acid-forming substances we can take in. It is of paramount importance that if you are a meat-eater, that you eat plenty of foods from the alkaline-forming list, and that you greatly reduce your intake of other acid-forming foods to reduce the buffering load on the body.

Since you've already given up refined sugars (see chapter 3), grains (see chapter 4), dairy (see chapter 5), table salt (see chapter 12), cooked eggs (see chapter 9), and artificial sweeteners (see chapter 13), and you're already facilitating flushing at least once, if not twice a day (see chapter 8), you're clearly on your way to vibrant health. Choosing 8 out of 10 foods a day from this list will keep you on track to topping off your body's alkaline reserves, maximizing its neutralizing abilities:

Vegetables	Fruits	Herbs, Spices, Condiments
Kelp (7.0)	Lemons (7.5)	Parsley (7.0)
Watercress (7.0)	Watermelon (7.5)	Cayenne Pepper (7.0)
Endive (6.5)	Cantaloupe (7.0)	Garlic, raw (6.0)
Escarole (6.5)	Dates, dried (7.0)	Sea salt (5.0)
Asparagus (6.5)	Figs, dried (7.0)	Bay leaves (6.0)
Carrots (6.0)	Papaya (7.0)	Cilantro (6.0)
Celery (6.0)	Mango (7.0)	Marjoram (6.0)
Swiss Chard (6.0)	Lime (7.0)	Sage (5.5)
Leaf Lettuce (6.0)	Pineapple (6.5)	Dill (5.5)
Spinach (6.0)	Kiwis (6.5)	Cloves (5.0)
Peas, fresh (5.5-6.0)	Pears (6.0-6.5)	Curry Powder (5.0)
Squash (5.0-6.0)	Pomegranate (5.5)	Raw Apple Cider Vinegar (5.5)
Cabbage (5.5)	Strawberries (5.5)	Vanilla (5.0)
Beets (5.5)	Raspberries (5.5)	
Broccoli (5.5)	Peaches (5.5-6.0)	
Cauliflower (5.5)		
Ginger, fresh (5.5)		AKEA Fermented Whole Food Supplement plus Probiotics and Enzymes is an Alkaline-forming Food with a pH of 8.54
Potatoes, with skin (5.5)		
Bell peppers (5.5)		
Sweet potatoes (5.5)		
Kale (5.5)		
Green beans (5.5)		
Cucumber (5.0)		
Brussel sprouts (5.0)		
Leeks (5.0)		
Onions (4.5-5.5)		
Sauerkraut (4.5)		
Tomatoes (4.5-5.0		

Adapted from Alkalize or Die: Foods that are known to be acid-forming include all of the following:

- Any sugars (including honey and agave nectar), salts, and foods that have been refined, processed, enriched, chemically- altered, or preserved
- Meat (all of it)
- Dairy products (all of them, but especially the pasteurized versions)
- Grains (all of them, but especially wheat)
- Cooked eggs (raw eggs and runny yolks are actually alkaline-forming!)
- Liquor, wine, and beer (all of them, though Dr. Baroody notes that "high quality, additive-free red wine used judiciously (no more than 4 oz. per day) becomes an important food for building the blood".
- Coffee (always choose organic, and try not to exceed 4 oz. per day)
- Artificial sweeteners

If you're going to eat beef, insist on only that from non-conventional ranches, where the animals have been grazing on green grass, not silage . Where they're not pumped full of steroids and hormones to maximize their yield, and not dosed with antibiotics to prevent illnesses that would surely result considering the conditions in which they're raised. You're on the hunt for 100 percent grass-finished beef, not just grass-fed. All cows have eaten grass at some point in their lives (or maybe not if the depiction of commercial cattle ranching is anything like that depicted in the movies Fast Food Nation and Food Inc). Grass-fed is a term that has lost all meaning since that "grass-fed" cow can spend the last 30 days of her life at a feed lot chowing down on gruel of soy and grains.

If you're going to eat chicken, insist on pasture-raised, preferably without the use of soy-based feed and without antibiotics administered. Understand that packaging is littered with meaningless rhetoric meant only to confuse the consumer into frustration and consequently resorting to playing "eenie meenie miney moe" as they try to pick the "best" one. That's a game that should be reserved for choosing players on a softball team, not what you're going to nourish your body with. Realize also that the main poultry producers in the country, Tyson, Perdue, Cargil and Pilgrim's, are no better than the other and all are playing the game of confusion in labeling and pollution of your body. Conventionally-raised chicken and turkey are loaded with antibiotic and other drug residues, and estrogens from the soy-based feeds meant to produce a slaughter-ready animal in half the time. They're also cramped and stressed to the max as all of their natural instincts of roosting, scratching, and stretching out while dust bathing to cool themselves are completely impossible considering their living arrangements.

Meat chickens are raised in "poultry houses" that can hold upwards of 40,000 adult chickens. These chickens never see the light of day or feel the softness of green grass beneath their feet. Stressed-out animals are fraught with stress hormones that you can't "cook out". As if you didn't have enough of your own stress. If you're going to eat fish, choose wild caught, and stay far away from the farmed variety, which is unfortunately the kind you're going to find at most restaurants. They're just as polluted with antibiotics as other conventionally-raised animals, and in the case of salmon, artificial color added to their food to hide the abnormal lack thereof indicative of ill-health. Limit your intake of large-breed fish like tuna and swordfish, since mercury bio-accumulates as they eat smaller fish, and those smaller fish eat smaller fish.

If you decide that you'd like to try removing the meat from your diet altogether, beware of the potential withdrawal symptoms. As George D. Pamplona-Roger, doctor of medicine and surgery at the University Of Granada in Spain notes, the sensation that "something is missing" always results from abruptly removing meat from the diet, "...stimulant hypoxanthine, not any special properties of its protein, vitamins, or minerals is responsible for the satisfying and stimulating effects of meat...It has been known since antiquity that those who regularly eat meat experience some degree of enervation [a feeling of being drained of energy or vitality; fatigue] when they are deprived of this food for some time.

Actually, both hypoxanthine and inosine are naturally present substances found in the muscle tissues of animals and humans alike (they are considered purines-substances that break down into uric acid in the body). As such, they are termed endogenous ligands, since they originate from within the organism's own body (a ligand is basically just a molecule that is able to bind to another). In the late 1970s both hypoxanthine and inosine were further identified as endogenous ligands for the benzodiazepine receptor in the brain , meaning they could "fit" in certain sites of the brain that had been identified as benzodiazepine receptors. Several nonbenzodiazepine exogenous ligands have been identified for the benzodiazepine receptor, with a few being the essential amino acid tryptophan, caffeine, melatonin, and the bronchodilator theophylline, used to treat symptoms of asthma and other lung problems such as emphysema and on-going bronchitis. Melatonin is actually the hormone- synthesized by the body from tryptophan- involved in regulating the sleep cycle or circadian rhythm. That leaves an essential amino acid (must be taken in from the diet), two substances found in meat, caffeine, and a pharmaceutical drug used to "treat asthma" as potential activators of something called a benzodiazepine receptor.

To truly understand the significance of both hypoxanthine and inosine and the potential for withdrawal symptoms resulting from the elimination of meat from the diet, we need to understand the significance of the benzodiazepine receptor to begin with. For anyone who has ever had trouble sleeping or has been plagued by anything from muscle spasms to chronic anxiety, a trip to the good doctor could yield a prescription for a sleep aid, muscle relaxant, or anxiolytic respectively. Anxiolytics are drugs categorized as benzodiazepines, their actions being among reducing feelings of anxiety and panic, but some have the added bonus of being anticonvulsants, muscle relaxants and hypnotics, so they're also prescribed for seizures, muscle spasms, and insomnia, respectively. Valium (diazepam), Xanax (alprazolam), and Klonopin (clonazepam) are three anxiolytic drugs prescribed for their both their anti-anxiety and muscle-relaxing effects.

Benzodiazepines are extremely addictive due to their effect on the function of one of the brain's own inhibitory neurotransmitters, GABA (gamma-aminobutyric acid). GABA's job is to slow or calm things down. Benzodiazepines increase the efficiency of GABA, thus causing greater inhibition or calming of a specific action (like muscle contraction or worrying). This effect is demonstrated in numerous areas of the brain including those responsible for affecting emotional reactions, memory, consciousness, muscle tone and coordination. An individual with not enough GABA may exhibit signs of stress and anxiety and an individual with too much may be overly relaxed. The confusing thing is that benzodiazepines are chemically synthesized and therefore not found in nature. So, if there is a receptor site where a chemical not found in nature, or exogenous ligand, could exert its actions, there must certainly be an endogenous ligand for which the receptor site was naturally intended, right? Well, scientists really haven't been able to identify any others besides hypoxanthine and inosine, and those are present in our own muscle tissues! So, since we're hopefully not eating the muscle tissues of other humans, one could postulate that when any other muscle tissue is consumed (MEAT), the hypoxanthine and inosine in that meat could exert an activating effect on those benzodiazepine receptors- the same way Valium, Xanax, and Klonopin do.

What happens when you stop taking a benzodiazepine? You get benzo withdrawal, a cluster of symptoms that emerge when a person who has taken benzodiazepines and has developed a physical dependence undergoes dosage reduction or discontinuation. Benzodiazepine withdrawal symptoms are notable for the manner in which they wax and wane and vary in severity from day to day or week by week instead of steadily decreasing in a straightforward manner:

- Often severe sleep disturbance.
- Irritability
- Increased tension and anxiety

- Panic attacks
- Hand tremor
- Sweating
- Difficulty with concentration
- Confusion and cognitive difficulties
- Memory problems
- Dry retching and nausea
- Weight loss
- Headache
- Muscular pain and stiffness
- Perceptual changes (hallucinations, seizures, psychosis)
- Suicide

I'm not saying for a second that someone might attempt suicide after deciding to become vegetarian, but the effect of meat with its at least two known inherent brain-stimulating substances certainly has the capacity to create a level of addiction. That addiction would seem to manifest itself, in certain susceptible individuals, when meat is given up abruptly. Because of this, it is recommended that those wishing to replace meat with plant-based foods follow a transition diet, possibly switching to fish in the meantime, to help avoid the effect of sudden deprivation. Why would anyone want to give up meat? It happens (see Appendix A).

So basically, the most important aspect of consuming any flesh or animal meat is balancing the acid formation in the body with plenty of alkaline-forming foods, especially raw vegetables, and making sure you're obtaining meat that is as "clean" as possible. "Clean" meat will be obtained from animals that are actually eating what nature meant for them to eat, in the habitat nature intended them to be living in. For example, cows don't graze in corn fields so "corn-fed" shouldn't be a selling point when buying steaks. Chickens are not vegetarians, so depriving them of the ability to scratch for grubs and worms in a lush green field adversely affects their health. Sunshine is as healthy for animals as it is for you and me. Keeping them in an artificially-lit "house" is not going to promote health. The use of antibiotics as prophylactics has also polluted animals raised for meat and as a result, we inadvertently keep dosing ourselves with those unwritten prescriptions. Try to purchase meat from a local, small-scale rancher, who stakes his reputation on raising his animals in as principled a way as possible. If that's just not a possibility for you, visit my website at SatFatRox.com for quality suppliers that will ship across the country. These suppliers vow to feed their animals the way God intended, right up to the time of slaughter, and to not routinely administer antibiotics or growth factors.

You may also want to consider keeping your own laying hens. They're easier to take care of than you might think, and there's really nothing quite like walking out to your backyard to pick up a freshly laid half dozen eggs every couple of days. The key to hens is to make sure they have plenty of green grass to pasture in, and to obtain a high quality, soy-free layer feed in addition to other organic grains from them to scratch for. Countryside Organics in Virginia has been our supplier for quality chicken feed for almost 5 years, and has provided our hens the wholesome organic grain supplementation with which to make the most beautiful, superfood-like eggs I could ever imagine. Only birds can efficiently digest grains, by the way!

If you are going to get your daily protein requirement from meat, keep in mind that shooting for one gram of protein for every pound of body weight you weigh is extraordinarily excessive. As Dr. Mercola describes in an article on his site, www.Mercola.com, actually related to gut flora and exercise, rarely is there a reason to consume more than 40 to 70 grams of protein per day:

> In fact, it's worth noting some other research when discussing the role of protein in gut health. Earlier this year, Science News ran an article about how local diets dictate the bacterial balance found in residents. For example, despite living on opposite ends of the earth, people in Malawi and the Guahibos of Venezuela have similar microbial makeup, courtesy of the similarities between their native diets. "Americans, on the other hand, have a distinctive microbiome with about 25 percent less diversity than indigenous Venezuelans," the article states.
>
> One of the primary differences between the diets is meat consumption. Malawian and Guahibo diets are high in corn and cassava, with an occasional piece of meat. Americans, on the other hand, are far more carnivorous, and also eat far more bread, lettuce and tomatoes, potatoes, pasta, milk, and dairy products. The microbial makeup of the three groups reveals these dietary differences. Granted, your body needs protein. It's a main component of your body, including muscles, bones, and many hormones. As you age, consuming adequate amounts of high-quality protein is especially important, as your ability to process protein declines with age, raising your protein requirements.
>
> That said, you do need to be careful to not consume too much. The average American consumes anywhere from three to five times as much protein as they need for optimal health. I believe it is the rare person who really needs more than one-half gram of protein per pound of lean body mass.

Those that are aggressively exercising or competing and pregnant women should have about 25 percent more, but most people rarely need more than 40-70 grams of protein a day...

The rationale behind limiting your protein is this: when you consume protein in levels higher than recommended above, you tend to activate the mTOR (mammalian target of rapamycin) pathway, which can help you get large muscles but may also increase your risk of cancer.

He goes on to point out that most people are actually consuming too much low quality protein [soy!] and carbohydrates, and not enough high quality fat. Does that mean that we should all be resorting to the Atkins diet? Not at all. Substantial amounts of protein can also be found in fish, legumes, nuts, and eggs!

Censored Nutritional Gem #16:
Excessive Protein Fertilizes the Acid Meadow
(One gram per pound of body weight at a time.)

Suggested Reading:

Alkalize or Die, Dr. Theodore A. Baroody

Foods That Heal, Dr. George D. Pamplona-Rogers

Diet for a Small Planet, Frances Moore Lappé

Animal Machines, Ruth Harrison

Conscious Eating, Gabriel Cousens, MD

Survival in the 21st Century, Viktoras H. Kulvinskas, MS

Patient Heal Thyself, Jodan S. Rubin, NMD, PhD

The Maker's Diet, Jordan Rubin, NMD, PhD

Notes

17
Honor Your Cravings
(Don't fight or control them.)

Have you ever seen some version of that "motivational" chart floating around the social media sites that teaches you how to "control your cravings"? The one that tells you to eat "this good food" if you're craving "that bad food". Substituting fat-free foods when our bodies crave full fat versions is a huge part of what has led us on this ill-fated journey to the "Town of Allopath" (visit www.Mercola.com to watch the video about the town that was afraid a solution to their problem would put everyone out of a job). Scan the charts on the next two pages and see if you can attest to ever craving any of those "bad" foods. Figuring out the truth about what you really should be eating, why, and how it's going to help you really start living, is going to free your mind to embrace your new-found wellness. The Censored Nutritional Gems have already debunked several of the myths in that motivational chart but I'm going to go through it briefly so you're never again tempted to replace chocolate with anything but organic raw cacao powder!

Now, it clearly makes sense to avoid all of the non-food items in those charts like, alcohol, tobacco, and recreational drugs (say "Yes, it does."), but certain foods have been wrongly implicated in contributing to an unhealthy physical state simply because of the ingredients that typically accompany them. For example, chocolate is most often found in the presence of sugar, a partially-hydrogenated oil, some type of dairy ingredient, and soy lecithin. In previous chapters, we've discussed the ill effects all four of those accomplices have on the immune system, and yet "chocolate" is named number one on that list!

Learning to identify your body's nutritional deficiencies through the hints it provides you via your cravings can open the door to a deliciously vibrant life. Craving chocolate, salt, and fat, is not something you should be ashamed of. The right forms of all of those foods will provide fundamental vitamins, minerals, and brain food that can actually heal you. Honoring your cravings also means learning to differentiate between your body's cries for nutrients and your brain's withdrawal symptoms from inflammatory and addictive substances such as glutens, caseins, hypoxanthine and inosine, and artificial food additives.

If you're craving chocolate, it could very well be that your body needs magnesium, but it could also be demanding iron, fiber and protein, plus a flurry of antioxidants and phytonutrients (epicatechin) that would never even be listed in the nutrition facts! If the body truly did need magnesium, as the chart indicates, organic raw cacao powder would be the perfect source for it. Just half an ounce (14 grams) of organic raw cacao powder gives you this abundance of nutrients, including almost a quarter of your recommended daily intake (RDI) of magnesium:

- Magnesium: 92 milligrams (mg) (23% RDI)
- Iron: 8% RDI
- Calcium: 2% RDI
- Potassium: 243 mg (7%)
- Dietary fiber: 4 grams
- Protein: 3 grams
- Fat: 1.5 grams, 1 gram saturated (yay!!)

But the truth is that if you're craving the "chocolate" most people crave, you're looking for the sugar normally accompanying it- or possibly even the milk solids that help neutralize real chocolate's edge. A true chocolate craving would be satisfied easily by a square or two of 70-80 percent dark or bittersweet chocolate, its taste almost an acquired one due to the bitterness of the naturally present polyphenols and catechins. Fifty grams (about 2 squares) of dark chocolate usually contains no more than 12 grams of sugar, where a regular size Snickers bar (52.7 grams), contains 27 grams of sugar, as well as "skim milk, lactose, milkfat, artificial flavor, skim milk, and more lactose (all in order of appearance on the ingredients label). Don't tell me you think reaching for a Snickers® bar means you're craving chocolate.

The real culprit of 50 percent of cravings: sugar. If you've acknowledged that what you were really looking for in that Snickers® bar or Dove® square was sugar, chances are your serotonin levels are low and your brain cells themselves are starving. As we learned in chapter 3, Censored Nutritional Gem: *Sugar is the Root of all Nutritional Evil*, simply eating foods containing tryptophan, the precursor to serotonin, is not going to mean that your levels will increase. In order for tryptophan to successfully cross the blood-brain barrier and start producing serotonin, other larger amino acids are going to have to be diverted from the barrier to the muscle tissues with a slow release of insulin, that's where organic potatoes with the skin on become heroes.

Potatoes are rich in complex carbohydrates that, when eaten in the presence of high quality fats like coconut oil and extra virgin olive oil give that perfect trickle of insulin to the blood so that tryptophan can sneak into the brain and work its serotonin-synthesizing serendipity. Sugar cravings also hit throughout the day because of the vicious cycle of simply eating sweet foods, refined and not. Oat beta glucans has been proven to lower the glycemic index of any of the food it's eaten with, thereby preventing spikes and dips in insulin, and the resulting cravings for yet more sugar. Ensuring the right amount of quality fat intake will also give your body the raw materials it needs to synthesize all of your feel-good brain chemicals, as well as stress-coping hormones.

If you're craving "bread, toast, pasta, and other carbs", again your serotonin levels are probably low and the consumption of all of those refined carbohydrates and grains is going to yield that brain pleasure-center stimulation with the gliadorphins that are partial digests from gluten contained in wheat and other grains. Remember from Censored Nutritional Gem: No Grains, No Pains, that gliadorphins are have opiate-like effects on the brain that leave you with withdrawal symptoms once their effects begin to wear off.

Just realize that if you're craving carbs, you're not craving prolamines like the avenin in oatmeal you can't digest, you need more fat like coconut oil, egg yolks, and avocados. The craving imposter is actually the gluten digest (partially digested protein, varying in amino acid chain length) that your brain usually receives opiate-like stimulation from. Akea Fermented Superfoods powder has also consistently been reported to drastically reduce cravings for carbs, sugar, and junk food. This would make sense since it contains the cultured minerals chromium, magnesium, zinc, selenium, calcium, and manganese, in the perfect ration of maximum absorption. And because Akea is a *fermented food*, any traces of avedin from the oat bran, quinoa, amarinth, millet or buckwheat (the last four of which are all complete proteins, by the way) would have already been predigested into single or double-chain amino acids, thereby *preventing* the activation of an immune-mediated response (better known as inflammation)!

If you're craving *fatty foods*, for your own sanity and the love of all that's good in the world, please eat more saturated fat! You're craving it because your brain is *dying* for it. You're craving it because your ccll membranes need to be repaired. You're craving it because your sex hormones are out of whack. You're craving it because your vitamin D3 production can't proceed to full capacity without cholesterol from raw egg yolks! Now, if you're craving *oily foods*, eat extra virgin olive oil and avocados, both great sources of the balanced amounts of polyunsaturated fatty acids (omega- 3 and 6) as well as the monounsaturated omega-9). According to the website, www.OliveOilSource.com, olive oil is on average 10% linoleic acid (an omega-6 oil) and less than 1% linolenic acid (an omega-3 oil). Bake up some SatFatRox Biscuits and dip them in extra virgin olive oil to your heart's content! There will be times you crave unsaturated fatty acids and other times you crave saturated fatty acids- listen to your body and take in the fat that you are most drawn to. Only then will you have given your cells the raw materials it needs to do what it does best without you consciously thinking about it: heal.

If you crave this...	What you really need is...	Healthy foods that have it:
Chocolate	Magnesium	Raw nuts and seeds, legumes, fruits
Sweets	Chromium	Broccoli, grapes, cheese, dried beans, calves liver, chicken
	Carbon	Fresh fruits
	Phosphorus	Chicken, beef, liver, poultry, fish, eggs, dairy, nuts, legumes, grains
	Sulfur	Cranberries, horseradish, cruciferous vegetables, kale, cabbage
	Tryptophan	Cheese, liver, lamb, raisins, sweet potato, spinach
Bread, toast	Nitrogen	High protein foods: fish, meat, nuts, beans
Oily snacks, fatty foods	Calcium	Mustard and turnip greens, broccoli, kale, legumes, cheese, sesame
Coffee or tea	Phosphorous	Chicken, beef, liver, poultry, fish, eggs, dairy, nuts, legumes
	Sulfur	Egg yolks, red peppers, muscle protein, garlic, onion, cruciferous vegetables
	NaCl (salt)	Sea salt, apple cider vinegar (on salad)
	Iron	Meat, fish and poultry, seaweed, greens, black cherries
Alcohol, recreational drugs	Protein	Meat, poultry, seafood, dairy, nuts
	Avenin	Granola, oatmeal
	Calcium	Mustard and turnip greens, broccoli, kale, legumes, cheese, sesame
	Glutamine	Supplement glutamine powder for withdrawal, raw cabbage juice
	Potassium	Sun-dried black olives, potato peel broth, seaweed, bitter greens
Chewing ice	Iron	Meat, fish, poultry, seaweed, greens, black cherries

If you crave this...	You really need this...	Healthy foods that have it:
Burned food	Carbon	Fresh fruits
Soda and other carbonated drinks	Calcium	Mustard and turnip greens, broccoli, kale, legumes, cheese, sesame
Salty foods	Chloride	Raw goat milk, fish, unrefined sea salt
Acid foods	Magnesium	Raw nuts and seeds, legumes, fruits
Preference for liquids rather than solids	Water	Flavor water with lemon or lime. You need 8 to 10 glasses per day.
Preference for solids rather than liquids	Water	You have been so dehydrated for so long that you have lost your thirst. Flavor water with lemon or lime. You need 8 to 10 glasses per day.
Cool drinks	Manganese	Walnuts, almonds, pecans, pineapple, blueberries
Pre-menstrual cravings	Zinc	Red meats (especially organ meats), seafood, leafy vegetables, root vegetables
General overeating	Silicon	Nuts, seeds; avoid refined starches
	Tryptophan	Cheese, liver, lamb, raisins, sweet potato, spinach
	Tyrosine	Vitamin C supplements or orange, green, red fruits and vegetables
Lack of appetite	Vitamin B1	Nuts, seeds, beans, liver and other organ meats
	Vitamin B3	Tuna, halibut, beef, chicken, turkey, pork, seeds and legumes
	Manganese	Walnuts, almonds, pecans, pineapple, blueberries
	Chloride	Raw goat milk, unrefined sea salt
Tobacco	Silicon	Nuts, seeds; avoid refined starches
	Tyrosine	Vitamin C supplements or orange, green and red fruits and vegetables

Source: Adapted from www.NatureWorksBest.com

If you're craving "salt", your body is screaming for minerals and "salty" is the taste it associates with minerals (because that is how they are found in nature!) That means that you must give it mineral salts! Chapter 12 discussed the Censored Nutritional Gem, *The Right Salt is Pink*. Don't be afraid to start adding salt into your cooking and baking repertoire, as long as it's the right salt (pink!), your food is going to start satisfying you more readily, and in reduced quantities. This is especially the case if you accompany pink salt with a high quality oil such as coconut oil or extra virgin olive oil.

If you find yourself "generally overeating", you must still be in the pre-contemplative state of figuring out whether or not to believe a word I've said. Don't doubt yourself. You've come this far for a reason and what is written in this book is not my own pipedream (yes, I said pipedream), theory or method. All of the information in this book has been gleaned from veritable heroes in this tragic day and age. The physicians, PhDs, chiropractors, scientists, and holistic health practitioners have put their information out there for the world to access; I have merely attempted to bridge the gap and bring it all to you in one cohesive package. Your body has an amazing propensity to heal itself and will do so if you just listen to it and honor your cravings. Basically, you're not going to have any desire to "overeat" once you start SatFatRockin' out! Don't forget your Akea! It will arm you with the cellular nutritional stores to let go of those addictive foods, while experience minimal backlash from their elimination.

One last idea that has recently come to mind is the true nature of craving the *taste* of alcohol, especially that of beer and wine. If you think about it, both beer and wine were traditionally fermented foods that cultures consumed most often in precise moderation. It is my (as far as I know) hypothesis, that when you crave beer or wine, what your body is truly begging for is fermented food. Food that has been predigested by friendly microorganisms, and that contains the necessary enzymes to further assist the digestive process. A remarkable decrease in the craving of wine and beer has been noticed by too many of my clients (none of whom, to my knowledge, have alcohol addiction issues) to be dismissed as random. The remarks have been quite nonchalently mentioned, thus leading me to believe that the individuals themselves do not realize what their bodies are requesting and requiring from them when they do "feel like a glass of wine".

Censored Nutritional Gem #17: Honor Your Cravings
(Don't fight or control them.)

The Last Word on Chocolate goes to…

The authors Leonardo Nogueira, Israel Ramirez-Sanchez, Guy A. Perkins, Anne Murphy, Pam R. Taub, Guillermo Ceballos, Francisco J. Villarreal1, Michael C. Hogan and Moh H. Malek, for their collaborative work on the article, *Epicatechin Enhances Fatigue Resistance and Oxidative Capacity in Mouse Muscle*, from the Journal of Physiology, published first online July 25th, 2011. The abstract:

During exercise, skeletal muscle performance depends in great part on the use of aerobic metabolism to supply the energetic demand of contractions. Endurance training increases the muscle aerobic capacity, which is not only associated with enhanced exercise performance, but also with a decreased risk of cardiovascular and metabolic diseases. Recently, it has been shown that regular use of small doses of dark chocolate may result in similar health benefits to exercise training. We show here that mice fed for 15 days with (–)-epicatechin (present in dark chocolate) had improved exercise performance accompanied by:

(1) an increased number of capillaries in the hindlimb muscle; and
(2) an increased amount of muscle mitochondria as well as signalling for mitochondrial biogenesis. These results suggest that (–)-epicatechin increases the capacity for muscle aerobic metabolism, thereby delaying the onset of fatigue. These findings may have potential application for clinical populations experiencing muscle fatigue.

Read the complete article at www.jp.physoc.org/content/589/18/4615.short

And for more studies on the phenomenal health benefits of epicatechin, the antioxidant found abundantly in raw cacao powder and dark chocolate, search: epicatechin and exercise on scholar.google.com, and instead of gearing up for the gym with a sugary "energy drink" or a Snickers bar that will wreak havoc on all your body systems, grab a square of two or 80 percent dark chocolate, and fly like the wind!

18
Herbs and Spices are Superfoods
(And they're here to heal.)

Did you know you had your very own "farmacy" right in your kitchen? Herbs such as parsley, oregano, basil, cilantro, and spices like turmeric, cinnamon, cayenne pepper, cloves and coriander all have well-documented abilities to provide potent antioxidant protection and even alkalize the acid meadow. They all have a place in your medicine cabinet in addition to your pantry! Preparing your meals with herbs and spices that have healing reputations and a plethora of antioxidants, bioflavonoids, and other organic compounds, will provide your cells with the raw materials to perform and heal at a level beyond our comprehension.

Must haves for immune-boosting properties are oil of oregano and fresh, raw, organic garlic. Just 1-2 drops of oil of oregano under the tongue followed by 6 ounces of filtered water helps annihilate any bug or virus attempting to plant roots in the acid meadow (a.k.a. Your tired, stressed out body.) Crushing and mincing organic garlic increases the surface area exposed to oxygen. It is this oxygen exposure that triggers a catalyzation of certain elements in the garlic into the healing compound allinase. Use a sharp-edged knife to chop it into very small pieces, or crush it in a garlic press. Before using the fresh-cut garlic, it should be allowed to sit for at least fifteen minutes to allow the chemical conversion to take place.

Cayenne pepper, has long been used for its antifungal and antibacterial properties; detoxifying and alkalizing effects; digestion support, as well as providing analgesic (pain relieving) and anti-inflammatory benefits from cayenne's key substance, capsaicin. Using cayenne pepper instead of black pepper will alkalize the body while enhancing the taste of any dish. For therapeutic benefit, 1-2 capsules once or up to three times daily improves digestion and can even help curb your appetite, according to a 2010 study at Purdue University in West Lafayette, Indiana. The study found that cayenne pepper also decreased appetite, especially in people who said they didn't already eat spicy foods. Cayenne can also be used as an endocrine system stimulator when taken in supplement form.

Ginger has also been widely used to promote efficient digestion, reduce nausea and vomiting related to chemotherapy. Anti-inflammatory effects have been seen in respiratory dysfunction such as asthma and bronchitis, arthritis and muscle pain, as well as inflammation of the colon. Raw and traditionally pickled ginger are superior to powdered or heated forms, as enzymes are maintained intact and the integrity of the myriad of other compounds are also preserved. Ginger shares a family tree with turmeric, cardamom, and galangal.

Chinese medicine and Ayurveda have used this spice for everything from indigestion and cramps to improving energy, vitality and circulation. Cinnamon actually comes in four varieties, but not all are created equal. Three of them also come with varying amounts of a substance called *coumarin* that can cause liver damage or complete failure. Only Ceylon or Mexican cinnamon has low levels of coumarin, while all other varieties have slightly to significantly higher levels. Cassia (Chinese) cinnamon, the most common cinnamon on grocers' shelves, has twice the amount of coumarin as Ceylon, where Indonesian contains over a hundred times the amount. Saigon cinnamon maxes out at over 400 times the amount of coumarin than the mild tasting Ceylon.

According to an article on www.CinnamonVogue.com, at one point the German government even banned the cassia type of cinnamon. I'm thinking Saigon should have actually received the axe more readily… All coumarin aside, cinnamon is known for its ability to stabilize blood sugar levels helping curb cravings, but also helps increase the body's own production of insulin. Just half a teaspoon of cinnamon per day can give you the anti-inflammatory benefits to lighten the body's need for cholesterol (a steroid hormone precursor that is also a powerful anti-inflammatory substance). Cinnamon also has antifungal and antimicrobial properties helping combat candida (yeast) and other potentially disruptive microorganisms.

Common Name	Scientific Name	Coumarin Content
Ceylon Cinnamon True Cinnamon Mexican Cinnamon	Cinnamomum Zeylanicum, Cinnamomum Verum	0.017 g/kg
Indonesian Cinnamon Korintje Cinnamon Padang Cassia	Cinnamomum Burmanni	2.15 g/kg
Saigon cinnamon, Vietnamese Cassia. Vietnamese Cinnamon	Cinnamomum Loureiroi	6.97 g/kg
Cassia Cinnamon or Chinese Cinnamon	Cinnamomum Aromaticum	0.31 g/kg

Cilantro, also known as coriander, and parsley are two related leafy herbs from the botanical family Apiaceae, and both are loaded with vitamins, antioxidants, and even "chemoprotective" qualities. Although parsley is synonymous with "garnish", the herb's anti-inflammatory properties will help flush out excess fluid from the body, subsequently supporting kidney function, relieving joint pain, and promoting normal blood pressure. Studies have indicated that a component of the essential oil of parsley, *myristicin*, may play a significant role in the reduction of risk of cancer. Per study authors, all of whom are members of the International Society for Horticultural Science, many of these phytochemicals [myristicin] are known to cause the induction of the Phase II drug metabolizing enzymes such as Glutathione S-transferase (GST) and NAD(P)H: quinone oxidoreductase (QR). It is the induction of the phase II enzymes that is believed to be "an effective and sufficient strategy for achieving protection against toxic agents including carcinogens".

Parsley is recommended for lactating mothers to stimulate milk production and is rich in many vitamins, including Vitamin C, B 12, and K, as well as beta caro-tene, the precursor to vitamin A, an antioxidant that can help protect the body against free-radical damage and fight the effects of aging. Parsley is also a source of the carot-enoids lutein and *zeaxanthin*, which help to preserve vision. Zeaxanthin, along with its relative lutein, has been suggested for preventing macular degeneration. Cilantro, also known as Asian parsley or coriander, is a frequent garnish in Latin and Asian cuisines. In research studies, cilantro's remarkable components have shown the potential to help promote detoxification, reduce high blood sugar and lower levels of cholesterol. Cilantro is a source of Vitamin A and beta carotene.

According to FoodFacts.Mercola.com, ancient medicinal uses for turmeric began when it was noted as an anti-inflammatory agent, and then to treat a variety of conditions, such as jaundice, menstrual cramps, hemorrhaging, toothaches, chest pain, and even digestive issues like flatulence and colic. An ounce of turmeric yields 26 percent of your RDI of manganese, a trace mineral found mostly in bones, the liver, kidneys, and pancreas. It is involved in formation of connective tissue, bones, blood clotting factors and sex hormones. Manganese is also necessary for normal brain and nerve function.

The antioxidant content within turmeric comes from active compounds called curcuminoids and recent research has even suggested that curcumin, has the ability to mediate its effects against cancer. The activity of curcumin reported against leukemia and lymphoma, gastrointestinal cancers, breast cancer and ovarian cancer to name but a few reflects its ability to affect multiple targets from cell mutation as well as free radical damage. These curcuminoids deliver antioxidants that may be 3 times more powerful than grape seed or pine bark extract, and strong enough to anhialate what is considered by many to be the most reactive of all oxidants, the hydroxyl radical. So cook up some curry or supplement with encapsulated curcumin to support important blood and liver functions, healthy joints, and your overall well-being, all while nourishing your skin and balancing the effects of skin flora.

With over 200 studies on the adaptogenic herb ashwagandha, its ability to improve thyroid function, support adrenal glands, reduce anxiety and depression, as well as combat the effects of stress and reduce brain cell degeneration has been well-documented. Ashwagandha, is an herb popular in Ayurvedic medicine (the medical system practiced for thousands of years in India)that has shown incredible results for lowering cortisol, balancing thyroid hormones, and stabilizing blood sugar. It is known in India as the "strength of the stallion" since it has traditionally been used to strengthen the immune system after illness.

There's no denying we're stressed to the max! Ashwagandha offers your body a chance to rejuvenate itself and restore balance. It has also been referred to as "Indian ginseng" because of its ability to enhance stamina and has extraordinary stress relieving properties. A tablet before bed will help you wind down your nervous system and prepare your brain and body to rest and restore itself through a good night's sleep.

Censored Nutritional Gem #18: Herbs and Spices are Superfoods (And they're here to heal.)

19
Nuts and Seeds are Fragile
(Handle them with care.)

I do not recommend heating seed meals such as flax or chia, nor do I approve of baking with almond meal or any other nuts in any form, which seems to be the go-to in all the Paleo cookbooks. Paleo-style cooking and diet guidelines refer to patterns of nourishment we believe were common in the Paleolithic era when our ancestors, the "cavemen", roamed around running from saber-toothed tigers and wearing the characteristic Fred Flintsone garb. Realistically though it basically suggests two very reasonable ideas:

1. Eat the types of food our ancestors would have eaten before agricultural times,

2. Eliminate foods (both processed and natural) that were introduced to the human diet so rapidly (due to agriculture and industrialization) that you may have trouble properly digesting and absorbing the nutrients.

Paleo enthusiasts refer to the way the majority of us are eating today as "Neolithic" and strict Paleo folk adhere to the following rules of thumb:

• Only eat foods that pre-date agricultural times to avoid disease
• Avoid dairy because we are the only animal who drinks the milk from other animals
• Avoid seeds because humans have yet to adapt the ability to digest them
• Avoid certain plants due to toxicity and anti-nutrient content

I actually like these rules, although I'm not totally sure which vegetables I currently eat that "pre-date agricultural times". My opinion on dairy is no secret to you by now, and seeds are high in unsaturated fatty acids so they need to be consumed as fresh and unaffected by heat as possible. Even though cavemen didn't know much about organic chemistry and heterocyclic aromatic amines back then, they ate what was available and as far as we know weren't dropping like flies from cancer and heart disease. I think one of the many benefits of modern science is being able to use all that lab work to identify the processes that hinder health in both modern man as well as our Paleolithic kinfolk (like eating plenty of meat).

Basically, the Paleo way of eating involves eating whole foods, like vegetables, and meats, and nuts and berries. And staying away from grains and seeds. Agreed! Now, when modern Paleo uses almond meal to bake, that's when we're coming to blows. You don't want to be baking with almond meal for two very important reasons:

1. Almonds are nuts and nuts are full of unsaturated fatty acids that are readily damaged by heat and oxygen.

2. You're not supposed to cook or bake with unsaturated fatty acids (pourable oils).

That seems to be one of the big reasons conventional nutritional dogma loves them so much since their campaign insists that those are the fatty acids that we should be eating the bulk of to ward off heart disease. The problem with unsaturated fatty acids, as I've explained before but I'm more than happy to say it again, is that they are not structurally stable in the presence of heat and oxygen. So, the first step in damaging the oils comes when the shell of the almond, or any nut for that matter, is cracked open. Yes, that nut is hermetically sealed in that shell, meaning without any air, and as soon as it's cracked, the shelf life of those oils begins to decrease rather rapidly. But then think about what happens when you grind up the almonds to make that fine, flour-like substance that's priced at around $8 per pound. You've just increased the surface area millions of times over so that those unsaturated fatty acids are being attacked by oxygen molecules so much more readily.

I implore you to not cook or bake with unsaturated fatty acids from nuts and seeds (pourable oils). Almonds contain almond oil, which would be a pourable oil after processing, and heating it at 350 to 425 degrees Fahrenheit is not what you want to be doing with it, especially since that this point in the game, it's probably already gone rancid. Yes, that's what happens to pourable oils or nuts and seeds when they've been out of their shells or hulls for an extended period of time. So, please don't bake with almond meal, it can render it extremely inflammatory and we're looking to eliminate those instances drastically in order to heal our cells and tissues, and to reduce the toxic load of the liver and other detox organs in the body. The same goes for roasted nuts and even "raw" nuts that are somply shelled sans roasting. When the shell of the nut is cracked and the meat is exposed, the oxidation process begins. Consuming the oxidized oils in those nuts is inflammatory.

If I sound like a broken record it means I'm doing my job. Changing the course of our health involves relearning the rules about what's right and what's monetarily motivated. The same issue arises when we talk about seeds like flax and chia. Both are phenomenal sources of omega-3 fatty acids, but omega-3s are *unsaturated,* and therefore not stable in the presence of oxygen. Grinding up flax and selling it months after the fact is giving consumers a false sense of security that they're doing something healthy, when in fact, they're contributing to the inflammation potential in the body. The solution? Purchase organic flax and grind it fresh right before you use it. And don't bake with it!

Censored Nutritional Gem #19: Nuts and Seeds are Fragile
(Handle them with care.)

20
Your Skin is a Bigmouth
(With no filter.)

For part of this chapter, I'm going to borrow a considerable amount of information from a fabulous lady I know and admire, Gina Zeiger, founder of the safest skincare line I have ever brought into my spa or had the pleasure of personally using: Pretty Mommies. After years in the clinical skincare industry, Gina did a complete 180 and formulated the first line of its kind for doctors so they could finally offer their patients pregnancy-safe products. Failure was not an option! She brought the best minds together to determine which all natural ingredients would be both safe and effective for moms and their babies. Significant research and development weeded out the toxic options and focused on elements that had science-backed safety and efficacy.

Gina knows skincare ingredients the way I know dietary supplement ingredients. Basically, the woman is a maven when it comes to what you should and shouldn't be putting on your largest organ, since it really does act like a *big mouth.* If it didn't have the absorption potential we're speaking of, pharmaceutical companies would not have invested millions in formulating drugs that can be dosed transdermally (the patch!) The following has been adapted from the *Frequently Asked Questions* page *on* www.PrettyMommies.com. You don't have to be pregnant or nursing to use and benefit from this unprecedented 3-Step System. You don't even have to be a woman (my 10 and 9 year olds use it!) Because as Gina puts it, "Don't we *all* deserve safe skincare?" Unequivocally.

Aren't all products that say "natural" ok for pregnant women to use?

Not only are some all natural products not recommended for pregnant or nursing women due to contraindications during pregnancy, but the term "natural" is also being frequently misused! It is very common for brands to only list their natural ingredients but to completely omit the dangerous chemicals also found in their products. Unfortunately, this is incredibly misleading to consumers; you believe you're using something that is safe for you and your baby but in reality you're not. Each ingredient — along with the skin care benefit and, in most cases, dietary benefit — is listed on our website, so you know exactly what you are putting on your skin.

Many skin care lines are changing their formulations to be paraben free by using a popular inexpensive preservative – Phenoxyethanol. Phenoxyethanol appears to be acceptable to other cosmetic companies and is also used by other maternity lines.

Why did Pretty Mommies decide not to use it?

Simple. Back in 2008, the FDA gave this warning against Phenoxyethanol:

"Phenoxyethanol is a preservative that is primarily used in cosmetics and medications. It can also depress the central nervous system and may cause vomiting and diarrhea."

Most importantly, they named a pregnancy cream in the warning. Knowing this information and deciding to use this ingredient anyway would go against our mission and everything we are trying to promote - Safe Maternity Skin Care.   Remember, the FDA does not regulate cosmetics and they also continue to allow Phenoxyethanol in products; so the fact they made this warning was a very big deal to us.

Do natural products work as well as their chemical counterparts?

Natural skin care products used to be perceived as lines that smell good and feel good– but show no measurable results. Today we know this is completely untrue. There are many key and active topical, natural ingredients that have amazing skin care benefits. Pretty Mommies put in years of research finding the perfect synergistic blend of active ingredients. We worked with top cosmetic chemists to ensure not only safe but also highly effective products. We initially launched as a safe replacement skin care system for expecting women, sold and recommended by physicians, so our products had to work.

I'm not digesting anything; why is it important to have natural ingredients just for my skin?

Here's a great analogy about synthetic vs. natural that should resonate with you:

We all know that a diet of whole natural foods provides rich vitamins and nutrients and results in amazing health benefits. But a diet loaded with processed food makes us lethargic, weak and generally sick. A healthy diet not only affects your physical well-being but you also see benefits in your hair, nails and skin. So let's apply the same logic to topical products. Wouldn't using natural nutrients and vitamins in our skin care products have the same impact and results topically as it would digestively? And wouldn't that mean skin care products that contain synthetic fillers also have similar results as processed food? Of course. So if you refuse to eat processed food, you probably want to treat your skin with the same care as you treat your digestive system. [Larger font intentional]

It's only going on my skin; how can that be dangerous to me and my baby?

Skin is our largest organ and what we apply to it is absorbed into our bloodstream – and that means it gets to your baby, too. In fact, that quick absorption is why more and more drugs are being dispensed topically, from hormones to pain management. It's also why before Pretty Mommies was an option, doctors were not recommending skin care products to their pregnant patients.

Many cosmetic companies claim that the toxins in their ingredients are way below harmful levels. So aren't they safe to use?

That statement may be true, but nobody goes on to explain the bio-accumulative effects of toxic ingredients. Bioaccumulation is the accumulation of a substance, such as a toxic chemical, in various tissues of a living organism. So these ingredients store in your body and reach toxic levels over time. The first 100 times you use that product you are probably fine, but what happens after 200 applications, 300, and so on?

More and more, toxins are being discovered in many common synthetic cosmetic ingredients. That's why consumers are demanding natural products. In fact, chemical ingredients that have long been used to treat certain skin conditions and considered beneficial are now showing long-term effects of damage to the skin. A perfect example of this is hydroquinone.

Hydroquinone can be found in many prescription skin care lines and it can be effective, at first, at lightening the hyperpigmentation that occurs as a result of sun damage and hormones. (Of course, this is completely off limits during pregnancy due to developmental and reproductive toxicity, organ toxicity, neurotoxicity and many other potential dangers.)

But hydroquinone was never indicated for long-term use because extensive exposure to this chemical can cause a condition called Ochronosis. When Ochronosis occurs the skin becomes permanently darker in color and thicker than normal. Furthermore, since hydroquinone causes frequent irritation and inflammation to the skin, it can accelerate the aging process.

What is the most dangerous topical ingredient that pregnant women are being exposed to?

Unfortunately, there are many harmful ingredients found in products that expecting women use daily, but we made sure to avoid them: formaldehyde, phthalates, dimethicones, parabens, etc. Many consumers have heard about the dangers associated with these common cosmetic ingredients, however, based on our research, we feel Oxybenzone might be the most alarming — and not many people know about it. Oxybenzone, or a derivative of it, is found in almost all mainstream sunscreens today. Organizations like the Environmental Working Group have been on a long mission to change the regulations and use of this ingredient. We find it particularly alarming to expecting women because it is a synthetic estrogen and hormone disruptor.When you're pregnant you do not want to use anything that causes estrogenic effects because it is dangerous to the fetus. In addition, a recent study came out from Georgetown Lombardi Comprehensive Cancer Center stating that women who had high levels of estrogen during pregnancy increased the chance of their daughter developing breast cancer.

What other ingredients should we be wary of?

Soy and all soy peptides, which are very common in cosmetic formulations today, is not recommended in the diet of pregnant women due to estrogenic effects.

Licorice, Mulberry and Bearberry are all great natural skin lighteners, however they can cause uterine stimulation and potentially premature contractions.

Surfactants help spread the product on the skin, emulsifiers hold the ingredients together and preservative systems help prevent dangerous microbes from forming.

Unfortunately, this is where other companies who may use natural key ingredients fall short…because some of the most dangerous cosmetic ingredients can be found in surfactants, emulsifiers and preservative systems.

Surfactant. Chemical surfactants such as dimethicone are silicone based and have shown links to storing in your lymph nodes and causing tumors. Instead, we used an all natural ingredient derived from macadamia seed oil.

Emulsifier. Our emulsifier is made from Sweet Orange Pulp, which was made for the all natural food industry.

Preservative Systems. Instead of using parabens, which thousands of studies have shown to be a carcinogen, or phenoxyethanol, which replaced parabens (even though it has an FDA warning), we used a three-part natural sugar enzyme as our preservative system.

Two dangerous ingredients and what we use instead:

Sodium Lauryl Sulfate. This is a common ingredient in many skin care lines, even though it is a known skin irritant and has restrictions in every health ministry. We refused to use it in our products.

Our solution: Instead, we used Vegetable Glycerin which is a non-toxic, colorless and odorless liquid produced from vegetables. It has emollient and lubricating properties and helps to cleanse and moisturize the skin. Glycerin has antimicrobial effects, helps to heal wounds and also helps to restore skin's elasticity.

Oxybenzone. In our opinion, this is one of the most alarming ingredients being used daily by some pregnant women. Oxybenzone is a chemical sunscreen found in almost ALL mainstream sunscreens on the market today. It is a synthetic estrogen and hormone disruptor and many studies show links to low birth weight in babies. A more recent study from Georgetown Lombardi Comprehensive Cancer Center shows that high levels of estrogen during pregnancy increases the chances of a daughter developing breast cancer.

Our solution: Our sunscreen is chemical FREE. We use pure non-nano zinc oxide. Since it has not been micronized it cannot penetrate the skin – truly the safest on the market.

Since bringing Pretty Mommies into my office in the summer of 2012, sales of our other lines grinded to a veritable halt- and I'm totally alright with that. I don't want to sell anything that is remotely questionable when it comes to safety or long-term hazardous effects, and Gina brought some information to my attention that I simply couldn't overlook. I want my clients to know that outward beauty can only come as a result of optimal nutrition and internal wellness. The healthier you are, the better your skin looks, the more lustrous your hair becomes and the brighter your eyes shine. We approach beauty from the inside out and recognize that although a cleanser or lotion may not erase fine lines the way laser skin tightening might, the last thing it should do is contribute to dysfunction and imbalance of the body's own systems. Everything you put on your skin has the potential to enter your body. Which brings me to the last part of this chapter; the use of essential oils to derive therapeutic benefit from their absorption through the skin, as well as from their scent.

Visit www.PrettyMommies.com and use code SATFATROX at checkout to receive 10% off your first order of the Pretty Mommies 3-Step Skin Care System

From the *Essential Oils Desk Reference*, compiled by Essential Science Publishing:

Essential oils are some of the oldest and most powerful therapeutic agents known. In their pure state, essential oils are some of the most oncentrated natural extracts known, exhibiting significant and immediate antiviral, anti-inflammatory, antibacterial, and hormone-balancing effects. In clinical practice they have been shown to have a profound influence on the central nervous system, helping to reduce or eliminate pain, release muscle tension and provide astrong emotional uplift.

The chemical structure of an essential oil is such that it can rapidly penetrate cell membranes, travel throughout the blood and tissues, and enhance cellular function... it has become very clear that there is a powerful life force inherent in these substances, which gives them an unmatched ability to communicate and interact with cells in the human body. They could very well be the missing link of modern health care, bringing allopathic and holistic practice together for optimal health in the 21st century.

Healthy-minded people the world over have learned the value of using high quality natural herbs... most therapeutic herbs can be distilled into an essential oil. The key difference is one of concentration. The essential oil can be from 100 to 10,000 times more concentrated- and therefore more potent- than the herb itself.

It is my belief that pairing the nutritional guidelines in this book with the daily consumption of a high quality whole food supplement, like Akea Fermented Whole Food, along with the therapeutic use of quality essential oils as preventive measures, can bring you a level of health you never thought possible. Use your skin to introduce benefit into your body, not burden. Visit www.YoungLiving.org/SatFatRox to learn more about the healing potential of essential oils.

Censored Nutritional Gem #20: Your Skin is a Bigmouth.
(With no filter.)

20
For More Life, Eat Less Food

Don't dig your grave with your own knife and fork.
                                    -English proverb

It's time for us to learn from cultures around the world that have mastered the art of living well, for a longer period of time. The vast majority of us don't need "an average of 2000 calories a day", every day! It's time we realized that the more we eat, even of good food, the more wear and tear we subject our body systems to and the faster they wear out. The phenomenal aspect to this is that when we actually do eat good food, we just naturally need less of it. This is the basis of superfoods: foods that are relatively low in bulk and calories, yet loaded with vitamins, minerals, and phytonutrients to give us vibrant life, naturally.

René Descartes, the French philosopher, mathematician, and writer said, "The senses deceive from time to time, and it is prudent never to trust wholly those who have deceived us even once." When it comes to food, our tongues are here but to taste and our noses to facilitate the endeavor. The trouble is, both can deceive us. It is the brain that truly knows; that can reason and demand action or resistance. It is my hope that the information in this book gives you the tools to stop being deceived and misled by your tongue and nose. ndustry only serves the purpose of deceiving both, and they in turn deceive your brain and body.

Hara hachi bun-ni ishia shirazu is Japanese for *He who has his stomach full only 80% will not need a doctor.* Many ancient cultures pay proverbial homage to the act of eating *less* while eating *well.*

From the Japanese still:

Sanri shihou-no yasai-wo taberu. Eating local vegetables will strengthen health

Satougui-no wakaji. Sugar eaters die young.

It is food that leads us to extremes in behavior, and it is food that can summon healing, the likes of we never imagined. Hippocrates, the Greek physician and philosopher, may be known for being "The Father of [Modern] Medicine", but he honored Mother Nature's potential when he wrote, "Everyone has a doctor within him... The natural healing force within each one of us is the greatest force in getting well. Our food should be our medicine. Our medicine shoud be our food." As we move on to the second part of the book, the *medicine,* if you will, I leave you with some parting words of the greatest minds in the history of mankind.

> *When the disease is at its height, it will then be necessary to use the most slender diet.* -Hippocrates.

> *Everything in excess is opposed to nature.* -Hippocrates

> *The reasonable man adapts himself to the world; the unreasonable one persists in trying to adapt the world to himself. Therefore, all progress depends on the unreasonable man.* -René Descartes

> *It is important to know what sort of person has a disease than to know what sort of a disease a person has.* -Hippocrates

> *A wise man ought to realize that health is his most valuable possession.* - Hippocrates

And some wisdom from tables around the world:

Japan- Nokorimono ni wa fuku ga aru *Luck exists in the leftovers.*

Japan- Hara-no kawa-ga hareba me-no kawa-ga tarumu.
Stomach skin stretching – eye skin sagging.

Libya – Eat too much honey and it becomes tasteless

Africa – Water is colourless and tasteless, but you can live on it longer than eating food.

Notes

Part II

The Foundation:
Akea Fermented Superfoods and Probiotics

Akea's Roots

William King

The history of Akea is a most serendipitous one. The brain-child of William King, a native North Carolinian whose vision and experience in the areas of health and wellness formed the inspiration for the company Akea LLC, "Akea Essentials" was brought to market in the summer of 2010. It was to be the nutritional foundation of the company's lifestyle wellness education program called "The Blueprint For Life". Mr. King was inspired by Longevity Hot Spots during his first visit to Nicoya, Costa Rica, in 2006 when a longtime friend and now-resident of Nicoya, pointed out the notably high local population of 80, 90, even 100 year olds, all living vibrantly in the community. Beginning to research the reasons behind the stark differences between the United States and this slice of paradise, he came to discover that Nicoya was one of nine areas of the world known for the excellent health of its people, absence of chronic diseases, all topped off with their significantly longer lifespans. Look for Mr. King's book *The Blast Fast,* discussing the benefits of intermittent fasting and the use of Akea as a detox-cleanse, coming October 2014. www.TheBlastFast.com

Sally Beare

Along the way, British nutritionist and author Sally Beare, became a phenomenal resource and contributor to the project. An accomplished author and expert in the areas of nutrition, health and wellness, Ms. Beare provided much of the research and insight on Longevity Hot Spots that fueled inspiration for the Akea concept, and the educational components of the Blueprint For Life. She is a nutritional therapist who has traveled and lived around the world studying exceptionally healthy, long-lived populations. Ms. Beare has authored two books based on her findings: *50 Secrets of the World's Longest-Living People* (Avalon, USA, 2006) and *The Live-Longer Diet* (reprinted as The Anti-Aging Diet, Plaktus, UK, 2003). She studied nutritional therapy at one of the UK's foremost nutrition colleges, the UK College of Nutrition and Health (BCNH), where she also lectures onanti-aging.

Maurice Werness, ND

As Mr. King also called upon his own personal doctor, Dr. Maurice Werness, a naturopathic physician who has dedicated his life to the research and prevention of chronic illnesses, it was clear that a revolutionary nutraceutical, second-to-none, was about to be born. With Dr. Werness as the lead architect of the formulation,

Akea researched the global food market and nature's gardens to discover which foods provide the healthiest benefits—the foods that are shared across tables in the world's key Longevity Hot Spots. No otherproduct was composed of so many indisputably beneficial factors. Organic, fermented, whole food based, enhanced probiotics, enzymes, cultured minerals, AND based on the diets of the healthiest, longest-living people on the planet, *Akea Essentials* offered consumers a convenient, comprehensive way to supplement their Standard American Diet with the very next best thing to picking it from a tree, organically grown no less.

Dr. Werness received his undergraduate degree from George Washington University and his Doctorate in Naturopathic Medicine from Bastyr University. He is a Board Member and former President of the Institute for Natural Medicine, has co-authored four books on natural healing and has long studied the effects of nutrition on wellness and longevity. He has developed an expertise in treating and preventing heart disease, high blood pressure and all forms of cardiovascular disease. Dr. Werness is the Lead Architect of Akea and was a Key Member of the Akea Science Advisory Board.

Gordon Koltis, MD

Dr. Koltis is a highly educated medical doctor certified by the American Board of Radiology and Radiation Oncology, and by the National Board of Medical Examiners. He has a background in oncology, human anatomy, human pathology and zoology. Dr. Koltis earned his undergraduate degree in Zoology from the University of Wisconsin in Madison. He then worked as a graduate student with a combined appointment in the Departments of Human Pathology and Human Anatomy doing research on congenital malformations.

During that time he was also an instructor at the University of Wisconsin MedicalSchool,teachinghumananatomy,andsubsequentlyattendedthatsameinstitution, receiving his Medical Degree in 1981. He completed four years of specialty training in Radiation Oncology at the University of Wisconsin Hospitals and Clinics in 1985, and since then had been in practice full-time as a radiation oncologist.

In 1989 he moved to Greenville, North Carolina, and has been on the active medical staff at Pitt County Memorial Hospital and Lenoir Memorial Hospital. He continues to serve as the Chairman of the Department of Radiation Oncology at the Lenoir Memorial Hospital Cancer Center, and is the Medical Director at the Carolina Radiation Medicine Cancer Treatment Center since that facility opened in August 1998.

Dr. Koltis is certified by the American Board of Radiology and Radiation Oncology and by the National Board of Medical Examiners. He also has the distinction of being a Fellow of The American College of Radiation Oncology (FACRO) and was a Key Member of the Akea Science Advisory Board.

Michael C. Fajgenbaum, MD

Dr. Michael C. Fajgenbaum is a Board Certified Orthopaedic surgeon who specializes in Sports Medicine and Arthroscopic Surgery. He has been with the Bone and Joint Surgery Clinic since 1988 and was the team Orthopaedic Surgeon for North Carolina State University Football for 20 years. He was born and raised in Trinidad in the West Indies. After graduating from Trinity College in Trinidad with a certificate from Cambridge University, he attended Tulane University and graduated with a Bachelor of Science degree in Chemistry in 1978. He was honored as a Tulane scholar and was a member of Phi Eta Sigma.

Dr. Fajgenbaum went on to Tulane Medical School and graduated in 1982, earning a residency position at the University of Florida in Gainesville. He completed his Internship in General Surgery and then directly entered the Orthopaedic Department in 1983. During his residency, Dr. Fajgenbaum received additional Sports Medicine training with Dr. Fred Allman of the Sports Medicine Institute of America, at that time the team physician for Georgia Tech and a former Olympic team doctor. Dr. Fajgenbaum also served as Chief Resident, and then joined the faculty as a Clinical Instructor in 1987. Upon leaving the University of Florida, Dr. Fajgenbaum joined the Bone and Joint Surgery Clinic in Raleigh, North Carolina. He is Board Certified and has recertified with a subspecialty in Sports Medicine.

Shortly after arriving in Raleigh, he was approached by the head coach of the North Carolina State University Football team and asked to become the team Orthopaedic Surgeon. At 30 years old, that made him the youngest Orthopaedist ever to be in charge of an NCAA Division I football program. Over the years he has also served as team physician for Methodist College, the Carolina Mudcats, the Carolina Cobras and Ravenscroft School. Dr. Fajgenbaum was a Key Member of the Akea Science Advisory Board.

James Stevens, MD

Dr. Stevens earned a Bachelor of Arts in Zoology from UNC-Chapel Hill and a Doctor of Medicine from East Carolina University School of Medicine. He completed a Family Practice Residency at the Fairfax Family Practice Program at the Medical

College of Virginia and a Sports Medicine Fellowship at the University of North Carolina, Chapel Hill. He is board certified in both Family Practice and in Sports Medicine. In 2003 he founded Carolina Family Practice & Sports Medicine with locations in Cary, Raleigh, and Holly Springs NC. He serves as Head Medical Team Physician for the National Hockey League's 2006 Stanley Cup Champion Carolina Hurricanes, a position he has held since 1997. In addition, he is Head Company Physician for the Carolina Ballet, and provides sports medicine services to many area high schools. Dr. Stevens was a Key Member of the Akea Science Advisory Board.

February 2014: A New Day Dawns on Akea

Akea thrived as a direct sales company, marketing Akea Essentials through independent consultants and educating their customers on how to incorporate the guiding principles of Hot Spot health through daily educational emails that comprised the "60 Day Challenge" of the "Blueprint Jumpstart".

In February 2014, Akea LLC merged assets and rights with *Asantae*, a direct sales company with interests in health and wellness products based out of Scottsdale, Arizona, and publicly-held by Avidus Management Group, Inc. (ASNHF:US on the OTCBB; AVD.V on the TSX Venture Exchange). Asantae's leadership is first rate. Their experience in marketing and business growth equally so. As with any company that wishes to see their product reach new heights and markets, Akea has become part of something bigger, stronger, and is ready to build on the foundation its visionaries poured their time, talents, and hearts into.

A new name, a new home, still the same old soul:
Akea Whole Food Supplement by Asantae.

www.SatFatRox.com/Share-Akea

What is Akea?

Akea is a high-performance therapeutic food. Its components work together, in synergy, to activate the major physiologic processes of the body:

- The probiotics prepare the body to digest and assimilate food efficiently.
- The enzymes activate digestion.
- Fermentation enhances the synergy of the ingredients and delivers enhanced health benefits.

Fermentation improves the body's ability to absorb and assimilate nutrients (bioavailability) and introduces probiotics, the good bacteria essential for healthy digestion.

- The complexity of the whole-foods matrix in Akea enhances the ability of the genome to adapt to changes in the environment.
- The herbal elements can help modulate the inflammatory system.

What is the difference between Akea and other nutritional companies?

The primary difference between Akea and other nutraceuticals is that Akea is based on the diets of the world's healthiest people (those living in Longevity Hot Spots). It is a unique whole food, organic, fermented nutritional supplement- created to support those with busy lives, enabling them to easily and conveniently incorporate fermented foods consumed by the healthiest people on the planet into their daily lives. The main differentiator between Akea and other nutritional supplements is that Akea is a fermented, organic, plant-based whole food.

The vast majority of nutritional supplements on the market are synthetic, or at the very least, contain synthetics. Second, Akea includes the specific foods consumed by the world's healthiest people. Third, Akea is organic (96%), vegan, dairy free, gluten free, and GMO free. The only ingredients that are not organic are those for which there is no organic certification, such as probiotics, enzymes and minerals. And last, but probably most importantly, Akea is fermented. The process of fermentation breaks down the nutrition for us, so it becomes highly bioavailable to the body, without significant effort on the part of our own digestive system.

Why was Akea created?

Akea was created to bridge the nutritional gap between the Standard American Diet (SAD) and what individuals in Longevity Hot Spots have consumed for millennia. When you take Akea as recommended, you give your body the nutritional support to help you reach optimal health—the kind of health enjoyed by Hot Spot residents.

Why is Akea fermented?

Akea is fermented to maximize absorption of the nutrition. The fermentation process begins to break down the nutrients making them easier for the body to digest and assimilate. A good analogy is milk and yogurt. Most people who are allergic to milk can have yogurt with no ill effects. Why? After all what is yogurt? Fermented milk. The process of fermenting the milk breaks down the proteins (casein) and sugars (lactose) making it easier for the body to absorb. Humans have utilized fermentation to preserve and optimize the nutritional value of food since we have been on the planet.

Fifty years ago, with the introduction of modern refrigeration and chemical preservatives, we interrupted the habit of canning fruits and vegetables so we would have something to eat over the winter. In so doing, we mitigated the consumption of fermented foods and deprived our body from of the essential benefits that can only be attained through the consumption of fermented foods. Here are some of the benefits of consuming fermented foods:

- Probiotics predigest food, taking macro molecules (carbohydrates and proteins) of food turning them into micro molecules (saccharides and amino acids) that can be consumed by our cells.

- Probiotics also configure the nutritional molecules contained in food into the right size, shape and form to fit into receptors on the surface of the cells, allowing activation of these receptors; in other words, turn on the cells.

- Fermentation creates hundreds of nutritional metabolites not in the original food. This greatly magnifies the nutritional density of the food. Fermentation provides the body with nutritional metabolites that cannot be attained through any other means. The body's access to these nutritional metabolites is essential for optimal biologic function.

Does fermenting the ingredients make them easier or more difficult to digest?

Fermentation makes foods much easier to digest.

What is the shelf life of Akea?

Akea is a very stable nutritional supplement and is best used within two years of purchase. Because it is live food, it should be stored in a cool, dry place.

Does Akea need to be refrigerated?

For maximum freshness, once opened, refrigeration is appropriate.

Why is Akea provided in powdered form as opposed to a capsule or liquid?

If Akea was encapsulated it would take 22, 500mg capsules per scoop, so the daily recommendation of 2 scoops would equate to 44, 500mg capsules per day. That's a lot of great high quality nutrition, but no one would choose to take 44 capsules a day. The powder mixes easily in a variety of juices, flavored water and smoothies.

When I mix Akea with juice, what is the stuff at the bottom/top of the glass?

Akea is a whole food, meaning it contains all the vitamins, minerals, fiber and co-factors that naturally exist in the whole plant. Any product that is comprised of a blend of whole food ingredients will inevitably result in some visual residue that appears on the bottom of the bottle. This separation is completely normal. Simply shake well and drink immediately. Think of the difference between whole pulverized apples (apple sauce) and apple juice. If there's no sediment a lot of nutrition has been extracted.

Are the probiotics in Akea coated or protected to survive the hydrochloric acid in the stomach?

Some people believe that probiotics taken in supplement form are destroyed by hydrochloric acid in the stomach. We believe this concept originates with some probiotic manufacturers who manufacturer proprietary capsules that are said to be resilient enough to make it through the harsh stomach acid to the colon. If this were true, how would we ever get probiotics into our digestive tract? We get our probiotics from food. We ingest living probiotics from a variety of foods that we eat like yogurt and pickled vegetables. The majority of our probiotics live in our colons. If stomach acid destroys probiotics, how would they make it all the way through the digestive tract (and stomach) to the colon? Physicians commonly recommend eating yogurt after taking antibiotics to replenish our probiotics. This would be ineffective if they were killed in the stomach. We believe live probiotics DO make their way through the stomach to the small and large intestines.

The probiotics, enzymes and minerals in Akea are not labeled as organic. How are they obtained?

There is no true classification for "organic" probiotics, enzymes and/or minerals. The probiotics and enzymes used in Akea are sourced from one of the world's leader in enzyme and probiotic production. Similarly, there is no organic certification for minerals as they are a natural substance.

What is the source of the probiotics that are included in Akea?

The probiotics and enzymes in Akea are sourced from one of the world's leaders in enzyme production.

How do the probiotics in Akea stay alive?

The probiotics in Akea are produced by cryo-freezing and freeze drying under tightly controlled conditions. The cryo-freezing process maintains and preserves the integrity of the bacterial cells, while freeze drying then removes any remaining moisture through evaporation, which increases the stability of the cultures. We include enough live cultures to assure a count of 3,000,000,000 (billion) per serving through the "use by" date on the can.

How can the probiotics stay alive being exposed to heat during shipping and over a long period of time, considering a two year shelf life?

We are experiencing tremendous results with Akea all over the country, so we are very pleased with the efficacy of our product. Heat is introduced during the process of fermentation, therefore any additional heat exposure during shipping can only possibly affect the ingredients added after fermentation, which are probiotics and enzymes. For living organisms such as probiotics to be affected, the temperature would need to be over 114 degrees, which would rarely happen, if ever.

Is dairy used during the production of the probiotics?

The probiotics used in Akea are grown in a non-dairy medium.
Akea is completely dairy- free.

Is Akea considered raw?

Akea is fermented, which requires heat, so it is not considered to be raw. We believe the process of fermentation increases the nutritional value of the foods in Akea.

What is the source of the enzymes that are included in Akea?

Akea contains plant based enzymes which are created as a byproduct of fermentation.

Where are the ingredients grown?

Our manufacturer is a US company and has thousands of acres of organic farmland in the Midwest and California. The vast majority of ingredients are grown here in the US, and some are sourced abroad from time to time depending on growing seasons and availability. Some of the more exotic ingredients such as goji, for example, are grown outside the US.

Juice products vs. Akea

Fresh juice from fruits and vegetables are filled with very healthy nutrition such as vitamins, minerals and antioxidants. Unfortunately, the vast majority of juice on the market is pasteurized, which is detrimental to the valuable nutrition. Additionally, the average serving (1/2 cup) of fruit juice contains around 30 grams of carbohydrates in the form of simple fruit sugar, which can elevate blood sugar and contribute to weight gain. Akea, by comparison, is a whole food containing the entire scope of nutrition including fiber and important co-factors.

The best analogy is to consider a juicer vs. a blender. Think of an apple. Let's say you put the apple in the juicer, what will you have? Apple juice. What is missing? A lot of fiber, vitamins, minerals, antioxidants and other vital nutrition. Now let's say you put the apple in the blender and liquefy it. Now you have the complete nutrition of the apple. In making Akea, we start with over 30 fruits, vegetables, herbs, etc., and we wash them, dehydrate them (extract the water), then we grind it down to a powder, add minerals, ferment, add active enzymes and probiotics, and package for use. The vast majority of the valuable nutrition is still intact.

What's the difference between a green food supplement and Akea?

Although Akea contains green superfoods, it is not specifically a green superfood product. Akea contains fruits, vegetables, herbs, beta glucans, minerals, enzymes and probiotics. It is also fermented, and most green superfoods are not.

How does Akea compare to other nutritional supplements (nutrition)?

Akea is the only Organic, Fermented, Whole Food nutritional supplement derived from the diets of the healthiest people on earth. The vast majority of nutritional supplements on the market are synthetic, meaning their ingredients were manufactured in a laboratory rather than grown on a farm. Even the vast majority of "Whole Food" nutritional supplements contain synthetic ingredients along with the "whole food" ingredients and most are not organic or fermented. When comparing Akea to other nutritional supplements, you must consider three primary factors:

- Whole Food: The food ingredients in Akea are "whole foods", which means that the ingredients were not created in a laboratory and pressed out millions per day on a conveyor belt. The ingredients were once a seed which was planted into the ground, nurtured, harvested, taken to market, cleaned, dehydrated, etc.

• Organic: The ingredients in Akea are organic, which means that they are grown without the use of pesticides, synthetic fertilizers, sewage sludge, genetically modified organisms, bioengineering or ionizing radiation, and the farmers use renewable resources and conserve soil and waste. If you've ever purchased organic produce at the grocery store, you're certainly aware of the dramatic difference in cost. Typically, producing organic fruits and vegetables over conventional produce adds approximately 30% to the overall cost.

• Fermented: Ingredients in Akea have been fermented for maximum bioavailability. The process of fermentation is delicate, and requires very specialized equipment and a great deal of expertise.

How does Akea compare to other nutritional supplements (cost)?

Comparing cost per gram there is no organic, completely whole food nutritional supplement (no synthetics, fillers or sweeteners) on the market that has a lower price per gram for nutrition delivered. Akea is also fermented, which adds an additional layer of expense. Akea delivers 11 grams of nutrition in every scoop and contains no synthetics, sweeteners or binders, all of which are very inexpensive to produce. We recommend two scoops daily which equates to 22 grams of nutrition per day.

If Akea were delivered in capsule form it would require 42 capsules daily. There is really no comparable product on the market. Products that are "whole food" usually suggest taking 2 to 4 capsules once or twice daily. This equates to around 1-4 grams of nutrition per day compared to 11-22 grams of nutrition with Akea. Once volume of nutrition is considered, Akea is clearly the better value. We have nothing more valuable than our health but it's important to spend our dollars on health wisely. All things considered, Akea is an exceptional value when compared with either actual food or "comparable" nutritional supplementation.

What is the pH of Akea?

Akea has a pH of 8.53 and is considered an alkaline-forming food.

What is Akea's ORAC (Oxygen radical absorbance capacity) value?

Akea was not created specifically to be a high ORAC product although it has a fairly high ORAC simply because it contains very nutrient dense fruits and vegetables. Some companies play an ORAC game of "how high can we go". However, most recent studies show that extremely high ORAC products reach a point of diminished returns and can even be counterproductive for health, since we actually need some free radicals in our immune system. Additionally, some antioxidants in supplement form are not natural (synthetic) and can become free radicalsthemselves, which does not happen when consumed from whole food form (an antioxidant becomes a free radical as soon as it donates its electron to neutralize another free radical.

Another antioxidant then comes along and neutralizes the new free radical, and so on in a chain. In a food, the antioxidant power will happen and then it will all get neutralized). However, there is no research suggesting the same of high ORAC food. As per usual, if it's something that would be part of a natural diet, it's almost certain to be healthy. Each scoop of Akea has an ORAC of approximately 1250, so two scoops would be around 2500. Where Akea differs from most HIGH ORAC products is that Akea is not an isolated nutrient such as a synthetic vitamin supplement or juice. It is estimated that average ORAC in the Hot Spots range between 10,000 to 15,000. The FDA recommended daily ORAC amount is 3500-6000.

Is Akea FDA Approved?

Under the Dietary Supplement Health and Education Act of 1994 (DSHEA), dietary supplement manufacturers are responsible for ensuring that a dietary supplement is safe before it is marketed. There is no FDA requirement to register products with the FDA nor get FDA approval before producing or selling dietary supplements. Manufacturers must make sure that the product label information is truthful and not misleading, and the FDA is responsible for taking action against any unsafe dietary supplement. The FDA does regulate the types of claims that can be made about supplements and food. One serving of Essentials qualifies for the FDA's "heart health" claim.

How does Akea go from its natural food state to a powder? Does it go through some sort of chemical process to get into a powder form?

When the foods (fruits, vegetables, herbs, grains etc.) arrive at the manufacturing facility, they are cleaned and dehydrated , which is a process of evaporating the water from the plant material. Then the foods are put through a mesh at our specification of fineness. Then the ingredients that are fermented are put into the fermentation vat to be fermented. After fermentation, the probiotics, minerals and enzymes are added and the material is put into the container. Akea is a combination of plant foods that are dehydrated, turned into powder, fermented and packaged. Of course, there are no chemicals used in the process.

Where is Akea manufactured?

The manufacturing facility is in the US, and the vast majority of ingredients are sourced from organic farmland in the mid-west United States and California. Some ingredients are sourced outside the US. Goji, for example, does not grow in the US.

Can I buy Akea in health food stores?

Asantae is not simply in the nutritional supplementation business. Asantae's mission is to foster a global community dedicated to the health and wellbeing of all participants. In offering Akea, we do everything we can to keep costs low. Selling direct is the most efficient method. Our goal is to make Akea cost effective so the benefits can be experienced by as many people as possible.

Visit www.NCSuperFood.com/Share-Akea
to learn more about becoming an
Asantae Affiliate

What's In Akea?

Is Akea 100 percent vegetarian?

Yes.

Is Akea organic?

The term organic is used to refer to the way a plant is grown or an animal is raised. Plants that are "certified organic" originated from seeds that have not been genetically modified (GMOs), and that were grown without the use of chemical pesticides, herbicides, or fertilizers, Akea uses the freshest and very best ingredients available. The whole food ingredients in Akea are 100% organic, and they account for just over 90% of the entire product. The remaining 10% of the product is comprised of the cultured minerals, probiotics, and enzymes, all of which the FDA does not have an organic classification for.

Is Akea gluten-free?

Yes.

How can Akea be considered gluten-free when it contains even ancient grains and oats?

First it is necessary to clarify that the term "gluten free", as it applies to food labeling, refers to the gluten present in traditional grains such as wheat, rye, barley, malt. To be considered gluten free a product must be below 20PPM (parts per million) of gliadin. We test every production run of Akea, and since those those traditional grains are not contained in Akea, it has always tested below 20PPM.

Are there any allergens in Akea?

Akea contains NO: soy, yeast, egg, preservatives, MSG, glutamate derivatives, artificial flavoring, salt, starch, intact proteins, or dairy.

Are there any tree nuts or tree nut derivatives in Akea?

There are no tree nuts or tree nut derivatives in Akea.

What sweeteners/sugars does Akea use? Are they natural?

No sugars or sweeteners are added to Akea.

What vegetables are included in Akea?

Beet juice powder, organic sweet potato, organic Brussels sprouts, organic chicory, organic broccoli sprouts, organic green cabbage, organic kale, organic spinach, organic okra.

What fruits are included in Akea?

Organic pomegranate, organic cranberry, organic mango, organic grape, organic papaya, goji berry, organic blueberry, organic noni, apricot and elderberry.

How many servings of fruits and vegetables do I get taking Akea?

Our daily recommendation of 2 servings (scoops) of Akea has the ORAC (Oxygen Radical Absorbance Capacity) or antioxidant equivalent of 5 servings of fruits and vegetables as well as the probiotics of 6 servings of yogurt, the Oat Beta Glucans of 8 servings of oatmeal and the resveratrol of 28 glasses of red wine.

What herbs and/or spices are included in Akea?

Organic chicory, organic turmeric, organic parsley, organic cinnamon, ginger and organic ginseng.

What are beta glucans and why are they in Akea?

Beta glucans are polysaccharides. They occur most commonly as cellulose in plants, the bran of grains, the cell wall of bakers' yeast, certain fungi, mushrooms, and bacteria. Beta glucans have been shown to be very supportive to the immune system. Numerous studies have also found they have a role in balancing blood sugar and regulating blood lipids as well as providing a host of additional positive effects on health.

What are phytonutrients?

Phytonutrients are nutrients contained within plants [phyto is a term used to refer to plants]. They have been shown to be very beneficial to a wide variety of biological processes. Many pharmaceuticals use phytochemicals as models upon which drugs are designed and produced. When you consume the phytonutrient in its natural state, as you do with Akea, the plant source still contains all the surrounding molecules that help modulate the effects of the phytochemical. This benefit is why herbal and nutritional medicine has very few side effects when taken properly.

What are probiotics? Which ones are included in Akea?

Probiotics mean "pro-life." They are, in many ways, the essence of life. These microbes are the only thing in nature with the capacity to turn inorganic elements into organic, life-giving nutrients. Probiotics help your digestive tract digest and absorb food. They are crucial; without probiotics, digestion would be impossible. Akea uses probiotics in the processing of our nutritional supplement. This unique process puts the supplement in the optimal form for the body to digest and assimilate. Akea contains the following probiotics: B. bifidum, B. breve, B. longum, L. acidophilus, L. casei, L. paracasei, L. plantarum, L. rhamnosus, L. salivarius, S. thermophilus. These have been shown to be the most beneficial organisms in supporting optimal digestive and overall health. To keep the probiotics alive and functioning, please keep Akea in a cool, dry place and do not cook foods containing Akea. Cooking will kill the probiotics.

What are enzymes? Which ones are in Akea?

Enzymes are mainly proteins that catalyze (i.e., increase the rates of) chemical reactions. Almost all processes in a biological cell need enzymes to be present at significant rates. Enzymes are known to catalyze about four thousand biochemical reactions within the body. You need enzymes to assist in the digestion of your food—to break down what you eat to its constituent parts (amino acids, vitamins, minerals, etc.). Akea contains the following enzymes: amylase, lactase, lipase, Nattozimes®, and protease. These enzymes are essential for optimizing the digestive process.

- Protease breaks proteins down to amino acids.
- Amylase breaks starches and carbohydrates down into simple sugars.
- Lipase breaks fats and oils down into fatty acids.
- Lactase breaks down lactose, making it readily absorbed by the body.

• Nattozimes ® are enzymes extracted from nattokinase, a protease (enzyme that breaks down certain proteins) compound formed during the fermentation process of natto. Natto provides benefits for the circulatory system, such as increasing blood flow. Natto has been shown to be able to breakdown plaque in the vascular system.

Why does Akea contain enzymes?

Enzymes are added to aid in digestion as well as to aid in the digestion of other foods that are consumed, as most people eat very few live foods.

What are superfoods? Which ones are included in Akea?

Superfoods for humans are the equivalent of high-octane fuel for automobiles. These nutrient-dense, low calorie foods that have been found to be very potent in promoting health. Akea provides the following superfoods in every serving: beet juice powder, cacao, reishi mycelia, goji berry, ginseng, red grapes, sweet potato, turmeric, noni, elderberry, green tea, ginger, buckwheat, blueberry, apricot, chlorella, spirulina and resveratrol.

What is cacao?

Cacao is the bean from which chocolate is derived. Raw cacao has been found to provide strong health benefits, including powerful antioxidant and anti-inflammatory functions. Raw cacao powder contains 955 ORAC units per gram. ORAC (Oxygen Radical Absorbance Capacity) is a rating scale the USDA uses to measure the ability of antioxidants to absorb cell-damaging free radicals. Tryptophan, a naturally occurring substance in cacao, enhances relaxation and promotes better sleep. Researchers have discovered that phenylethylamine (PEA) has a positive effect in enhancing feelings of affection and love. And cacao is an excellent source of PEA. Cacao also contains more magnesium than any other common food. Magnesium is the number one mineral that assists and supports healthy heart functioning. Arginine, the aphrodisiac-like amino acid believed by body builders to build muscle and aid in recovery, also occurs naturally in cacao.

What is ginseng?

Ginseng is an herbal medicine that has been taken for thousands of years as an adaptogen, aphrodisiac, and nourishing stimulant.

What is turmeric?

Turmeric is a plant from the ginger family. Various nutritional studies have shown turmeric to have a positive effect on liver and cardiovascular function well as being anti-inflammatory.

What is goji berry?

Goji berry has been eaten for thousands of years in China and Tibet as a medicinal food. Published studies have reported a wide variety of medicinal benefits of its antioxidant properties.

What are micro-algae chlorella and spirulina?

Spirulina is one of the most nutrient-dense foods on the planet. This form of blue-green, single-celled super-algae offers a concentrated source of complete, balanced protein. Spirulina also offers high levels of the antioxidants beta-carotene and zeaxanthin,plus unique immune-supportive elements. Spirulina has also been shown to offer potent blood-purification properties. It is one of the only sources of the anti-inflammatory, joint-strengthening super Omega-6 fatty acid, GLA (Gamma-linolenic acid).

Chlorella is a genus of single-celled green algae. Studies have shown that chlorella has anti-tumor properties in mice. Another study found enhanced vascular function in hypertensive rats who were fed chlorella. Chlorella is a complete protein. It is also packed with calories, fat, and vitamins.

What is molybdenum and why is it included in Akea?

Molybdenum is a trace mineral found in most plant and animal tissues. Molybdenum is an essential cofactor for many of the enzymes involved in protein synthesis and the mobilization of iron use in the body. Molybdenum helps with metabolism of fats and carbohydrates. It plays an important role in the enzyme process for the use of iron in the body, by mobilizing iron from the liver reserves. Molybdenum is absorbed from the gastrointestinal tract and excreted in the urine. It helps prevent anemia and enhance a general feeling of well-being.

What is resveratrol?

Plants—most famously, grapes—produce resveratrol naturally as a defense against fungi and other threats. In humans, it has shown to be effective in reversing symptoms of aging. It's believed to be a significant factor behind the French Paradox—why the French can consume diets heavy on calories and saturated fats, yet live longer with a lower incidence of heart disease. The source for the resveratrol in Akea is Japanese knotweed, which is considered to be the most nutritious source.

Does Akea contain essential amino acids?

Amino acids are the building blocks of proteins, and essential amino acids are the amino acids the body cannot produce on its own and that must be obtained from dietary sources. Most plants are deficient in one or more of the essential amino acids, although quinoa, amaranth and buckwheat are exceptions because their protein matrix includes all 8 of these essential amino acids. They are considered complete proteins and are all in Akea.

The fermentation process that Akea undergoes has broken down those proteins into amino acids and therefore minimizes the effort the digestive system has to put forth when Akea is consumed. So Akea contains a complete complement of all amino acids, and they are already in a form that will not trigger adverse immune system action.

In the ingredients list, under Enzyme Composition, "Nattozimes" includes a trademark symbol. What exactly is Nattozimes™?

Nattozimes™ is an extract of nattokinase, a protease compound formed during the soybean fermentation process that is very beneficial for health. Nattokinase was first discovered in the fermented soybean cheese known as natto. This cheese has been a staple of the Japanese diet for over a thousand years. Today it is popular as a traditional therapy to support a healthy cardiovascular system.

Modern research initiated by Dr. Hirouki Sumi identified the active principle in natto to be a protease produced by the fermenting organism, Bacillus natto. They named the enzyme nattokinase and began using it therapeutically in Japan. Nattokinase is frequently consumed in Okinawa and has been shown to cause a reduction in atherosclerotic plaque and blood clots.

Nattozimes is formulated to provide a blend of proteases which have been shown to break down standard fibrin substrates in a manner similar to nattokinase. In vitro research has shown that the proteases used in Nattozimes possess fibrinolytic activity. Nattozimes proteases support healthy protein metabolism, both within the digestive track and systemically.

Nattozimes™ is a registered trademark of National Enzyme Company, Forsythe, Missouri

How to Take Akea

What can I mix it in?

Akea can be mixed into a liquid of your choice or blending into a smoothie. We highly discourage the use of soy milk, cow's milk, carbonated beverages, and drinks containing artificial sweeteners, colors or flavors, due to the high potential for adverse reactions of those beverages alone. Akea does not contain sweeteners or flavorings and has a neutral, natural flavor that takes on the taste of whatever you mix it in. We recommend using 6-8 oz. of liquid followed by an additional 6-8 ounces of water.

If mixing in juice, it is recommended to dilute with water since fruit juice still contains a large amount of simple sugar. Though studies have shown that the beta glucans contained in Akea reduces the glycemic index of foods it is consumed simultaneously with, for diabetics and those wishing to lose weight, it is especially important to avoid over-consumption of simple sugars.

For one scoop of Akea, pour just 3-5 ounces of juice in the BlenderBottle and add another 2-4 ounces of water. This will be enough juice for flavoring without the additional unwanted calories of sugar. Don't forget to follow with another 6-8 ounces of filtered water.

How much should I take?
Is it OK to take more than is recommended on the container?

Two scoops (22 grams) is recommended as the optional daily dosage. Since Akea is a whole food, individuals can take as much as desired. Check out the website, *www.TheBlastFast.com* for directions on how to use Akea as a weight loss cleanse and to order the book of the same name by Akea founder, William King.

When should I take Akea?

Ideally Akea should be taken in two separate servings; one, first thing in the morning and the second, mid- to late afternoon. Two separate servings are recommended; however, they can be combined into one serving if a second serving time is not possible.

Should I take Akea with or without other food?

Akea can be taken either with food or away from food. Vitamin pills are suggested to be taken with food because they are void of certain co-factors required to assimilate the nutrition, and synthetic B vitamins can be harsh on the stomach especially taken away from food. Akea is fermented whole food nutrition and does not have to be taken with food.

Can I drink Akea in coffee or tea?

Akea mixes well in most any liquid; however, it is not recommended to mix Akea in hot beverages (over 114 degrees Fahrenheit) as the high temperature may degrade the living probiotics.

What do you mean by absorption and bioavailability?

Human nutrition is affected by the body's ability to absorb the food, as well as by the bioavailability of the food. Absorption rates may be better or worse, depending upon the individual's capacity to absorb nutrients—which can be determined by the condition of the digestive tract and other factors. Bioavailability is a function of the nutritional element—how ready it is to be digested and assimilated by the body. Akea creates the right environment for optimal digestion and provides the nutritional substrate in the optimal form to be digested and assimilated.

Is Akea a meal replacement?

Akea contains less than 50 calories per serving, with only two grams of protein and virtually no fat. Akea is micronutrient dense (vitamins, minerals, phytonutrients), not macronutrient dense (carbs, proteins and fats). By adding high quality fat such as avocado, or coconut and protein such as fresh raw eggs from free-roaming hens, pea protein, or hemp protein powder, you'll enjoy a highly nutritious, high quality, convenient meal.

Does Akea have side effects?

The Standard American Diet has resulted in the decimation of the intestinal flora responsible for proper digestive function, immunity, even nervous system action (think gut-brain connection). Depending on the individual and the current state of their digestive tract, reintroducing probiotics and enzymes, along with soluble fiber can have varying effects. For some, the bowels may slow, while others might experience a slight laxative effect. This is a normalization process that should moderate over the course of several days as any "build-up" in the digestive tract is broken down and eliminated. Be sure to drink plenty of filtered, unchlorinated water [water filtered by reverse osmosis, for example]. Also for those who are not accustomed to eating vegetables and fruits, there can be an adjustment period in which it may be best to add Akea slowly and gradually.

Does Akea cause any digestion problems or discomfort?

Akea helps maintain healthy digestion. The soluble fiber Akea does add bulk to assist movement through the digestive tract. The probiotics and digestive enzymes restore balance to the gut.

Drink plenty of water to ensure proper hydration and to avoid any slowing of the bowels due to this increased fiber and accelerated detoxification. We encourage you to consider any diet or nutrition program as an adjunct to the care and monitoring of healthcare professional who has been educated in the use of nutrition as preventive medical practice.

Is Akea safe for kids? How much?

Akea comes with the FDA GRAS certification, which denotes that every ingredient in Akea has been deemed generally regarded as safe for human consumption. Akea is a whole food, so there is no problem giving it to children. Graduated dosages should be considered for children. Children over 12 can enjoy one scoop a day while children under 12 may enjoy 1/2 scoop a day with their favorite juice. Toddlers may enjoy a third of a scoop a day.

Part III

The Cookbook

Why Organic

There's something to be said for the satiation value of a baked potato and a big green salad- provided the potato is crowned with a spoonful of coconut oil and a sprinkling of pink salt, of course. There's also a reason that salads are "dressed". Leafy greens and other vegetables rich in color are loaded, in varying ratios, with fat soluble vitamins A, D, E, and K. A dressing made with high quality extra virgin olive oil will facilitate the body's absorption of those vitamins so they can quickly be put to necessary use. Avoid commercial dressing at all costs, even if they're "organic", as they are most likely littered with poor quality, rancid oils like canola (bioengineered rapeseed oil), soybean, and sunflower.

I'm giving you free reign to have potatoes *every day,* if you so desire (honor your cravings!) Make sure you always have a few prebaked organic russets in the fridge so you can whip up some Country Fried Potatoes in a few minutes, satisfying any craving (sign of deficiency!) that might sneak up on you unexpectedly.

You're going to find yourself at the grocery store several times a week now, restocking your fridge with fresh produce, organic as often as possible, especially for those "Dirty Dozen". Don't make the mistake of seeing that as a chore. This is how we're meant to nourish ourselves, with fresh food that goes bad if you don't eat it in a few days. Gone are the days of going to the mega mart once a month "so you can stock up and not have to waste your time on another trip to the store". Your number one priority from the moment you open your eyes in the morning to the moment you shut them at night is to feed your body cleanly and efficiently with macromolecules (fat, proteins, carbohydrates), and abundantly where micronutrients (vitamins, minerals, bioflavonoids, catechins, antioxidants, enzymes) are concerned.

One thing to note about organic produce: the use of pesticides is only one factor that differentiates organically-grown produce from conventional. Herbicides, fertilizers, fungicides, genetically modified seeds, and "growth regulators", are all hazards that conventionally grown plants could have been exposed to.

The Environmental Working Group (EWG) creates an annual resource list that helps consumers identify which of approximately 40 vegetables and fruits test for highest pesticide residues. They then categorize 27 of those foods into two parts they cleverly named, the "Dirty Dozen™", and the "Clean 15™". From the 2014 *EWG's Shopper's Guide to Pesticides in Produce™*:

Why Should You Care About Pesticides?

The growing consensus among scientists is that small doses of pesticides and other chemicals can cause lasting damage to human health, especially during fetal development and early childhood. Scientists now know enough about the long-term consequences of ingesting these powerful chemicals to advise that we minimize our consumption of pesticides.

What's the Difference?

EWG research has found that people who eat five fruits and vegetables a day from the Dirty Dozen™ list consume an average of 10 pesticides a day. Those who eat from the 15 least contaminated conventionally-grown fruits and vegetables ingest fewer than 2 pesticides daily. The Guide helps consumers make informed choices to lower their dietary pesticide load.

Will Washing and Peeling Help?

The data used to create these lists is based on produce tested as it is typically eaten (meaning washed, rinsed or peeled, depending on the type of produce). Rinsing reduces but does not eliminate pesticides. Peeling helps, but valuable nutrients often go down the drain with the skin. The best approach: eat a varied diet, rinse all produce and buy organic when possible.

How the List was Created

EWG analysts have developed the Guide based on data from nearly 89,000 tests for pesticide residues in produce conducted between 2000 and 2008 and collected by the U.S. Department of Agriculture and the U.S. Food and Drug Administration. You can find a detailed description of the criteria EWG used to develop these rankings and the complete list of fruits and vegetables tested at our dedicated website, www.FoodNews.org.

My issues with this "guide" are numerous, not the least of which is the false sense of security consumers are given when choosing conventionally-grown versions of foods on the Clean 15 list. What about the other dangers present in conventionally-grown produce? Corn, papaya, and more recently, pineapple, are some of the most genetically-modified crops in the produce section! Not to mention that most conventional watermelon, with its absence of those beautiful black seeds, also runs the risk of coming from GMOs as well as being sprayed with various "growth accelerators".

An MSNBC report in June of 2011 told of a Twilight Zone-type happening where watermelon fields in eastern China were covered in exploded fruit. "Farmers used growth chemicals to make their crops bigger, but ended up destroying them instead... The farmers used the growth accelerator *forchlorfenuron*. Even the melons that survived tended to have fibrous, misshapen fruit with mostly white instead of black seeds." The story also reported that, "Chinese regulations don't forbid use of the substance. It is also allowed in the United States for use on kiwi fruit and grapes ... About 20 farmers and 115 acres of watermelon around Danyang were affected ... Farmers resorted to chopping up the fruit and feeding it to fish and pigs". You'd certainly be hard-pressed to find a conventional farming outfit that didn't use fertilizers (growth accelerators)or herbicides (see next paragraph)to maximize their yields and profits.

And cue "Bud Nip"! Google "bud nip sweet potato video" to see how a third grader introduced the masses to a little ditty called *chlorpropham*. According to the EXTOXNET*[see page 234], chlorpropham, also known as Bud Nip, Beet-Kleen, and Sprout Nip, is a "plant growth regulator used for preemergence control of grass weeds in alfalfa, lima and snap beans, blueberries, cane berries [raspberries and blackberries], carrots, cranberries, garlic, onions, spinach, sugar beets, tomatoes, safflower, soybeans... *It is also used to inhibit potato sprouting* and for sucker control in tobacco. Italics are mine to underscore the fact that it is the sweet potato that the little girl chose to use in her experiment. Acute toxicological effects are outlined as follows:

> Chlorpropham is moderately toxic by ingestion. It may cause irritation of the eyes or skin. Symptoms of poisoning in laboratory animals have included listlessness, incoordination, nose bleeds, protruding eyes, bloody tears, difficulty in breathing, prostration, inability to urinate, high fevers, and death. Autopsies of animals have shown inflammation of the stomach and intestinal lining, congestion of the brain, lungs and other organs, and degenerative changes in the kidneys and liver.
> Chronic exposure of laboratory animals has caused retarded growth, increased liver, kidney and spleen weights, congestion of the spleen and death. Long-term exposure to chlorpropham may cause adverse reproductive effects. Chlorpropham may cross the placenta. Long-term exposure to chlorpropham may cause tumors.

EWG's Shopper's Guide to Pesticides

2011		2012	
Dirty Dozen	**Clean 15**	**Dirty Dozen**	**Clean 15**
Apples	Onions	Apples	Asparagus
Celery	Corn	Bell Peppers	Avocado
Strawberries	Pineapples	Blueberries	Cabbage
Peaches	Avocado	Celery	Cantaloupe
Spinach	Asparagus	Cucumbers	Corn
Nectarines	Sweet peas	Grapes	Eggplant
Grapes	Mangoes	Lettuce	Grapefruit
Sweet bell peppers	Eggplant	Necatrines	Kiwi
Potatoes	Cantaloupe	Peaches	Mangoes
Blueberries	Kiwi	Potatoes	Mushrooms
Lettuce	Cabbage	Spinach	Onions
Kale/collard greens	Watermelon	Strawberries	Pineapples
	Sweet potatoes	PLUS	Sweet Peas
	Grapefruit	Grean Beans	Sweet Potatoes
	Mushrooms	Kale/Greens	Watermelon

2013		2014	
Dirty Dozen	**Clean 15**	**Dirty Dozen**	**Clean 15**
Apples	Asparagus	Celery	Avocados
Celery	Avocados	Peaches	Pineapple
Cherry Tomatoes	Cabbage	Strawberries	Sweet Peas
Cucumbers	Cantaloupe	Apples	Kiwi
Grapes	Sweet Corn	Blueberries	Eggplant
Hot Peppers	Eggplant	Nectarines	Watermelon
Nectarines	Grapefuit	Bell Peppers	Sweet Potato
Peaches	Kiwi	Cherries	Onions
Potatoes	Mangoes	Kale/Collard Greens	Asparagus
Spinach	Mushrooms	Grapes (Imported)	Mangoes
Strawberries	Onions	Spinach	Cabbage
Bell Peppers	Pineapple	Potatoes	Cantaloupe
PLUS	Sweet Peas (frozen)		Grapefruit
Kale/Collard Greens	Sweet Potatoes		Honeydew Melon
Summer Squash	Papaya		Sweet Corn

Buy All of Your Produce Organic as Often as Possible, if Not Always

I've included the last four years of the EWG's guide to illustrate a very important point. Every year where "pesticide residues" are concerned, some items bounce off both lists, and several seem to be permanent fixtures. In 2011 and 2012, lettuce was "dirty", but in the last two years, it wasn't on either list. The same went for cucumbers in 2012 and 2013. Does that mean I can make a lettuce and cucumber salad with the conventionally-grown versions in 2014 without exposing my children to list-worthy amounts of pesticide residues? And do crops like onions, spinach, and sweet potatoes, that can be sprayed with chlorpropham for "preemergence control", and to prevent sprouting after cultivation, really deserve to be called "clean"? In 2012, upon the June release of that year's guide, a CNN Health report warned:

> Apples and celery are still agriculture's dirtiest pieces of produce, according to the Environmental Working Group's annual "Dirty Dozen" report. The report names the fruits and vegetables ranking highest in pesticide residue. Cucumbers were added to the 2012 Dirty Dozen, while Kale and collard greens were moved from the list to join green beans in a new "Plus" category. The category was created this year to highlight crops that did not meet traditional Dirty Dozen criteria but are still commonly contaminated with organophosphate insecticides, which are toxic to the nervous system.

The confusion from year to year this guide has the potential to cause, simply where pesticides are concerned, should be the first reason that people take it for what it's worth: a drop in the bucket. Raising awareness is a noble goal, except when it runs the risk of causing frustration as the rules seem to keep changing. Using words like "dirty" and "clean" to categorize food based on *one criterion alone* is, in my opinion, an irresponsible practice, no matter how good the intention. Adding to the confusion on a completely different note is the fact that corn is the only grain on a list otherwise comprised of only fruits and vegetables. Now I know why so many people think it's either a fruit or a vegetable- the Clean Fifteen list told them so!

On February 19th, 2014, the EWG introduced their first-ever *Shopper's Guide to Avoiding GE [genetically engineered, aka GMO] Food*. A few of the offenders implicated in the new guide are previous Clean 15 darlings, papaya, summer squash, and sweet corn! Per the guide, "Most sweet corn sold in supermarkets and farm stands is not grown from genetically engineered seeds, but a few varieties are, so it's best to buy organic sweet corn". Less than two months later in April of 2014, sweet corn appears on the list labelled "clean", vice on the "Buy Organic" one. Are you confused yet?

Papayas must have bribed their way on to the 2013 Clean 15 list because how else could you give trusting consumers the nod of approval to buy them conventionally-grown that year when over 10 years ago in 2004, the organization GMO Free Hawaii designed a study to look at the extent of GMO contamination around the state only to be slapped in the face with this:

> The results indicate massive GMO contamination of papaya seeds on Hawaii Island, of the order of 50%, substantial GMO contamination on Oahu (<5%) and thankfully, only traces of contamination on Kauai (0.0%). Both organic farms tested had no GMO trees unintentionally planted, but sadly, were discovered to have air contamination of the seeds in their fruits (<5% on Hawaii Island and 0.01% on Kauai). Most shocking was the GMO contamination of the University of Hawaii's non-GMO papaya seed supply (Waimanolo Solo variety) at greater than 0.01% but less than 0.1%.

Confusion breeds frustration and frustration breeds capitulation. Capitulation to the idea that trying to eat right is a battle we have no hope of winning. The Clean 15 is a misleading misnomer, and the Dirty Dozen should be renamed the Filthy 48. All conventionally-grown produce runs the risk of being "dirty" because of ALL of the chemicals copiously doused on it, not just pesticides. Below is the entire EWG-ranked list of 48 foods that tested positive for pesticide residue per testing data from the U.S. Department of Agriculture USDA) and Food and Drug Administration (FDA), starting with the apple as the "dirtiest", and ending with the avocado as the "cleanest". Note that nectarine, snap peas, and blueberries have both a domestic and an imported rank.

1. Apples	14. Blueberries, Dom.	27. Raspberries	39. Cantaloupe
2. Strawberries	15. Lettuce	28. Broccoli	40. Grapefruit
3. Grapes	16. Kale/Collards	29. Snap Peas, Dom.	41. Eggplant
4. Celery	17. Plums	30. Green Onions	42. Kiwi
5. Peaches	18. Cherries	31. Oranges	43. Papayas
6. Spinach	19. Nectarines, Dom.	32. Bananas	44. Mangoes
7. Sweet Bell Peppers	20. Pears	33. Tomatoes	45. Asparagus
8. Nectarines, Imp.	21. Tangerines	34. Watermelon	46. Onions
9. Cucumbers	22. Carrots	35. Honeydew	47. Sweet Peas, Frozen
10. Cherry Tomatoes	23. Blueberries, Imp.	36. Mushrooms	48. Cabbage
11. Snap Peas	24. Green Beans	37. Sweet Potatoes	49. Pineapple
12. Potatoes	25. Winter Squash	38. Cauliflower	50. Sweet Corn
13. Hot Peppers	26. Summer Squash		51. Avocados

Source: Environmental Working Group (EWG)

Buy All of Your Produce Organic as Often as Possible, if Not Always

Perhaps the final reason you should insist on organic produce, as well as herbs and spices, has to do with something called *irradiation*. Some time ago you may have heard the term "irradiated" as it was briefly tossed around the media to inform consumers about yet another way toway to help keep our foods squeeky "clean". According to the United States Environmental Protection Agency (EPA):

Food irradiation is a technology for controlling spoilage and eliminating food-borne pathogens, such as salmonella. The result is similar to conventional pasteurization and is often called "cold pasteurization" or "irradiation pasteurization." Like pasteurization, irradiation kills bacteria and other pathogens, that could otherwise result in spoilage or food poisoning. The fundamental difference between the two methods is the source of the energy they rely on to destroy the microbes. While conventional pasteurization relies on heat, irradiation relies on the energy of *ionizing radiation* [italics are mine]. The FDA emphasizes that no preservation method is a substitute for safe food handling procedures.

How is food irradiated?

Bulk or packaged food passes through a radiation chamber on a conveyor belt. The food does not come into contact with radioactive materials, but instead passes through a radiation beam, like a large flashlight.

How much radiation is the food exposed to ?

The type of food and the specific purpose of the irradiation determine the amount of radiation, or dose, necessary to process a particular product. The speed of the belt helps control the radiation dose delivered to the food by controlling the exposure time. The actual dose is measured by dosimeters within the food containers. Radiation doses vary for different foodstuffs. For the vast majority of foods, the limit is less than 10 kilo Gray. The U.S. Food and Drug Administration (FDA) sets radiation dose limits for specific food types:

Food Type	Dose (kilo Grays)
fruit	1
poultry	3
spices, seasonings	30

How does irradiation kill bacteria?

When ionizing radiation strikes bacteria and other microbes, its high energy breaks chemical bonds in molecules that are vital for cell growth and integrity. As a result, the microbes die, or can no longer multiply causing illness or spoilage. [As in, anything living to include but not limited to: enzymes, friendly microorganisms and the cells of the plant itself.]

You may be wondering why the radiation dose limit is so much higher for herbs and spices than for poultry or fruits. Very simple. According to the EPA, "they [herbs and spices] are consumed in very small quantities". I'm not even sure how to wrap my mind around that rationale. But don't worry, because "Irradiating food protects people in this world -- and out of this world as well! NASA astronauts eat food that has been irradiated to avoid any chance of food-borne illness in space."

FDA has approved food irradiation methods for a number of foods. Irradiation can be used on herbs and spices, fresh fruits and vegetables, wheat, flour, pork, poultry and other meat, and some seafood. FDA requires that irradiated food labels contain both a logo and a statement that the food has been irradiated.

USDA works with FDA to promote food irradiation where it is appropriate. USDA also controls the use of the word "organic" on food labels. Foods which have been irradiated, no matter how they are grown or produced, cannot be labeled as USDA certified organic.

Well, thank God for that!

* EXTOXNET: A Pesticide Information Project of Cooperative Extension Offices of Cornell University, Michigan State University, Oregon State University, and University of California at Davis. Major support and funding provided by the USDA/Extension Service/National Agricultural Pesticide Impact Assessment Program.

Buy All of Your Produce Organic as Often as Possible, if Not Always

Salads, Spuds and Veggies

Bruschetta Salad
Serves 3 to 4

1/3 cup California extra virgin olive oil*
2-3 Tbsp balsamic vinegar*, without caramel color or added sulfites
pink salt to taste (about ¼ tsp)
1 tsp organic salt-free herb seasoning* OR Mrs. Dash
3 vine-ripened tomatoes, cut into bite-sized wedges
1/2 cup cucumber, thinly sliced
1 small red onion, thinly sliced (about 1/2 cup)
1/4 cup chopped fresh basil leaves

Whisk the vinegar, salt, and herb seasoning in a large bowl and allow to rest for about 10 minutes while chopping the veggies. Add the olive oil and veggies to the vinegar and toss gently. Serve immediately.

Cucumber Salad
Serves 3 to 4

1/4 cup California extra virgin olive oil
2-3 Tbsp combination of Bragg's Raw Apple Cider Vinegar*
and red wine vinegar
1 pepino or English cucumber, thinly sliced
1/2 small red onion, thinly sliced (about 1/4 cup)
1Tbsp chopped fresh dill weed or ½ Tbsp dry dill weed
pink salt to taste (about ¼ tsp)

Whisk the vinegar, salt, dill, and finely sliced onion in a large bowl and allow to rest for about 10 minutes. Cut the cucumber in half length-wise and slicc thinly using a Börner or Mandolin slicer (be careful!). Add the olive oil and cucumbers to the vinegar and toss gently.

* Refer to Appendix B: Restocking Your Pantry

Salad For Dinner
Serves 3 to 4
Who needs a main course when you've got this powerful meal-deal to satisfy you!
Warm up some SatFatRox Biscuits to soak up all of that luscious dressing.

Dressing:
¼ cup Bragg's Raw Apple Cider Vinegar
1 Tbsp balsamic vinegar, without caramel color
2 cloves fresh garlic, quartered
½ teaspoon ground pepper
pink salt to taste (about 1/2 tsp)
1 tsp organic dry dill[weed] or finely chopped fresh dill
1/2 cup California extra virgin olive oil

1 romaine lettuce heart, torn into bite-sized pieces
1 cup baby spinach
1 cup cherry tomatoes, halved
1 cup cucumber, halved, quartered and sliced
1/2 cup chopped scallions or green onions
½ red bell pepper, cut into bite-sized pieces
1 cup cooked garbanzo beans or black-eyed peas
1 ripe avocado, halved, peeled and sliced

In a small food processor, puree garlic cloves, vinegars, salt, pepper, and dill until garlic is minced. Pour mixture into a large bowl and allow flavors to blend for about 10 minutes while preparing the veggies. You can reserve the avocado for garnishing just before serving or slice it into half inch pieces and incorporate it into the salad, allowing it to give the dressing a creamy consistency. Add the olive oil to the vinegar and whisk to combine well. Add the rest of the veggies and beans to the bowl and toss until they are thoroughly coated with dressing. Serve immediately.

Notes:
Can the can! Refer to page for how to cook your own dry beans.

Buy All of Your Produce Organic as Often as Possible, if Not Always

Two Easy Ways to Cook Potatoes

1. Baked

You can either bake potatoes for immediate enjoyment or for later use in any recipe calling for "pre-baked potatoes". Begin by washing and gently scrubbing desired number of organic Russet potatoes and placing them in an oven-safe glass baking dish arranged in a single layer. Prick each potato once and loosely cover the dish with aluminum foil (ideally your dish will be deep enough so that when you do cover it, no contact with the potatoes will be made.) Bake in the center rack of a preheated 350°F oven for 60 to 90 minutes, depending on their size, and flipping them over half way through the baking time to faciliate faster, even baking.

Freshly baked potatoes can be topped with coconut oil and then any number of non-dairy toppings such as Salsa, Guacamole, or Hummus, or sauerkraut. For a heartier meal, warm up some leftover Stewed Lentils, Green Curry and Garbanzos, or Veggie Chili. and turn that potato into a protein powerhouse.

If you're baking for later use, allow them to cool individually on a baker's cooling rack and store them in tightly sealed container in the refrigerator for up to 4 days.

2. Boiled

To make perfect boiled potatoes, begin by rinsing them with warm water, and arranging them in a single layer in a lidded pot large enough to accomodate them. Do not peel or scrub them aggresively; the peel will hold in the valuable minerals the potato is rich in (chapter 11). Cover with an inch of filtered water and sprinkle with half to a whole teaspoon of pink salt (1-2 pounds; 3 pounds of potatoes). Cover pot with lid and cook on medium heat for about 30 minutes, turning potatoes over half way through cooking time. Once the water comes to a full boil, lower heat to low/medium. To test for doneness, insert a toothpick into the middle of the largest potato seeking tenderness but not overcooking to the point of splitting. For boiling purposes, any organic potato variety will work, although my personal favorites are red. Freshly boiled potatoes can either be mashed, used to make any of the potato salads on the next few pages, or saved for later use covered in the fridge for up to 4 days.

California Potato Salad
Serves 4 to 6

When my husband and I were first married, we were stationed in Barstow, California. We lived in base housing and I had a gas range with a broiler underneath, just like the one I grew up with. I used to slice fresh red bell peppers and onions and roast them under the broiler right before adding them to the salad. The original version also had (gasp!) bacon in it. It was extremely tasty but we have since given up meat and I haven't had a broiler since 2002. But even if I did, I now know too much to enjoy using it ever again (chapter 15). This salad is named partly for the fact that I created it while we were in Cali and partly because I associate anything with avocados with that beautiful state.
"I give you, the Mighty Mojave!" -JKN

Dressing:
1/4 cup raw honey
1/4 cup Grey Poupon Dijon Mustard
1/4 cup California extra virgin olive oil
1 Tbsp dry dill weed
1 tsp pink salt

3 pounds red potatoes
3/4 cup roasted red peppers, drained and chopped into bite-size pieces
1 small red onion, chopped in half, and sliced thinly
2 avocados, ripe but still firm with no brown spots inside

Boil potatoes as outlined on page 218. Once cooked, drain immediately; cut lengthwise and then in third inch slices into a large mixing bowl. In a small bowl, whisk together the dijon mustard, dill weed, and pink salt, and allow to rest for about 10 minutes while chopping the onions, and red peppers. In a large bowl, slice potatoes into bite-sized pieces, leaving the skins on; add the onions and red peppers. Slice the avocados just before you're ready to dress the salad and add them to the potatoes. Whisk the honey and olive oil into the mustard mixture and pour over the potatoes. Toss gently and serve while still warm.

Notes:
Southern California produces approximately 80 percent of the avocados on the US market. The most common variety is the Hass avocado, with rough, bumpy skin. Visit www.WikiHow.com/Choose-Avocados to learn how to choose the best avocados for your specific recipe.

Buy All of Your Produce Organic as Often as Possible, if Not Always

Salată Orientală
Serves 4 to 6

Why Romanians call this creation "Oriental Salad", I have no idea. I just know that growing up, I absolutely loved it when my mom used to make it. For the record, I don't cook the yolks of our eggs anymore, so when I do make Salată Orientală, I don't use eggs. It's a slight variation on the traditional American potato salad, only this one is served warm, and dressed without mayo (because it's full of rancid oils, soy and sucralose).

3 pounds red potatoes
6 warm soft-boiled eggs
(preferrably pastured, but at least organic or from a local supplier)
1 small white onion
1/2 cup Niçoise* or Arbequena olives*, or more if you wish
1/3 cup California extra virgin olive oil
1/3 cup Bragg's Raw Apple Cider Vinegar
Pink salt and black pepper to taste

Boil potatoes as outlined on page 218. Prepare soft-boiled eggs as outlined in notes below. Once potaoes are cooked, drain immediately; cut lengthwise and then in third inch slices into a large mixing bowl. Peel and chop the onion, first in half, then in thin slices; add to the potatoes. Peel the eggs and slice widthwise with a serrated knife or an egg slicer*. Add the eggs, olives, and at least 1/2 teaspoon of sprinkled pink salt and pepper to taste, to the potatoes. Generously drizzle the vinegar and olive oil over top and toss gently. Serve warm or cold.

Notes:
Adapted from the American Egg Board, your instructions for the perfect *soft-boiled* egg (please don't overcook them!) Step 1: PLACE eggs in saucepan large enough to hold them in single layer. ADD cold water to cover eggs by 1 inch. HEAT over high heat just to boiling. REMOVE from burner. COVER pan. Step 2: LET EGGS STAND in hot water about 8-9 minutes for large eggs (5-6 minutes for medium eggs; 9-11 minutes for extra large). Step 3: DRAIN immediately and serve warm. OR, cool completely under cold running water or in bowl of ice water, then REFRIGERATE.
*Do not use canned black olives (ever). They are processed (cured) by being submerged in vats filled with a lye solution. Although the alkaline lye quickly leaches out the glucosides from the olive, also takes with it much of the olive's natural flavor, leaving behind a slight chemical aftertaste. Plus, they contain notable amounts of acrylamide (see chapter 15 for more information on acrylamide.)

Mediterranean Potato Salad
Serves 4 to 6

Dressing
3 to 4 cloves raw garlic, peeled and quartered
1/2 teaspoon pink salt
1/2 tsp black pepper
1/3 cup balsamic vinegar (no added sulfites or caramel color)
1/3 cup California extra virgin olive oil

3 pounds red potatoes
1 (9.5) ounce jar organic roasted red peppers, drained and sliced
1 small red onion, half and thinly sliced
1/2 cup Kalamatta olives (or more if desired)
1/4 cup fresh basil, chopped

Place garlic in a small food processor and pulse until minced. Allow to sit for 10 minutes with lid removed before adding pink salt, pepper and vinegar. Pulse again for about 30 seconds to incorporate; set aside. Boil potatoes as outlined on page 218. Once potaoes are cooked, drain immediately; cut lengthwise and then in third inch slices into a large mixing bowl. Peel and chop the onion, first in half, then in thin slices. Chop the basil and add to the potatoes along with the onion and roasted red peppers. Drizzle the garlic and vinegar, and olive oil over everything, tossing gently to mix. Serve while while warm or at room temperature.

Sautéed Shrooms
Serves 2, depending on use

1 pint fresh mushrooms of your choice, rinsed well
1/2 medium onion, halved and thinly sliced
2 Tbsp coconut oil
pink salt and black pepper to taste

After rinsing, cut off bottom quarter inch of mushroom stems to remove tough portion. Cut shrooms in half and then slice into desired thinness, or just leave halved. In a stainless steel sauté pan, warm coconut oil on low-medium heat until melted. Add the onions and cook for about 5 minutes, stirring often to promote fast and even cooking. Add the mushrooms and stir to coat evenly with onions and oil. Sprinkle with pink salt and pepper and cover, reducing heat to low until shrooms are tender, about 10 to 12 minutes.

Spaghetti Squash
Serves 4 to 6, with leftovers

Can be pre-baked and reheated on stovetop when ready to serve. After washing the out-side of the squash with vinegar and water, pat dry and use a heavy chopping knife (be careful!), to cut the squash in half. Spoon out the seeds and stringy mass and place cut side-down in an oven-safe glass pan. Bake on center rack at 350°F for 35 to 45 minutes. Squash wiil be done when a knife is easily inserted. and rind gives slightly to pressure. Use a heavier fork to scrape the inside the of shell, "fluffing" small sections of it at a time. Toss each half of the squash with:

2 Tbsp coconut oil
pink salt to taste
1 Tbsp organic salt-free herb seasoning

or

with Marinara Sauce (page 243)

*If you plan on using the other half of the squash later in the week, cook it closer to the 35 minute time to maintain the shape of the flesh when reheating. Remove the flesh from the shell as above and after it has cooled, place in a container with a tightly-fitting lid and refrigerate for up to 3 days. When ready to prepare, warm 2 tablespoons coconut oil on low-medium heat in a stainless steel or ceramic-coated sauté pan until melted. Add the squash and sprinkle with pink salt and non-salt seasoning; toss to coat evenly with oil, for about 10 minutes or until warmed.

Notes:
Coconut oil should be consumed as unrefined, preferably organic- unless purchasing the Expeller-pressed variety produced by Tropical Traditions (TT), available on my site www.SatFatRox.com/The-Store. If you dislike the scent of virgin, unrefined coconut oil, the Expeller-pressed will still give you a wonderful degree of benefit without the (awe-some) trademark scent of the virgin unrefined oil.

Easy Garlic and Herb:
Green Beans OR Broccoli OR Cauliflower

Steaming veggies is a wonderful way to create a fast and filling snack or side dish, as long as you're not doing it in the microwave! Microwaving can destroy vitamins and enzymes and leave your vegetables seriously lacking in the nutrients they once possesed. Remember that purchasing the organic versions in frozen form will allow you to consume the necessary variety of plant foods your cells need, on a year-round basis, if the fresh versions are out of season.

Using a stainless steel steamer basket inside a 2-quart saucepan, place about half an inch of filtered water in the a pot and cover with a tight-fitting lid, heating on medium heat until it begins to simmer. Place desired amount of veggies in the basket and cover with lid.

Make sure to not exceed a stack of over 1 inch, as you'll end up over-cooking the bottom part. Beans and broccoli are optimally steamed when just tender, and their color has turned a rich, bright green- about 5 to 7 minutes. Chopping frozen green beans into 1-inch sections and fresh broccoli into smaller florets will yield shorter cooking times., while cauliflower may need a little more- about 8 to10 minutes.

Once the veggies have steamed to desired tenderness, remove steamer basket from pot (carefully!) and empty them into a serving dish. Toss with a generous table-spoon or two of coconut oil, or olive oil if you allow them to cool to the point of not giving off any steam, and season with pink salt and salt-free herb seasoning.

Creamed Spinach
Serves 2

You can serve this side partially through the process simply as *sautéed spinach* or go all the way by completing the last two steps for the "creamed" version.

1 container ready-washed baby spinach
1/2 small onion, finely chopped
2 cloves raw garlic
2 Tbsp coconut oil
1/4 cup full fat coconut milk
pink salt and black pepper to taste

In a stainless steel sauté pan, warm coconut oil on low-medium heat until melted. Add the onions and garlic and cook for about 5 minutes, stirring often to promote fast and even cooking. Add the spinach, pink salt and pepper, and cook for another 8 to 10 minutes until leaves are wilted. Stir in the coconut milk and mix to warm. Transfer the entire mixture to the food processor and pulse for 30 seconds. Can be served as a side or as a dip with toasted SatFatRox Biscuits.

Garbanzo Bean Tabouli
Serves 3 to 4
My take on a Mediterranean restaurant favorite, minus the gluten!

2 cups cooked garbanzo beans
1/2 medium onion, finely chopped
2 cloves raw garlic, peeled, crushed and minced
3 cups fresh parsley, minced
2 tomatoes, chopped
1/3 cup California extra virgin olive oil
juice of 1 or 2 lemons, freshly squeezed (about 2 to 4 Tbsp)
1/2 tsp pink salt or to taste

Chop all vegetables and allow garlic to sit for 10 minutes to increase its benficial properties (chapter18). Combine all ingredients and mix well. Use desired amount of lemon juice for your own taste.

Black-Eyed Pea Gazpacho
Serves 3 to 4

I realize that genuine gazpacho is made in a blender but I'm going to buck the system (surprise!) and borrow the name for this refreshing creation that is just as satisfying as it is delicious. You will need to have pre-soaked the black-eyed peas before cooking them.

1/2 bag dry black-eyed peas
2 Turkish bay leaves
4 cloves raw garlic
2 avocados, firm but ripe
4 tomatoes, diced and individually portioned
1 large red onion, chopped medium, divided into 4 portions
4 cloves raw garlic, peeled, crushed and minced
2 cubanelle peppers, chopped medium
1/2 cup fresh cilantro, chopped
California extra virgin olive oil
Bragg's Raw Apple Cider Vinegar
pink salt to taste

After soaking peas according to package, cover with 2 inches of filtered water, add 1 teaspoon pink salt, 4 cloves of garlic and 2 whole Turkish bay leaves and cook until tender. Allow peas to cool and do not drain cooking liquid, refrigerate until ready to use. To assemble gazpacho, laddle 1 cup of chilled cooked peas and broth into individual bowl and top with 1 crushed and minced garlic clove, one quarter of the chopped red onion, 1 chopped tomato, half of one diced cubanelle pepper, and 1/2 of an avocado, sliced. Drizzle gazpacho with 2 tablespoon olive oil and 1 to 2 tablespoons of vinegar. Garnish with chopped cilantro and serve.

Quick Pan-Fried Potatoes
(Country Fried Potatoes)
Serves 1 to 2
Now's your chance to use those pre-baked potatoes for the fastest way to the most satisfying "side that eats like a meal".

Warm 2 to 3 tablespoons of coconut oil in a ceramic-coated frying pan (throw your Teflon out right now), on low-medium heat until melted. Cut 2 pre-baked potatoes in half lengthwise and then slice into third inch pieces. Add potatoes to oil and sprinkle with pink salt and generously with organic salt-free herb seasoning. Warm through for 6 to 10 minutes; do not allow to over-brown (chapter 15). Enjoy any time of the day, every day if you wish (chapter 17).

Oven-Baked Ranch Fries
Serves 3 to 4

4 Russet potatoes, raw
3 Tbsp liquefied coconut oil
1/2 tsp pink salt
1/2 tsp garlic granules
1/2 tsp paprika

Preheat oven to 350°F, and line a 10 by 14 inch jelly roll pan with a silicone baking liner mat*. Rinse potatoes and slice into ranch fries by cutting them in half lengthwise and then each half into 3 to 4 wedges. In a large bowl, toss the potatoes with the pink salt, garlic granules and paprika until evenly coated and spread in a single layer in the jelly roll pan. Drizzle the liquefied coconut oil over them and loosely lay a sheet of aluminum foil over the pan. Bake on the center rack for 20 minutes and use a pancake flipper to turn the fries over gently. Return to oven for another 15 to 20 minutes, and bake uncovered until tender.

Mashed Potatoes
Serves 4 to 6

3 pounds red potatoes
1/2 cup coconut oil
2 or 3 raw eggs
1/2 Tbsp pink salt and pepper to taste

Begin by rinsing potatoes with warm water, and arranging them in a single layer in a lidded pot large enough to accomodate them. Do not peel or scrub them aggresively; the peel will hold in the valuable minerals the potato is rich in (chapter 11). Cover with an inch of filtered water and sprinkle with one teaspoon of pink salt. Cover pot with lid and cook on medium heat for about 30 minutes, turning potatoes over half way through cooking time. Once the water comes to a full boil, lower heat to low/medium. To test for doneness, insert a toothpick into the middle of the largest potato seeking tenderness but not overcooking to the point of splitting. Drain water immediately, add coconut oil and salt and mash with a potato masher. Make a well in the center and crack in the 2 raw eggs continue to mash quickly until well-blended. If you like your mashed potatoes creamier, just crack in another egg- pastured or organic , of course!

Garlic and Herb Mashed Potatoes

Prepare as above and mix in 1/2 Tbsp organic garlic granules and 1/2 Tbsp organic dry dillweed.

Notes:
Due to the fact that there are egg yolks in the mashed potatoes, they should only be eaten fresh and not reheated, especially in the microwave.

Buy All of Your Produce Organic as Often as Possible, if Not Always

Crustless Quiches

Scallion and Dill Quiche
Serves 4 to 6

This is a recipe adapted from that of an omelette my mother used to make on the weekends for us. She used to send me to our garden to pick fresh dill and green onions for it right before she made it. I believe fresh dill vice dry makes all the flavor difference. I have reduced the egg yolks in all of these recipes in an attempt to limit the amount of cholesterol oxidation from cooking. I believe the coconut oil and lower oven temperature also lessens the blow. The pot of water on the bottom rack of the oven lends an almost custard-like consistency to the egg, and the insulated cookie sheet under the baking dish reduces the risk of over-cooking and drying out.

1/4 cup coconut oil
1 bunch green onions, chopped
1/4 cup fresh dill, chopped
4 whole eggs
6 egg whites
3/4 cup full fat coconut milk
1 tsp pink salt

Preheat oven to 325 degrees and place a pan filled with 3 cups of water on the bottom rack. You'll also need an insulated cookie sheet on which to put the quiche dish to reduce over-browning of the quiche. Separate 6 eggs, reserving the yolks (make ice cream or mashed potatoes later in the day with them) and dropping the whites in a medium-sized bowl. Over the whites, crack in another 4 whole eggs; add the coconut milk, and 1 teaspoon of pink salt. Blend mixture on lowest speed of an immersion blender just until completely incorporated. Add the fresh dill and whisk in until evenly dispersed throughout the egg mixture. In a stainless steel sauté pan, warm coconut oil on low-medium heat and sauté the green onions for about 5 to 8 minutes until fragrant and wilted. Spread onions evenly in a round 12" quiche dish, using a spatula to get all of the coconut oil off the pan (to help prevent sticking). Gently pour egg mixture over the green onions. Cover tightly with aluminum foil and place on an insulated cookie sheet on the middle rack of the oven. Bake for 45 to 60 minutes and start checking for doneness at around 35 minutes. Dish will be ready when center is set. Resist the urge to over-bake.

Spinach and Shroom Quiche
Serves 4 to 6

1/4 cup coconut oil
1 small onion, finely chopped
3 cloves raw garlic, peeled, crushed and minced
2 cups fresh baby spinach, chopped
2 cups baby portabella mushrooms, washed and chopped
4 whole eggs
6 egg whites
1/2 cup full fat coconut milk
1/2 Tbsp pink salt
1/2 Tbsp organic salt-free herb seasoning

Preheat oven to 325 degrees and place a pan filled with 3 cups of water on the bottom rack. You'll also need an insulated cookie sheet on which to put the glass baking dish to reduce browning of the bottom. Separate 6 eggs, reserving the yolk (you know what to do with them) and dropping the whites in a medium-sized bowl. Over the whites, crack in another 4 whole eggs, and add the coconut milk. Blend mixture on lowest speed of an immersion blender just until completely incorporated. In a stainless steel sauté pan, warm coconut oil and sauté the onions and garlic on low-medium heat for 5 minutes, stirring often to prevent scorching. Add the mushrooms, pink salt and herb seasoning, stirring and cooking for another 5 to 6 minutes before adding the spinach. Continue to sauté the mixture until spinach begins to turn bright green. Remove from heat and spread evenly ina round 12" quiche dish, using a spatula to get all of the coconut oil off the pan (to help prevent sticking). Gently pour egg mixture over the vegetables. Cover tightly with aluminum foil and place on an insulated cookie sheet on the middle rack of the oven. Bake for 45 to 60 minutes and start checking for doneness at around 35 minutes. Dish will be ready when center is set. Resist the urge to over-bake.

Veggie Breakfast Bake
Serves 6 to 8

I struggled for some time with what to name this dish- quiche, bake, casserole? Whatever you decide to call it, it'll become an instant favorite! Whether for brunch, or breakfast for dinner, it's satisfying and full of color and flavor. Served with Bruschetta Salad (page 204) and Garlic and Herb Biscuits (page), it puts Sunday Brunch at "The Club" to shame. Use the 8 other yolks to make Mashed Potatoes, or Ice Cream or Peanut Butter Mousse for dessert.

4 small boiled red potatoes, halved and thinly sliced
1/4 cup coconut oil
1 small onion, finely chopped
1 red bell pepper, chopped
1 1/2 cup broccoli florets
6 whole eggs
8 egg whites
1 cup full fat coconut milk
1/2 Tbsp pink salt
organic salt-free herb seasoning

Preheat oven to 325 degrees and place a pan filled with 3 cups of water on the bottom rack. You'll also need an insulated cookie sheet on which to put the glass baking dish to reduce browning of the bottom. Separate 8 eggs, reserving the yolk (make ice cream for dessert with them) and dropping the whites in a medium-sized bowl. Over the whites, crack in another 6 whole eggs, and add the coconut milk, and 1 teaspoon of pink salt. Blend mixture on lowest speed of an immersion blender just until completely incorporated. Set mixture aside while prepping the veggies. In a stainless steel sauté pan, warm coconut oil and sauté the onions and red bell peppers on low-medium heat for 5 minutes (until onions become fragrant). Add the sliced potatoes and broccoli and season with ½ teaspoon of pink salt, and 1 tablespoon of herb seasoning. Cover and reduce heat slightly, allowing the broccoli to steam for about 8 to 10 minutes. Spread the veggie mixture into a 9x13" glass dish, using a spatula to get all of the coconut oil off the pan (to help prevent sticking). Slowly pour the egg mixture over the veggies and sprinkle the top with about another tablespoon of herb seasoning. Cover tightly with aluminum foil and place on an insulated cookie sheet on the middle rack of the oven. Bake for 50 to 75 minutes and start checking for doneness at around 45 minutes. Dish will be ready when center is set. Resist the urge to over-bake.

Beans, Soups, and Other Bowl Fare

Beans: The "magic fruit" that's good for your heart.

Do you remember those little rhymes about beans that would float around the playground when you were a kid? "Beans, beans, the magic fruit..." Or how about this one, "Beans, beans, they're good for your heart..." The ellipses are replacing references to flatulence, in case you had never heard, and both rhymes ended with, "... the more you eat... the better you feel, so eat beans for every meal." So much truth in childhood silliness, especially that last part- *the more you eat, the better you feel*. Eating beans doesn't have to leave your family donning gas masks to deal with the aftermath of *The Gas We Pass*. If you prepare beans carefully, and if you avoid unfermented SOYbeans, you could quite honestly eat beans for every meal, without having to yell, *Gas! Gas! Gas!,* after dinner.

The greatest way to buy beans is dry. Whether your favorite are black-eyed peas, garbanzos, or black beans, starting from scratch is much easier than you think and you can even freeze them for use later on. You can also add to their mineral content by adding pink salt to the cooking water, and the taste alone is reason enough to make the switch. Can the cans and stock up on dry beans instead.

Sort and Soak

All beans will have slightly different cooking times, but if you're cooking them on the stove top, they must be soaked. Follow the directions on the bag for specific cooking times. Start by sorting through the beans and remove any small stones or other debris. Wash the beans in cold water and drain. I prefer soaking beans at least overnight, and in the case of garbanzos, I've even kept them going for 24 to 36 hours to get a little fermentation going. Place the beans in a bowl large enough to accommodate swelling, then, add enough filtered water to cover them by at least two inches. Sprinkle about ½ teaspoon of pink salt over the beans and cover the bowl with a clean kitchen towel. Let them soak for at least 6 to 8 hours. After soaking is complete, rinse the beans well with filtered water.

Cook and Rinse

To cook, transfer the beans to a large pot after rinsing and cover with 3 times the amount of water. Bring the water to a boil, then reduce heat to a simmer, cover and let simmer for 45 min to 1 hour. Stirring them a few times throughout the process will ensure faster, more uniform cooking. Some stovetops are more powerful than others so start checking the beans for doneness at around the 40 minute mark. When they are tender, remove them from heat and drain them in a colander in the sink again. Rinse with cold water and allow to drain well before storing.

Store

Cooked beans can be stored in a covered container (with a good seal), in the fridge, for up to 5 days. Sprinkle over salads or make hummus and black bean dip. Freshly-cooked garbanzos are great on their own too just after you rinse them.

To freeze, let the beans cool completely and portion into freezer bags, making sure to lay them flat in the freezer until the beans are frozen. This will ensure easy separation when you're ready to use them. Just drop the bag on the counter to loosen them up and add directly to the pot or let them thaw in a covered container in the fridge to use them in salads or hummus.

Soups and Stews: Nutritious Bowl Fare

When I was growing up, my mom worked a lot. She had already left for work in the morning before I woke up for school; and more times than not, she wouldn't get home until after dinner. And then she would prepare our dinners for the next few days: beans, soups, and various other warm, wholesome one-bowl meal deals that she would make enough of to last us at least 3 meals. We all had our favorites from her repertoire, and we also had our not-so-favorites. But the versatility of "bowl fare" lends itself perfectly in our busy lives to give us quality nutrition in a fast and delicious format. Making a pot of soup or chili ahead of time will reduce the chances of having to "order out" or "pick something up" in response to, *I'm too exhausted to make dinner.*

Any of the recipes in this section can be made fresh for dinner tonight, or allowed to cool after cooking and refrigerated for quick meals over the next few days. Just make sure you don't reheat them in the microwave, please (Google it, or I'll never finish this book). You'll notice that all recipes start off pretty much the same way; onions and/or garlic sautéed in coconut oil. Nothing flavors a soup or stew quite like cooked onions and garlic, and we *know* this because there are shelves on top of shelves at the grocery store filled with various powders and mixes trying to imitate the real deal. In some recipes I have called for *granulated garlic,* a term which some brands use for garlic powder. Be sure you're only buying organic garlic whether it's fresh or in dehydrated form, and also avoid garlic powder that contains any other ingredients besides "garlic".

Mîncărică de Cartofi (Potato Stew)
Serves 6 to 8
Pairs well with chicken

Another staple I loved growing up. Make any of the following recipes on Sunday to help you eat wholesomely for the first couple of days of the week. They can even be pre-portioned in glassware with tight-fighting lids and frozen. To thaw, just dip the bottom of the container in hot water to release the meal and reheat on low on the stovetop for 6 to 10 minutes.

2 to 3 pounds potatoes of your choice
1/2 cup coconut oil
1 large yellow onion, peeled and finely chopped
4 carrots, peeled and thinly diced
1 (4 ounce) jar organic tomato paste
2 tsp pink salt
filtered water
2 Tbsp dry organic dillweed

Rinse potatoes well and remove any obvious blemishes; cube and set aside (you can peel them if you wish or just leave the skin on for extra fiber, calcium, iron, vitamin C, etc.) In a large stainless steel pot, warm coconut oil on low-medium heat until melted and add the onions. Cook for about 5 minutes, stirring often to prevent scorching and add the tomato paste, stirring until oil and paste are well-blended. Add the carrots, potatoes and enough filtered water to just cover the contents of the pot. Cover the pot and simmer for about 45 minutes until potatoes are tender. Remove from heat and stir in the dry dill weed. Serve warm or refrigerate once stew cools to room temperature. I have left it on the counter overnight to cool when I've made it late in the evening, and refrigerated it first thing in the morning without any worry of spoilage.

To reheat, laddle the desired amount into a glass or stainless steel saucepan and warm on low-medium heat until desired temperature is reached.

Ghiveci de Fasole Verde (Stewed Green Beans)
Serves 6 to 8
Pairs well with sausages and chocken

1/3 cup coconut oil
1 medium yellow onion, finely chopped
4 carrots, diced
1 (4 ounce) jar organic tomato paste
2 tsp pink salt
2 to 3 cups filtered water
2 1/2 pounds frozen organic green beans, chopped into 1 inch pieces
2 Tbsp dry organic dillweed

In a large stainless steel pot, warm coconut oil on low-medium heat until melted and add the onions. Cook for about 5 minutes, stirring often to prevent scorching and add the tomato paste and pink salt, stirring until oil and paste are well-blended. Add the carrots, and frozen green beans, and filtered water to barely cover the beans. Stir beans into tomato sauce. Cover and simmer for 35 to 45 minutes or until beans are tender. When done, remove from heat and add the dill. Serve warm or refrigerate once stew cools to room temperature. To reheat, laddle the desired amount into a glass or stainless steel saucepan and warm on low-medium heat until desired temperature is reached.

Panang Curried Lentils
Serves 6 to 8

1/3 cup coconut oil
1 medium onion, finely chopped
1 (4 ounce) jar red curry paste (Thai Kitchen)
1 (15 ounce) can full fat coconut milk (Thai Kitchen)
2 cups lentils, cooked per package instructions, and drained

In a 3 quart stainless steel saucepan, warm coconut oil on low-medium heat until melted and add the onions. Cook for about 5 minutes, stirring often to prevent scorching. Add the curry paste, stirring until oil and paste are well-blended. Add the coconut milk and pre-cooked lentils to the curry and stir to incorporate. The curry paste should provide the bulk of salt for this dish, but feel free pink salt it to your taste if it's too bland. Cover and simmer another 10 to 15 minute on low, stirring once or twice. Serve on its own with SatFatRox Biscuits or over a freshly-baked potato.

Green Curry and Garbanzos
Serves 6 to 8

1/3 cup coconut oil
1 medium onion, finely chopped
4 cloves raw garlic, peeled, crushed and minced
1 (4 ounce) jar green curry paste (Thai Kitchen)
1 (15 ounce) can full fat coconut milk (Thai Kitchen)
4 cups cooked garbanzo beans
4 small red potatoes, boiled
pink salt to taste

In a 3 quart stainless steel saucepan, warm coconut oil on low-medium heat until melted and add the onions and garlic. Cook for about 5 minutes, stirring often to prevent scorching. Add the curry paste, stirring until oil and paste are well-blended. Cube the cooked potatoes and add them, the coconut milk and the beans to the curry stirring to incorporate. Cover and simmer another 10 to 15 minute on low, stirring once or twice. Pair with Salad For Dinner. Full. Meal. Deal.

Mîncărică de Morcovi (Carrot Stew)
Serves 4 to 6
Pairs well with chicken.

1/3 cup coconut oil
1 medium onion, finely chopped
4 cloves raw garlic, peeled, crushed and minced
1 (4 ounce) jar organic tomato paste
8 medium carrots, peeled and coarsley grated
1 cup filtered water
2 tsp pink salt
1 Tbsp dry or fresh organic dillweed

In a 3 quart stainless steel saucepan, warm coconut oil on low-medium heat until melted and add the onions and garlic. Cook for about 5 minutes, stirring often to prevent scorching. Add the pink salt, tomato paste and water, stirring until oil and paste are well-blended. Add the grated carrots and simmer on low, covered, for about 35 minutes. Add more water if necessary to create desired amount of sauce. Remove from heat when carrots are tender and add dill, stirring to incorporate.

Buy All of Your Produce and Staples Organic as Often as Possible, if Not Always

Varsă Călită (Stewed Cabbage)
Serves 6 to 8

1/3 cup coconut oil
1 medium onion, finely chopped
1 (4 ounce) jar organic tomato paste
1 whole green cabbage, shredded
1 cup filtered water
2 tsp pink salt
1 tsp black pepper

In a 3 quart stainless steel saucepan, warm coconut oil on low-medium heat until melted and add the onions and garlic. Cook for about 5 minutes, stirring often to prevent scorching. Add the tomato paste, salt, and water, stirring until oil and paste are well-blended. Add the cabbage and pepper and stir well. Cover and simmer for 35 to 45 minutes or until cabbage is tender.

Vegetable Soup
Serves 6 to 8

1/3 cup coconut oil
1 medium yellow onion, finely chopped
4 stalks celery, diced
4 carrots, diced
6 medium red potatoes, raw, washed and cubed
1 (4 ounce) jar organic tomato paste
3 tsp pink salt
4 to 6 cups filtered water
1 1/2 pounds frozen organic green beans, chopped into 1 inch pieces
2 Tbsp dry organic parsley

In a large stainless steel pot, warm coconut oil on low-medium heat until melted and add the onions and celery. Cook for about 5 minutes, stirring often to prevent scorching and add the tomato paste and pink salt, stirring until oil and paste are well-blended. Add the carrots, green beans, potatoes and filtered water, stirring to incorporate everything. Cover and simmer for 35 to 45 minutes or until potatoes are tender. When done, remove from heat and add the parsley. Serve warm or refrigerate once soup cools to room temperature. To reheat, laddle the desired amount into a glass or stainless steel saucepan and warm on low-medium heat until desired temperature is reached.

SatFatRox Serendipity!

Thanksgiving Stuffing
Serves 4 to 6

You'll be making your own bread cubes with day-old biscuits, sliced down the middle and cubed. Arrange them in a single layer on a jelly roll pan and dry them out in the oven at 250 degrees Fahrenheit for about an hour, flipping them over midway through.

1 dozen SatFatRox Biscuits or SatFatRox Rolls
1/3 cup coconut oil
1 small onion, finely chopped
4 stalks celery, finely chopped
1 1/2 tsp pink salt
2 tsp dried sage
1/2 tsp poultry seasoning
1/2 tsp black pepper
2 - 2 1/2 cups filtered water

Preheat oven to 350°F and grease a 3 quart casserole dish with coconut oil or just use the stainless steel saucepan you will cook the onions in. In a 3 quart stainless steel saucepan, warm coconut oil on low-medium heat until melted, add the onions and celery. Cook for about 5 minutes until the onions are clear, stirring often to prevent scorching. Add the pink salt, sage, seasonings and water and simmer covered on low heat for another 8 to 10 minutes. Add the biscuit cubes and stir quickly and coat evenly with onion mixture. Place dressing in the greased casserole dish and cover with aluminum foil, or leave stuffing in the saucepan and cover with foil. Bake for 30 minutes on middle rack, and allow to sit for 5 minutes, covered before serving.

Banza™ Pasta Made From Chickpeas!

A week before the scheduled launch of this book, I had the unbelievably good fortune (thank you for following SatFatRox Radio on Twitter, guys!) of finding out about Banza, a pasta made from chickpeas, the phenomenal creation of Brian and Scott Rudolph, two brothers from Detroit, Michigan. I immediately ordered a 6-box pack of rotini and waited with bated breath for its arrival, as my daughters and I had not indulged in one of our favorite gluten foods in over almost 2 years.

Our order was one of a significant enough number of orders received that first week to delay its normal arrival. The brothers kept us in the loop though and we received our serendipity about a week and a half later. Every day leading up to the delivery date when we received a boxed delivery (we're Amazon.com folk), my girls would squeal *The Banza's here!* Even when the package was clearly too small to hold 6 boxes of pasta. The day it finally arrived, I found it on our doorstep, but didn't realize what it was until I tapped it gently with my foot (I had grocery bags in both hands), to reveal the melodious rattle that hadn't been heard in our house since we had gone grain-free. I open the door and squealed *The Banza's here!*

It was 11 in the morning and they couldn't wait for dinner, demanding the Banza even if I didn't have time to make my Marinara Sauce (page 229) to accompany it. I'm going to give you a couple quick tips to make sure you prepare your Banza beautifully from the very first box.

1. Banza doesn't have to be boiled the way grain pasta does, but you do have to make sure the water is about as close to boiling as possible before adding the pasta to it.

2. Make sure you have enough water in the pot to cover the Banza by about an inch and a half to ensure proper cooking, quickly.

3. So if you're going to prepare an entire box of Banza (8 ounces dry, 4 servings total), I personally recommend you use a 3 quart saucepan filled with about 2 1/2 quarts of water, salted with 1 teaspoon of pink salt.

4. As soon as the water is about to boil, turn the burner off and add the Banza to the water. Stir once and set the timer to 4 minutes. Stir again when the timer goes off and test a piece of pasta to see if the tenderness is to your liking. If it's not, add another 2- 4 minutes to the timer and retest.

5. Drain when cooked and use exactly the same way you would use the grain variety. In fact, we even substituted it for the potatoes in the Mediterranean Salad, and it was exceptional.

Banza currently comes in rotini and penne varieties and can be ordered online in multiples of 6. Visit www.EatBanza.com and don't forget to tell them who sent you! We've since placed another order for 24 boxes.

Breads and Biscuits

With all the awareness being raised about gluten intolerance nowadays, it's hard to imagine adopting the new lifestyle and forever giving up comfort foods like bread and rolls. When I first started scouring the net for "gluten-free" bread recipes, I came across one that called for rice flour and powdered skim milk. Needless to say, the skim milk never made it into my version, and as the months wore on and my study of gluten continued, the rice flour eventually found its way out too. This recipe has gone through so many revisions and modifications since the first time I made it in October of 2012 to make sure it was really ready for prime time. That being said, there are some key things to remember to make sure it turns out perfectly every time:

1. Make sure you preheat the oven, and then turn it off so that you can "proof" the rolls prior to baking. Proofing will ensure that the rolls bake evenly and aren't too dense.

2. Don't use the microwave to heat your water or melt the coconut oil. Research shows that the microwave can reach temperatures that can damage any kind of oil, including coconut, as well as disrupting the molecular structure of even water. Use your stove top and always heat or cook on low to low-medium.

3. Always pour the flour into your measuring cup as opposed to scooping it up. When you scoop you're actually compressing more flour into the measure than if you poured it in and that will definitely affect the consistency of the batter/dough, and subsequently the texture and density of your rolls.

4. Use silicone bakeware set on top of an insulated cookie sheet. Have a second cookie sheet ready to place on the rack above the rolls in case they brown too quickly. Remember the Maillard Reaction is responsible for the browning of baked goods and cooked foods, and the browner something gets, the greater the
carcinogenic acrylamide content.

5. Allow rolls to cool for at least 20 minutes before you smear some coconut oil on them to minimize the possibility of that "doughy" texture.

Visit www.SatFatRox.com for step-by-step pictures of the process and stay tuned for the webcast in the near future!

Buy All of Your Produce and Staples Organic as Often as Possible, if Not Always

SatFatRox Rolls
Makes about 24 rolls

Preheat oven to 350°F and turn it off once it has reached said temperature. While the oven is preheating, heat on stove top:

2 cups filtered water

Once it reaches about 105°F or the temperature of bath water, pour 1 cup of it into a 3 cup glass bowl and stir with a wire whisk to dissolve:

1 Tbsp raw honey
3 tsp dry yeast

Cover the yeast with a tea towel and place in a warm place to rise for about 10 minutes or until almost doubled in volume with foam. (I set mine on a trivet on the stove as the oven is heating.) In the remaining water you warmed in the saucepan, add the following and then remove from heat. (If the water is too hot, you'll end up killing the yeast when you blend it with the dry ingredients) :

1 1/2 tsp Himalayan Pink Salt
2 Tbsp raw honey

Whisk until totally dissolved, and add:

1/4 cup coconut oil

Measure in the bowl of a stand mixer (preferably a KitchenAid because they're still made in the USA!) and whisk until well incorporated:

1 1/2 cups tapioca flour
1 cup organic coconut flour
3/4 cup garbanzo bean flour
2 1/2 tsp xanthan gum

Add the yeast and the water/oil/salt/honey mixture to the dry ingredients, making sure you used a rubber or silicone spatula to scrape as much of the water and yeast out of the containers as possible. Attach the paddle and mix the dough on low speed for about 20 seconds and then medium for another 30 seconds. Scrape the bowl to make sure there is no flour remaining on the sides. If dough is too dry, slowly add another 1/4 of water until it's a little softer but not overly sticky. Using a spring-loaded 2.6 ounce ice cream scoop, fill a silicone muffin pan with the dough and place in the warm oven on an insulated cookie sheet, on the middle or upper middle rack. Set timer to 20 minutes. Once the timer goes off, turn the oven back on to 350°F and set timer for 30 minutes. Midway through the bake time, rotate the cookie sheet for even exposure and place the protective cookie sheet on the top rack if needed. Remove from oven and allow to cool for 5 minutes before transfering to cooling racks and allowing them to cool upside down. Store cooled rolls in an airtight container in the fridge for up to 5 days. To reheat, slice down the middle and warm in the toaster oven.

Focaccia

Grease a 10 by 13 inch glass baking dish with palm shortening and prepare the dough for SatFatRox Rolls. Spread the dough in the baking dish, smoothing the top with a rubber spatula. Brush the dough with Garlic Butter (page), and sprinkle 1/2 teaspoon of dried rosemary on top. Proof and bake as above.

For Roasted Garlic Focaccia:

Separate 2 heads of galric into cloves but do not peel them. Cut off the hard base of each clove (about 3 mm), just exposing the inside of the clove. Place cloves on a sheet of aluminum foil and gather the sides to seal the garlic inside (cinch and twist the foil just above the cloves). Roast in a 350°F oven for 35 minutes. Pop the softened cloves out of their shells and set aside. Grease a 10 by 13 inch glass baking dish with palm shortening and prepare the dough for SatFatRox Rolls, adding the roasted garlic cloves to the dough for the last 10 seconds of mixing. Spread the dough in the baking dish, smoothing the top with a rubber spatula. Brush with palm shortening and sprinkle with pink salt. Proof and bake as above.

Cinnamon Raisin Buns

Cover 1 1/2 cups organic raisins with warm water and soak for 20 minutes. Drain and set aside. Prepare the dough for SatFatRox Rolls, adding 1 teaspoon Ceylon or cassia cinnamon to the flour mixture, and 3 tablespoons of honey to the coconut oil water (keep the honey to raise the yeast at 1 tablespoon). Add the raisins to the dough during the last 30 seconds of mixing. Proof and bake as above.

SatFatRox Biscuits
Makes 18 to 20

This version of the traditional baking powder biscuit is going to become a staple in your house. We make them almost every day, and once a week spice it up with the Garlic and Herb modification.

1 cup coconut flour
1 ½ cup tapioca flour
1 cup garbanzo bean flour
½ cup potato starch
2 Tbsp Hain Featherweight baking powder
2 tsp xanthan gum
2 tsp pink salt
2/3 cup palm shortening or coconut oil
2 ½ to 2 ¾ cups filtered water

Preheat oven to 350°F and line two insulated cookie sheets with silicone baking mats. In a large bowl, whisk together all of the dry ingredients, making sure they are uniformly blended. Using a pastry blender, cut in the palm shortening until completely blended and the mixture looks mealy. Make a well in the center of the flour and pour the filtered water in all at once. Using a heavy metal serving or wooden spoon, quickly mix the flour into the water until well blended, but be careful to not over-mix. Drop by ¼ cup scoops onto baking sheets about an inch apart and bake for 35 minutes on middle rack. Allow to cool 10 to 15 minutes before serving.

Garlic and Herb Biscuits

Prepare as above and add 1 tablespoon organic garlic granules and 1 tablespoon organic dry dillweed to the flour before cutting in palm shortening.

Sun-Dried Tomato and Herb Biscuits

Prepare as above, soaking 1/2 cup organic sun-dried tomatoes in the 2 1/2 cups of water that you will use for the biscuits, for 20 minutes. Spoon out the tomatoes and chop. Add 1 teaspoon of each to the flour mixture before cutting in shortening: dried oregano, dried basil, garlic granules. Add the tomatoes back to the water and bake as above.

Grain-Free Potato Biscuits

For the people who believe they may be allergic to coconut, this recipe is for you. Although I whole-heartedly believe your reactions are coming from either the sulfites that shredded coconut is treated with or other allergens like soy, gluten, and casein.

2/3 cup potato flour
1 ½ cup tapioca flour
1 ¼ cup garbanzo bean flour
¼ cup potato starch
2 Tbsp Hain Featherweight baking powder
2 tsp xanthan gum
2 tsp pink salt
2/3 cup palm shortening
2 2/3 cup filtered water

Preheat oven to 350°F and line two insulated cookie sheets with silicone baking mats. In a large bowl, whisk together all of the dry ingredients, making sure they are uniformly blended. Using a pastry blender, cut in the palm shortening until completely blended and the mixture looks mealy. Make a well in the center of the flour and pour the filtered water in all at once. Using a heavy metal serving or wooden spoon, quickly mix the flour into the water until well blended, but be careful to not over-mix. Drop by 1/4 cup scoops onto baking sheets about an inch apart and bake for 35 minutes on middle rack. Allow to cool 10 to 15 minutes before serving.

Pancakes/Waffles

Whisk together in a medium mixing bowl:

1/2 cup tapioca flour
1/2 cup garbanzo bean flour
1/2 cup coconut flour
1/8 cup potato starch
1 Tbsp GRAIN-free baking powder (Hain Featherweight)
1/4 tsp xanthan gum

Bring the following ingredients to room temperature:

1 1/2 cups coconut milk, whisked with 1 Tbsp Bragg's Raw Apple Cider Vinegar
2 organic eggs, beaten well
2 tsp vanilla extract (not artificial!)

Melt on low heat in a heavy saucepan (turn burner on very low and remove pan from burner as soon as oil is melted):
3 Tbsp coconut oil
2 Tbsp honey

Pour the "sour" coconut milk into the saucepan and whisk with the oil and honey until smooth and blended.

Add the room temperature beaten eggs to the coconut milk mixture and whisk well again. Pour the contents of the saucepan (sour coconut milk, coconut oil, honey, beaten eggs, vanilla) into the dry ingredients and whisk until incorporated.

Heat coconut oil on low heat in a non-toxic, non-Teflon 10 inch frying pan, using about ½ tsp of oil for every three pancakes cooked. Use 1/4 cup of batter to cook 3 pancakes at a time, flipping pancakes over when the batter loses its gloss (about 2 to 3 minutes). Do not exceed low-medium heat, and do not over-cook.

Notes:
Make coconut milk using: 1 can full fat Thai Kitchen coconut milk and ½ can water. Whisk together well and refrigerate in a tightly covered in a glass mason jar for up to 5 days.

Notes

_____
_____
_____
_____
_____
_____
_____
_____
_____
_____
_____
_____
_____
_____
_____
_____
_____
_____
_____
_____
_____
_____
_____
_____
_____
_____
_____
_____
_____

Buy All of Your Produce and Staples Organic as Often as Possible, if Not Always

Notes

Dips, Dressings, and Spreads

Hummus

3 cups cooked, drained, garbanzo beans
1/4 cup lemon juice, freshly squeezed is best!
2 to 4 cloves garlic, peeled
2 tsp pink salt or to taste
2 Tbsp tahini (sesame seed paste)
1/2 to 1 tsp ground cumin, to taste
1/8 tsp ground cayenne, or to taste
1/4 cup California extra virgin olive oil
2 to 4 Tbsp filtered water, or more as needed
Paprika and dried parsley to garnish

In the bowl of a food processor, add the garlic and pulse to mince. Add in the beans, lemon juice, pink salt, tahini, cumin, and cayenne. Process until a paste forms and drizzle the olive oil in while continuing to process. Add in filtered water, a little at a time, until desired consistency is reached. Serve at room temperature drizzled with more olive oil, if desired, and sprinkled with paprika and parsley.

Kalamata Olive Hummus

Once desired consistency of hummus is achieved by the addition of the 2-4 tablespoons of filtered water, add 1/3 of a cup coarsely chopped Kalamata olives and pulse just enough to incorporate the olives.

Roasted Red Pepper Hummus

Instead of filtered water to thin the consistency, use the juice from Peloponnese brand Whole Roasted Sweet Peppers. Chop 2 whole peppers in smaller pieces and add to the hummus, pulsing just a few times to incorporate and reach your desired texture.

Sun-Dried Tomato Hummus

Coarsely chop ¼ cup sun-dried tomatoes and soak in ¼ cup filtered water for about 30 minutes. Add the entire mixture (tomatoes and soak water) to the bean paste after the first round of processing, omitting the addition of the plain filtered water.
weeks. Recipe can be doubled. Yes, it's that easy.

Guacamole

3 avocados, peeled, pitted, and mashed
1 lime, juiced
1 small red onion
3 Tbsp fresh cilantro, chopped
2 roma (plum) tomatoes, diced
3 cloves garlic, peeled, crushed and minced
1/8 tsp ground cayenne
1/2 tsp pink salt

In a medium bowl, mash together the avocados, lime juice, and salt. Mix in onion, cilantro, tomatoes, and garlic. Stir in cayenne pepper. Refrigerate 1 hour for best flavor, or serve immediately.

Tomato Artichoke Sauté

1/3 cup coconut oil
1 small onion, finely chopped
4 cloves raw garlic, peeled, crushed and minced
1 (4 ounce) jar organic tomato paste
1/2 cup filtered water
1/2 tsp pink salt
1 (6 ounce) jar of marinated artichoke hearts, drained and chopped
1 tsp dried parsley

In a 1 quart stainless steel saucepan, warm coconut oil on low-medium heat until melted and add the onions and garlic. Cook for about 6 to 8 minutes until onions are fragrant, stirring often to prevent scorching. Add the tomato paste, salt, parsley, and water, stirring until oil and paste are well-blended. Add the artichokes and simmer on low heat for 5 to 8 minutes. Serve with sliced and toasted SatFatRox Biscuits or Rolls.

Honey Mustard Dressing

1/2 cup California extra virgin olive oil
1/4 cup raw honey
1/4 cup Dijon mustard

Whisk together ingredients in 2-cup glass measuring cup, cover and refrigerate for up to 3 weeks. Yes, it's that easy.

Marinara Sauce
Perfect for dipping Foccacia and Biscuits and for BANZA! (page 290)

1/3 cup coconut oil
1 medium onion, finely chopped
4 cloves raw garlic, peeled, crushed and minced
1 (4 ounce) jar organic tomato paste
1 Tbsp dry organic oregano
1 Tbsp dry organic sweet basil
1 1/2 cups filtered water
1 tsp pink salt, or to taste
1/2 tsp black pepper

In a 2 quart stainless steel saucepan, warm coconut oil on low-medium heat until melted and add the onions and garlic. Cook for about 6 to 8 minutes until onions are clear, stirring often to prevent scorching. Add the tomato paste, salt, herbs, and water, stirring until oil and paste are well-blended. Cover and simmer on low for 20 minutes.

Spinach Artichoke Dip

1 Tbsp garbanzo bean flour
1 Tbsp tapioca starch
2 (10 ounce) bags frozen spinach, thawed
1/3 cup coconut oil
1 small onion, finely chopped
4 cloves raw garlic, peeled, crushed, and minced
1/2 cup full fat coconut milk
1/2 tsp pink salt
1 (14.5 ounce) jar artichoke hearts, MariaJesus brand
1 lemon, juiced
1/8 tsp cayenne

Buy All of Your Produce and Staples Organic as Often as Possible, if Not Always

Whisk flours together and set aside. Press water out of spinach and chop, removing any large stems. drain the artichoke hearts and process them in the food processor for about 45 seconds. In a 3 quart stainless steel saucepan, warm coconut oil on low-medium heat until melted; add the onions and garlic and cook for about 5-8 minutes. Whisk in the flour stirring constantly. Before the flour gets lumpy, whisk in the coconut milk and continue stirring until thickened, about another minute. Add the spinach, pink salt and pepper, tirring until well blended. Transfer the entire mixture to the artichokes in the food processor, add the lemon juice and pulse until creamy. Serve with toasted SatFatRox Biscuits or Rolls, or on top of a baked potato.

Roasted Garlic Butter

1 head roasted garlic
1/4 to 1/2 tsp pink salt
1 tsp parsley flakes
1/4 tsp paprika
1/2 cup palm shortening
1/8 cup coconut oil

Pop the garlic cloves out of their shells and process in mini food processor with salt, parsley and paprika. Let stand for 10 minutes to allow the salt for dissolve. Add the palm shortening and coconut oil and process for another 30 seconds. Empty butter into a 2 cup glass container, with a tight-fitting lid, and refrigerate. Keeps for up to a week. Use on SatFatRox Biscuits, rolls, baked or pan-fried potatoes.

Quick Garlic Butter

1/2 cup palm shortening
1/4 tsp pink salt
1 tsp garlic granules
1/4 tsp paprika
1 tsp parsley flakes

Whip shortening in a 1-cup custard cup with a spoon until light; add the salt, garlic, paprika and parsley and mix well. Store covered in the fridge for up to 3 weeks.

Cinnamon Butter

1 cup coconut oil
1/4 cup cinnamon*, (preferrable Ceylon but definitely not Saigon)
1 Tbsp raw honey (or Canadian Frontier)**

Mix all three ingredients together well and store on the counter in a glass container with tight-fitting lid indefinitely.

Peanut Butter

I know there's some concern out there about the aflotoxin that grows on peanuts, it happens to be on the Proposition 65 list of chemicals known to the state of California to cause cancer. Here's the deal: Valencia peanuts are the only variety that do not harbor aflotoxin. When a California Valenica peanut farmer decides to start making powdered Valencia peanut butter, angels will sing. Until then, ditch the conventional stuff that's loaded with oxidized polyunsaturated oil, and opt for still getting the fiber and protein of peanut butter, with a rock solid dose of coconut oil. Amen.

1 cup coconut oil
1 to 1 1/2 cups powdered peanut butter (TruNut or PB2)

Blend oil and powdered peanut butter until smooth in a 3-cup glass cotainer with a tight-fitting lid (or at least one big enough so you can mix it properly). Store on the counter for up to a week. Refrigerate if you're not going to consume it within that time frame. It will harden considerably in the fridge; just let it sit on the counter for about 5 minutes before you dig in.

* Order at www.CinnamonVogue.com
** Order at www.SatFatRox.com/the-store

Buy All of Your Produce and Staples Organic as Often as Possible, if Not Always

Coconut Nibtella

1 cup coconut oil
1/2 cup powdered peanut butter
1/2 cup unsweetened shredded coconut
1/2 cup raw cacao nibs
a splash of organic maple syrup
1 tsp alcohol-free vanilla extract (no corn syrup!)
6 to 8 drops liquid stevia, any flavor you'd like

Mix all ingredients together and store in a glass container with a tight-fitting lid in the fridge. Keeps for several weeks, but should be enjoyed often, by the spoonful or on sliced Granny Smith apples.

Desserts

All of the baked goods in this section have a few fantastic things going for them:

1. They're made with heat stable fats and oils that will protect the protein and natural sugars in the recipes, while also satisfying you with considerably fewer servings.

2. They're not made with almond meal, a source of oxidized unsaturated fatty acids.

3. They're loaded with protein and fiber from the garbanzo bean and coconut flours; and *pre*-biotics from the potato starch, making them way easier on the blood sugar than anything else dessert-like you could indulge in. The first five recipes are transitional recipes to getting you off of sugar, even "natural sweeteners" like honey. Enjoy!

Chocolate Chip Cookies
Makes about 4 dozen

I don't think I've ever made a cookie this true to the classic everyone imagines. Even when I used to bake with white flour, my chocolate chip cookies were mediocre at best. Be careful to not over-bake them, and make sure you let them cool on the cookie sheet completely before transferring them to a cooling rack.

1 cup organic palm shortening
3/4 cup raw honey
1/8 cup organic molasses
2 tsp real vanilla extract
1 egg, preferably organic
1 tsp Stevita Spoonable stevia
1/4 tsp pink salt
2/3 cup coconut flour
1/2 cup garbanzo bean flour
1 cup tapioca flour
1 1/2 tsp xanthan gum
1 tsp baking soda
1 tsp Hain Featherweight Grain Free baking powder
¾ cup semi-sweet chocolate chips (without soy or dairy ingredients)

Preheat oven to 350°F. Cream first four ingredients in the bowl of a stand mixer until light and fluffy. Add the egg, stevia, and pink salt and cream on medium for about a minute. Sift the flours, xanthan, baking soda and baking powder in a separate bowl and whisk together well until blended. Add the dry ingredients and the chocolate chips to the honey/shortening cream and mix on low until completely mixed. Be sure to scrape the bottom of the bowl with a spatula to ensure all the shortening has been incorporated with the flour. Drop by spoonfuls onto silicone baking mat lined cookie sheets, about an inch apart. Bake for 11 to 13 minutes on the middle rack. Insulated cookie sheets will require closer to 13 minutes.

Snickerdoodles
Makes about 4 dozen

The measurements of the flours look a little OCD but the alternative would require you owning a digital kitchen scale. Make sure you use potato starch, not potato flour as there is a difference between the two. Don't omit the cream of tartar as it gives the Snickerdoodle its signature bite. The organic sugar on top is optional- they're just as yum sprinkled only with cinnamon.

1 cup organic palm shortening
1 cup raw honey
2 tsp real vanilla extract
1 egg, preferably organic
1 tsp Stevita Spoonable stevia
¼ tsp pink salt
½ cup and 2 Tbsp coconut flour
½ cup and 2 Tbsp garbanzo bean flour
3/4 cup tapioca flour
¼ cup potato starch
1 ½ tsp xanthan gum
1 ½ tsp baking soda
½ tsp cream of tartar
1 Tbsp organic sugar
1 tsp ground cinnamon

Preheat oven to 350°F. Cream first three ingredients in the bowl of a stand mixer until light and fluffy. Add the egg, stevia, and pink salt and cream on medium for about a minute. Sift the flours, xanthan, baking soda and cream of tartar in a separate bowl and whisk together well until blended. Add the dry ingredients to the honey/shortening cream and mix on low until completely mixed. Be sure to scrape the bottom of the bowl with a spatula to ensure all the shortening has been incorporated with the flour. Drop by spoonfuls onto silicone baking mat lined cookie sheets, about an inch apart. Flatten one cookie with the bottom of a glass and then dip the glass in cinnamon sugar and proceed to flatten the rest, re-dipping the bottom of the glass before each one. Bake for 12 to 14 minutes on the middle rack. Insulated cookie sheets will require closer to 14 minutes.

Peanut Butter Cookies
Makes about 4 dozen.

1 cup organic palm shortening
¾ cup raw honey
1/8 cup organic molasses
2 tsp real vanilla extract
¾ cup powdered peanut butter
2 eggs, preferably organic
1 tsp Stevita Spoonable stevia
¼ tsp pink salt
¾ cup coconut flour
½ cup garbanzo bean flour
1 cup tapioca flour
¼ cup potato starch
1 ½ tsp xanthan gum
1 tsp baking soda
½ tsp Hain Featherweight Grain Free baking powder

Preheat oven to 350°F. Cream first five ingredients in the bowl of a stand mixer until light and fluffy. Add the egg, stevia, and pink salt and cream on medium for about a minute. Measure the flours by pouring into the measuring cups, not scooping/packing. Combine flours, xanthan, baking soda and baking powder in a separate bowl and whisk together well until blended. Add the dry ingredients to the honey/shortening cream and mix on low until completely mixed. Be sure to scrape the bottom of the bowl with a spatula to ensure all the shortening has been incorporated with the flour. Drop by spring-loaded mini ice cream scoops onto silicone baking mat lined cookie sheets, about an inch apart. Press with a fork to make the signature peanut butter cookie criss-cross pattern. Bake for 10 to 12 minutes on the middle rack. Insulated cookie sheets will require closer to 12 minutes.

Double Chocolate Chunk Cookies
Makes about 4 dozen.

1 cup organic palm shortening
3/4 cup raw honey
1/4 cup organic molasses
2 tsp real vanilla extract
2 tsp Stevita Spoonable stevia
3/4 cup organic raw cacao powder
1 egg, preferably organic
1/4 tsp pink salt
1/2 cup coconut flour
1/2 cup garbanzo bean flour
1 cup tapioca flour
1 1/2 tsp xanthan gum
1 tsp baking soda
1 1/2 tsp Hain Featherweight Grain Free baking powder
3/4 cup Enjoy Life chocolate chunks

Preheat oven to 350°F. Cream first four ingredients in the bowl of a stand mixer until light and fluffy. Add the egg, stevia, and pink salt and cream on medium for about a minute. Sift the flours, xanthan, baking soda and baking powder in a separate bowl and whisk together well until blended. Add the dry ingredients and the chocolate chunks to the honey/shortening cream and mix on low until completely mixed. Be sure to scrape the bottom of the bowl with a spatula to ensure all the shortening has been incorporated with the flour. Drop by spoonful onto silicone baking mat lined cookie sheets, about an inch apart. Bake for 11 to 13 minutes on the middle rack. Insulated cookie sheets will require closer to 13 minutes.

Chocolate Cupcakes
Makes about 24

Preheat the oven to 350°F and prepare 24 muffin liners (get the aluminum foil ones that can just be placed on top of a cookie sheet or invest in reusable silicone ones). When measuring the flour, pour it into the measuring cup, don't scoop it out of the bag or container.

Sift or whisk dry ingredients in the bowl of a stand mixer:

1 cup coconut flour
1 cup tapioca flour
3/4 cup garbanzo flour
3/4 cup cacao powder, preferably raw organic but Hershey's will work too
1 1/2 tsp xanthan gum
2 tsp baking soda

In a medium saucepan on the stove top, on low heat, combine and stir until everything is completely dissolved but do not allow to simmer:

1 cup filtered water
3/4 cup raw honey
1 Tbsp. Stevita Spoonable Powdered Stevia
1/2 tsp pink salt

Remove from heat and add, stirring until the coconut oil is melted:

2 Tbsp real vanilla extract
2/3 cup coconut oil

Then add and whisk well:

3/4 cup filtered water (yes, more water)
3/4 cup organic unsweetened applesauce
2 Tbsp apple cider vinegar

Pour the entire liquid mixture over the dry and use the paddle attachment to blend for about 30 seconds. Scrape the side and bottom of the bowl with a rubber spatula to make sure everything is well incorporated.Quickly get the batter into the liners and the muffins into the preheated oven so you don't lose the rising power of the baking soda.

Buy All of Your Produce and Staples Organic as Often as Possible, if Not Always

Using a 1/3 cup spring loaded scoop (Vollrath or Pampered Chef), fill the muffin liners and bake on the center rack for 25 to 30 minutes. Check for doneness when a toothpick inserted in the middle of the middle muffin comes out relatively clean. Wait no more than 5 minutes after taking muffins out of the oven to transfer to cooling rack. Allow to cool completely before eating (about 30 minutes).

Carrot Muffins (or cake!)
Makes 20 muffins or 2 (8 inch) rounds

15 pitted dates, soaked in hot water for 20 minutes
1 1/2 cups organic apple sauce
1 tsp Stevita Spoonable stevia
2/3 cup melted coconut oil
2 cups carrots, finely shredded

1/2 cup coconut flour
1/2 cup garbanzo bean flour
3/4 cup tapioca flour
1/2 cup potato starch
2 tsp cinnamon
2 tsp Hain Featherweight Grain Free baking powder
1 1/2 tsp baking soda
1 tsp xanthan gum
1/2 tsp pink salt

Preheat oven to 350°F. Sift dry ingredients together and set aside. Drain dates, chop coarsely and mince in mini food processor, scraping the sides to ensure even exposure. Add half of the applesauce to the dates and continue to process until smooth before adding the remainder. Peel and finely grate about 6 medium organic carrots. Turn date puree into the bowl of a stand mixer and add the coconut oil, carrots and flour, mixing on medium speed for about 30 seconds. Scrape the sides and bottom of bowl for evening mixing. Quickly get the batter into the liners and the muffins into the oven so you don't lose the rising power of the baking soda.Using a 1/3 cup spring loaded scoop (Vollrath or Pampered Chef), fill the muffin liners and bake on the center rack for 25 to 30 minutes.

Banana Muffins
Makes 20 or 4 mini loaves

5 very ripe bananas, medium size
2/3 cup palm shortening
1 tsp Stevita Spoonable stevia
1/2 tsp pink salt

1/2 cup garbanzo bean flour
1/2 cup coconut flour
3/4 cup tapioca starch
1/4 cup potato starch
1 tsp xanthan gum
1 tsp baking soda

Preheat oven to 350°F. Cream first four ingredients together on medium speed of stand mixer. Whisk flours together and add to the bananas; mix on medium speed for 30 seconds. Using a 1/3 cup spring loaded scoop (Vollrath or Pampered Chef), fill silicone muffin liners and bake on the center rack for 25 to 30 minutes.

Ice Cream

Yet another reason to add a KitchenAid stand mixer to your kitchen: whipping up homemade ice cream in 20 to 30 minutes. The KitchenAid Ice Cream Maker Attachment (KAICA) comes with a special bowl that you freeze about 24 hours before you're ready to churn out frozn treats using your KitchenAid stand mixer. If you already have a Cuisinart Ice Cream Maker, be sure to freeze the bowl for at least 24 hours beforehand to ensure adequate freezing potential.

Vanilla Ice Cream

2 cans full fat coconut milk (I like Thai Kitchen)
1/4 cup organic maple syrup
3 tsp alcohol-free vanilla extract and 1/2 tsp ground vanilla bean
4 raw eggs

In a wide-mouthed juice jug, whip first three ingredients on medium speed with an immersion blender for about a minute. Add the eggs and blend on low for 30 seconds. Pour into bowl of ice cream maker and allow to freeze for 20 to 30 minutes.

Buy All of Your Produce and Staples Organic as Often as Possible, if Not Always

Strawberry Ice Cream

1 pound frozen organic strawberries, thawed
2 cans full fat coconut milk
1/8 to 1/4 cup organic maple syrup
4 raw eggs
1/2 pound frozen strawberries, thawed in a separate bowl

Thaw first pound of strawberries in a widemouthed juice jug in the fridge overnight. When ready to assemble the ice cream, add the coconut milk and maple syrup to the thawed strawberries and blend with an immersion blender until smooth. Add the eggs and blend on low speed for 30 seconds. Drop the 1/2 pound of thawed strawberries into the mix and stir with a spoon. Pour into bowl of ice cream maker and allow to freeze for 20 to 30 minutes.

Chocolate Coconut Bars

40 pitted dates, soaked in hot filtered water (about 45 minutes)
1 cup organic raw cacao powder
2 tsp alcohol-free vanilla extract
1 1/2 cup cocoa butter, melted on very low heat
1 cup unsweetened coconut, finely shredded

Line an 8x8 baking pan with parchment paper. In a small saucepan, melt the cocoa butter or very low heat until entirely liquefied and wisk in the cacao powder. Cocoa butter looks like white chocolate and comes in a bucket, chips, or in chunks. If you've ordered yours in a bucket (www.BulkApothecary.com) use a strong spoon to scrape the cocoa butter into smaller chunks to measure roughly a cup and a half. Drain dates but reserve the water. Chop coarsely and process in a mini food processor until pureed, adding 1/4 cup of reserved water and pink salt to continue the process. Transfer to the bowl of a stand mixer. Whip dates for about a minute and reduce speed to low while adding vanilla extract and slowly incorporating the chocolate cocoa butter. Once blended, add the shredded coconut and whip on medium speed for 2 minutes, scraping the sides and bottom of the bowl a few times. Spread the batter in the baking pan and refrigerate for at least two hours. Cut into squares and store in an airtight container in the fridge for up to a week.

Peanut Butter Fudge

25 pitted dates, soaked in 1 cup hot filtered water (about 45 minutes)
1 cup powdered peanut butter
1 teaspoon alcohol-free vanilla extract (Trader Joe's brand)
1 1/2 cup cocoa butter, melted on very low heat

Line an 8x8 baking pan with parchment paper. In a small saucepan, melt the cocoa butter or very low heat until entirely liquefied. Cocoa butter looks like white chocolate and comes in a bucket, chips, or in chunks. If you've ordered yours in a bucket, (www.BulkApothecary.com) use a strong spoon to scrape the cocoa butter into smaller chunks to measure roughly a cup and a half. Drain dates but reserve the water. Chop coarsely and process in a mini food processor until pureed, adding 1/4 cup of reserved water to continue the process. Add 1/3 cup of the powdered peanut butter and the pink salt to the dates; process one last time before transferring to the bowl of a stand mixer. Add remainder of peanut butter powder, vanilla extract and the liquefied cocoa butter and mix on low speed for 2 minutes, scraping the sides and bottom of the bowl a few times. Pour the fudge into the baking pan and refrigerate for at least two hours. Cut into squares and store in an airtight container in the fridge for up to a week.

Peanut Butter Mousse
Serves 6 to 8

Prepare the peanut butter fudge as indicated but add the remainder of the reserved water and the pink salt and process one last time before transferring to the bowl of a stand mixer (total water should be 1 cup). Add the vanilla extract and the liquefied cocoa butter and mix on low speed for 2 minutes, cracking in 4 raw eggs and scraping the sides and bottom of the bowl a few times. Refrigerate for 2 hours and whip with the paddle of the stand mixer once more before piping into serving dishes.

Notes:
Dates can be soaked for less time depending on their hardness. I store my dates in the fridge, so they require a little more time to soften up.

Buy All of Your Produce and Staples Organic as Often as Possible, if Not Always

Smoothies and Sipables

Stevia Strawberry Lemonade
Makes 3 quarts

2 cups frozen strawberries, thawed
4 lemons at room temperature
1 teaspoon Stevita Spoonable Stevia OR 20-30 drops Stevita Liquid Stevia
6 to 8 cups filtered water

Place the frozen strawberries in a wide-mouthed 2 quart jug, cover, and allow to thaw either overnight in the fridge or on the counter for a few hours. When strawberries are ready, use a citrus juicer to juice the lemons, then add the juice to the thawed strawberries. Using an immersion blender, puree the strawberries and lemon juice until smooth and no chunks are present. Add the stevia and continue to blend. Top the mixture with filtered water and blend with immersion blender one last time. Chill covered until ready to serve. Keeps fresh for up to 3 days.

Berry Banana Akearita Mix
Makes 1 gallon

Building on the Stevia Strawberry Lemonade above, this is the mix that our entire family uses as the base of our daily Akea shake. It can be used on its own by adding one scoop of Akea to 6 to 8 ounces of the mix, or as the liquid medium when making a more meal-like Akea smoothie.

3 pounds frozen strawberries, thawed
2 bananas
6 lemons, room temperature, juiced
1 teaspoon Stevita Spoonable Stevia OR 20-30 drops Stevita Liquid Stevia
4 to 6 cups filtered water

Place the frozen strawberries in a wide-mouthed gallon jug, cover, and let thaw either overnight in the fridge or on the counter for a few hours. When strawberries are ready, peel and cut bananas into inch-wide pieces and add them to the strawberries. Use a citrus juicer to juice the lemons and pour the juice over the bananas and strawberries. Using an immersion blender, puree the strawberries, bananas and lemon juice until smooth and no chunks are present. Add the stevia and continue to blend. Top the mixture with filtered water and blend with immersion blender one last time. Chill covered until ready to serve. Keeps fresh for up to 3 days.

Buy All of Your Produce and Staples Organic as Often as Possible, if Not Always

Akea Breakfast Mug 'o Cream
Serves 1 to 2

Breakfast at the Norris house every morning consists of the Mug 'o Cream. It give us the nutritional foundation for a productive, energy-filled day, and makes cravings for refined foods and simple carbs a thing of the past.

Layer the following, in order, in a 1 quart jug:

1/2 cup Berry Banana Akearita Mix
1/2 cup frozen organic blueberries
2 to 3 scoops Akea Fermented Whole Food Supplement
1 avocado, peeled, pitted and quartered
1/2 to 1 banana, sliced
6 frozen organic strawberries, quartered
1/2 to 3/4 cup Berry Banana Akearita Mix (yes, again)

Blend with immersion blender on high until smooth. Add 3 organic, free-roaming raw eggs and blend on low until just incorporated (blending eggs on high can damage their proteins).

Peanut Butter Banana Blast Smoothie
Serves 1 to 2

Layer the following, in order, in a 1 quart jug:

1/2 cup filtered cold water
1/2 banana, sliced
2 to 3 scoops Akea Fermented Whole Food Supplement
2 Tbsp powdered peanut butter
1/2 banana, sliced
1/2 cup filtered cold water

Blend with immersion blender on high until smooth. Add 2 to 3 organic, free-roaming raw eggs and blend on low until just incorporated (blending eggs on high can damage their proteins).

Coconut Strawberry Milk
Makes 2 quarts
Perfect for blending with Akea Fermented Whole Food Supplement

2 pounds frozen, organic strawberries, thawed
3 cans full fat coconut milk (Thai Kitchen)
1/8 to 1/4 cup organic maple syrup
2 cups filtered water

Blend all ingredients together with immersion blender. Store covered in refrigerator for up to 4 days.

Akea Strawberry Milkshake
Serves 1

Combine in a 16 ounce BlenderBottle and blend with immersion blender:

8 ounces Coconut Strawberry Milk
1 scoop Akea Fermented Whole Food Supplement

Add 1 to 2 organic, free-roaming raw eggs and blend on low until just incorporated (blending eggs on high can damage their proteins).

Akea Chocolate Covered Strawberry Smoothie
Serves 1

Blend 1 to 2 tablespoons organic raw cacao with the Strawberry Milk and Akea before adding eggs. Sweeten with a few drops of Stevita Liquid Stevia to taste, if desired.

Buy All of Your Produce and Staples Organic as Often as Possible, if Not Always

Coconut Coffee Creamer
Makes about 20 ounces

1 can full fat coconut milk (Thai Kitchen)
1/2 cup filtered water
1/8 cup organic maple syrup
1 Tbsp alcohol-free vanilla extract

Blend with immersion blender and refrigerate, covered tightly, up to 5 days.

Coconut Chai Creamer
Makes about 20 ounces

1 can full fat coconut milk (Thai Kitchen)
1/2 cup filtered water
1/8 cup organic maple syrup
1 Tbsp alcohol-free vanilla extract
1 tsp cinnamon

Blend with immersion blender and refrigerate, covered tightly, up to 5 days.

Notes:
Avoid coconut milk with carragenan as the thickener, and do not purchase the "lite" version, as you can dilute the coconut milk on your own.
I do not recommend the flavored coconut milk available in the aseptic packs or refrigerated cartons as they're loaded with sugar and synthetic vitamins, particularly vitamin D2 (your body makes and needs the D3 original version).

Appendix A

Where's The Beef?

When I first started mapping out this book's contents in the spring of 2013, it was laden with meat recipes, just as my family's diet. I had a roast beef recipe that my husband would rave to his colleagues about, chicken wings that would rival those on the Hooter's menu, and a chicken Panang curry that made us stop frequenting our local Thai restaurant. The various meat dishes accounted for almost 30 percent of the cookbook section! I had been a meat-eater/lover for over 35 years, taking great pride in my ability to "digest it so easily" (since I have type-O blood and all). Our family would consume some type of meat with every main meal. I say "with" as though it was a side dish- it wasn't. It was the main focus, the whole reason we were eating to begin with.

After giving birth to my daughters, my number one responsibility was to provide them with the nourishment that would facilitate the creation of the highest-quality biological foundation possible. Can you find the error in that last statement? The highest-quality biological foundation for the construction of a human being begins with the health of the mother (and father!) months and years prior to conception, let alone birth. I was under the impression that I was pretty healthy when I conceived and took more than just a prenatal vitamin during my pregnancies, so all that was left after they were born was to continue with the framework. Now faced with the daunting task of figuring out how I was to go about it, I read, and googled, and read some more. It wasn't until they were toddlers that the subject of meat really had to be addressed as they began eating more (I nursed my youngest daughter until she was 2 and a half, so she really wasn't eating many solids yet).

In February of 2007, when my daughters were 3 (Abby) and almost 2 (Caroline), we moved (as we usually did every two to three years with my husband's job) from the Eastern Panhandle of West Virginia to Coastal North Carolina. We were freshly healing from Abby's almost two year struggle with eczema and all seemed right with the world since we had eliminated soy from all of our diets. The curious thing was that there were still times she would begin scratching in the same places she used to have her outbreaks, and sometimes the skin in those areas would even begin to show signs of irritation.

Having come across information that revealed soy as a huge part of the diets of commercially-raised chickens, I began wondering how much "soy protein residue" might be accumulating in the chicken and eggs I was feeding her almost every day. If my hypothesis was correct, and there were soy proteins in those foods, it would be extraordinarily difficult to eliminate those sources of allergic proteins. The only alternative would be to have our own hens for eggs and meat, and there was no way that I would ever kill another living thing, even if it was to feed my children. Frustration set in again and I started searching for sources of "uncontaminated" meat.

It was in April 2007 that I placed my first online order for grass-finished, soy-free meat, hoping to provide all of us with "clean", hormone-free protein that wouldn't speed up the rate of their sexual maturation, and that wouldn't induce an eczema reaction in my eldest. Even though it was more expensive than the meat I could buy at the grocery store, I was content with the idea that we would just have to consume less of it so we wouldn't have to sacrifice our health for quantity. It tasted great (although the girls really weren't that interested in it to begin with), and it gave peace of mind that I was doing a "good thing" by not buying mass-produced beef contaminated with e. coli, and chicken teeming with soy residue. I was even entertaining ordering our eggs online but the $7/dozen price tag drove me to start dreaming of the day we could finally start raising our own laying hens so we could ensure they wouldn't be fed soy.

While researching this section of the book I decided to have a look at my order history over the last 7 years from the two websites I had ordered our meat to quantify the financial impact on eating "clean" meat. The data revealed a significant amount of money spent on everything from whole pastured chickens ($25 each) and turkeys ($75 each) to grass-finished buffalo dogs ($10 for 5) and humanely-raised, steroid-free, nitrite-free bacon ($10 per pound). I even ordered butter and raw cheese made with milk and cream from strictly pasture-fed cows ($9 per pound of butter!) There were definitely times that I would pick up steaks from the local store but for the most part, we only ate what I could order online (it was the chicken that proved too pricey to consistently order online). About a year and half later, I began purchasing our eggs from a local farmer who allowed his hens to spend plenty of time out in the green grass (not certain if the feed he supplemented them with was free of soy but I do know supplementation was minimal).

In the spring of 2010, I finally got my wish of having our very own laying hens! I ordered a beautiful Amish-made coop straight from Pennsylvania, and their soy-free starter feed from Countryside Organics, a high quality feed and farming company in Virginia. We named our four sweet little Rhode Island Reds: Rose, Linda, Woodpecker, and Big Red, and waited patiently for their development and the ability to contribute to the nutrition of their eggs. It would be another five months before Big Red would be the first of the foursome to lay an egg, but when she did, it was a joyous day! After that, the race was on every day to see which one of girls could get to the coop first to collect the freshly-laid treasures.

Heartbreak struck us all about a week before Thanksgiving that same year, when a chicken hawk swooped down in our backyard, and upon sinking its talons into our Big Red, began to feast. My husband and the girls were able to get to scene quickly enough to only make the hawk release our Red, but the life had already left her. It was the first exposure my daughters had to losing someone dear to them. We all cried and grieved, and from that moment on, kept a very close watch on our three remaining little red hens while they enjoyed the pasture and roaming freely. They continued to lay their wonderful eggs, almost every day, and we were elated that we didn't have to wonder what they were eating. All was right with the world.

In June of 2011, we would end up moving from our roomy house, that was practically in the country and that we had spent the last four and half years in, to a smaller one practically in the middle of the city. Our three little hens would be coming with us, but the problem was that I wouldn't have room for my stand-up freezer and therefore, no place to store our thrice-yearly order of ground beef, hotdogs, and stew meat (all forty pounds of it). Sadly, my last order of grass-finished, never-an-antibiotic-administered, frolicking-happily-in-the-fields-of-Wisconsin-and-Minnesota beef was placed in February of 2011. It lasted us four months, and after that, we were denigrated once again to the grocery store meat department. My guilt about eating and feeding the girls "that" meat increased steadily with each weekly trip to the store, but it didn't stop us from continuing to eat it. The good thing was that we were only eating the eggs our hens laid, and in the spring of 2012 even added another five chicks to our flock to make sure we always had a spare dozen on hand.

It was the fall of 2012 that I would succumb to the effects of chronic stress and stress-induced insomnia. About a month into my illness, as I lain in bed for most of my only day off (Sunday), I tried to rest but couldn't help continuing my research to see how I could put an end to my symptoms and illness. I picked up a book one of my husband's colleagues had loaned me a couple years before (yes, I still have it and yes, I know that five years is long time to borrow a book), Survival In The 21st Century. The first edition was written in 1981, and the edition I have is the 48th, printed in 2002. I remembered that it had some sections on mucus and enzymes when I had flipped through it after he initially brought it home for me. But while I read the rest of it intently that Sunday afternoon, more fuel would be sprayed on the fire that was my guilt as I came across the section titled Food In Your Poison. From Survival In the 21st Century, by Viktoras H. Kulvinskas, P.O. Box 2853, Hot Springs AR 71914, www.Viktoras.org:

Meat, the most perishable (and most expensive) of all foods is also one of the most tampered with. To see exactly how meat is produced one should read the Animal Machines, by Ruth Harrison. It is the story of animal factories, where animals may live out their lives in darkness, immobile in steaming pen from birth to death, fed by conveyors containing drugs, antibiotics, tranquilizers, pesticides, and hormones…

After an animal is slaughtered, or dies from disease, it is shipped off to the processing house. The meat is doctored up for the benefit of the gullible public, with aesthetic beautifiers, stink reducers, taste accentuators, color additives, drug camouflagers, nutritive enhancers, bleaching agents, and death certificate. No corpse gets such a facelift by the embalmers, and with good reason, for the corpse is soon buried, whereas salami, hotdogs, bologna, and chicken may sit on the shelves for months.

Meat is colored red with sodium nicotinoate otherwise it would turn yellow-gray. Uneven or excessive application can result in severe sickness, even death. However, when such incidents occur they are seldom diagnosed correctly.

At the Congressional Hearing on Meat Inspection , it was reported that the sausages, ham, hamburgers, and hotdogs you eat, may be filled with hog blood, cereals, lungs, niacin, water, detergents, and/or sodium sulfide.

The FDA refuses to recognize tests conducted by Dr. Patrick Riley at a London Medical School, where it was shown that BHA, a widely used preservative is carcinogenic. This preservative appears in luncheon meats, such as salami, bologna, and pressed ham, canned meats, peanut butter, canned chicken and other foods. Senator Alan Cranston commented in 1970 that "perhaps they (FDA) consider food processor's interests more than the people's interests."

A typical Associated Press release occurred around Thanksgiving 1969: "U.S. finds pesticide in 90,000 turkeys at toxic levels." A few years ago cranberries were found to be unfit companions to the turkey. In Massachusetts alone , during a more active month for health inspectors, 250 tons of meat was seized because it was contaminated. Such meat is quite often resold as 4-D meat: dead, dying, disabled or diseased. The winter of 1969, Boston had a month long scandal over the pollution in the slaughter houses of Massachusetts...

ONLY TEN PERCENT of the meat adulterated with pesticides and chemicals, or contaminated with filth and diseased organs is condemned by food inspectors. The other 90 percent gets through to the unsuspecting consumer, so claims Leray Houser of the Health Education and Welfare Department , "In 1965, a total of 711 firms suspected of producing harmful or contaminated consumer products refused to let the FDA conduct inspection...The FDA does not have subpoena authority either to summon witnesses or authority to require firms to divulge pertinent records."

Well, one of the bones of contention I had with meat products before I made the decision to start ordering online was the use of MSG (monosodium glutamate, a known neurotoxin) and sodium nitrite/nitrate (known carcinogens) as flavor enhancers. The hotdogs and salami I used to buy online contained none of those questionable ingredients, and I felt a little relief when I began seeing conventional manufacturers remove them from some of their products. We were able to buy "naturally cured" nitrite-free bacon, hard salami, and ham without MSG or nitrites. Granted, the pork and beef used to make those lunch meats were still conventionally raised, I managed to repress my guilt a little more with the hope that we would soon be able to start ordering of the "good" stuff again.

By the spring of 2013, the whole family relied heavily on chicken, pork, and beef, especially since we had given up wheat and dairy 6 months earlier. We still ate salads almost every day, and potatoes, but it seemed as though we were now eating more animal protein than when I was ordering it online (because we were). And trying to figure out whose package "promises" to believe would prove even more of a stressor, with chicken being the most deceptive. You can still see things like "100% Natural" (whatever that means), and "No Hormones or Steroids Added*", with the asterisk clarifying that the "USDA prohibits the use of hormones and steroids in poultry". Well if that's the case, what are you bragging about? It's like saying "I didn't kill anyone today", and then following it up with "because, you know, it's illegal." Not to mention that there would be no reason to add steroids or hormones to meat, since the effects they're meant to facilitate can only occur if administered to the animal while it's alive (so it can grow bigger, faster).

The rhetoric about poultry and antibiotics was, and still is, equally ambiguous. Some growers give you meaningless assurances like "No Antibiotics Ever", and some are a little more specific by saying "No Antibiotics Administered". What consumers don't realize is that the major issue with commercially raised poultry is the use of antibiotics as preventive or prophylactic measures due to the deplorable living conditions the birds are subjected to. Those antibiotics remain in the meat and cannot be "cooked out". Also, their soy-heavy diets cause such rapid growth that their little legs can't support their body weight, so they just lie down and are trampled to death by the others. And anyone who has ever been tricked into thinking that chickens are vegetarians, you're about to get a reality check- they're not. They'll peck out the eyes of dead chickens in an instant. The living conditions of chickens have to be considerably roomy and the flock small enough, for the grower to not run the risk of losing his entire flock should he decide to not medicate.

All this internal conflict can really begin to wear a mother down, especially when you decide to watch Food Inc. because you heard what a revealing documentary it is. It went from bad to worse one evening in February 2013 when my eldest daughter informed me that she didn't want to eat chicken anymore (just as she was finishing up a chicken drumstick), because she didn't want to eat the relatives of our little hens. I was aghast. What would I feed her? I remarked that if that was the case, that drumstick she had just eaten would be her last, and that the chicken sausages we ate twice a week would also be off limits to her while the rest of us still indulged (I know, I'm horrible, but I panicked). As the evening wore on, I began feeling worse and worse. I couldn't believe I had guilted her into not "inconveniencing" me by having to adapt to her request. She moved on to another subject quickly enough, but my guilt began resurfacing.

My decision to stop eating meat, along with no longer feeding it to my family, is one that I never thought I would make. It involved a complex overlapping of circum-stances including but not limited to distrust of the industry, cost-prohibitive "clean" alternatives and anxiety if those alternatives were not accessible, and undoubtedly the most provoking of all, the emotional prodding of an animal-loving 8 year old. The straw that broke the camel's back would come on trip to visit a dear friend of mine in Charlotte. I was fresh off of an extremely indulgent party the night before, where it took five chefs to prepare the food. Three differently-themed "stations" showcased Italian dishes, Asian cuisine, and Tex-Mex fare with no fewer than 6 options at each station. I didn't hold back. Not even a tiny bit. I tried to stay away from gluten and dairy, and did so for the most part, until they brought out dessert.

Somehow, I was willing to accept the consequences of my actions on my asthma as long as I could indulge just that one gastronomically-luscious night. The following morning I felt nothing short of hung-over, repulsed even, by my gluttonous impulses. It was the perfect punishment as I boarded my flight later that evening. When I arrived in Charlotte, I hadn't eaten all day, by choice of course. As I sat in my friend's kitchen while she prepared dinner, she asked me for my take on a book she had recently purchased, *Conscious Eating*, by Gabriel Cousens, MD. I flipped through it, giving my "approval" on many subjects, but my attention came to rest on a page that would alter my life incredulously from that night forward. Rabbi Cousens, who is not just a medical doctor, but also a psychiatrist, as well as a naturopathic physician, noted how even though universal compassion for all God's creatures is the hallmark of many of the world religions, vegetarianism isn't universally practiced at the present time in Buddhism, Sikhism, Judaism, or Christianity, quoting Buddha from the Lankavatar as saying:

> *For the sake of love of purity, the bodhisattva should refrain from eating flesh...For fear of causing terror to living beings, let the bodhisattva, who is disciplining himself to attain compassion, refrain from eating flesh...It is not true that meat is proper food and permissible when the animal was not killed by himself, when he did not order others to kill it, when it was not specifically meant for him...*

> *Again, there may be some people in the future who...being under the influence of the taste of meat will string together in various ways many sophisticated arguments to defend meat-eating...But meat-eating in any form, in any manner, and in any place is unconditionally, and once and for all, prohibited...Meat-eating I have not permitted to anyone, I do not permit, and I will not permit.*

So I thought for a moment about the relevance of these words, and all the guilt from that evening when my daughter implored me to allow her to not eat chicken came rushing back. I continued perusing the book with an increasingly greater amount of energy feeding my heart and soul with each word I read, and came across Chapter 17 on the teachings on vegetarianism from the Old Testament (Torah), where the first dietary law of Judaism is:

> *Behold, I have given you every herb-yielding seed which is upon the face of all the earth, and every tree, in which is the fruit of a tree yielding a seed-to you it shall be for food. (Genesis 1:29)*

And the Lord God commanded the man saying: of
every tree of the garden, thou mayest freely eat...
(Genesis 2:16)

...and thou shalt eat the herbs of the field.
(Genesis 3:18)

Dr. Cousens went on:

In Exodus 20:13, it says, "Thou shalt not kill." This sixth commandment is basic in terms of its compassion and love for all of creation. The exact Hebrew translation reads "lo tirtzach." This word refers to any sort of killing, and not just humans. The practice of this commandment not only keeps the fundamental order in the world of nature, but supports the basic principle of compassion and love for all of God's creation that is taught in the Torah. It clearly supports the essential observance of vegetarianism.

Vegetarianism is the basic and unitary commandment on diet. It is a blueprint, in essence, of the basic diet needed to support a spiritual life in harmony with all of creation. It gives us a context to understand Genesis 9:3, the first of several concessions to people's lust for flesh:

Every moving thing that lives shall be food for you; as the
green have I given you all.

Vegetarian Rav Abraham Isaac Hacohen Kook, the well-respected Jewish spiritual leader and Torah scholar in the early part of the twentieth century and the first Chief Rabbi of the pre-state of Israel, said that the permission to eat meat was only a temporary concession to the people. He believed it was inconceivable that God would design a perfect plan of harmony for humanity and the Earth and find that it was imperfect a few thousand years later. Rabbi Kook thought that Genesis 9:3 was a temporary concession because people had sunk to such a low level of spiritual awareness that they needed to feel superior to the animals and to concentrate first on improving their relationship with each other.

He said that humanity's lust for meat was so strong that if they were denied they might even have reverted to eating human flesh. In his understanding, the permission to slaughter animals was a way to control the blood lust. He interpreted the permission to eat meat as a stopgap measure until a more enlightened era would be achieved and we would all return to vegetarianism. With the permission to eat meat, animals and people stopped existing in a peaceful harmony. It was a significant shift in the relationship of the human organism to the world ecology.

Kosher laws were seen as way to make meat-eating tolerable, yet not particularly convenient. A renowned Torah scholar, Rambam, said, "Be holy by abstaining from those things which are permitted to you. For those drink wine and eat meat all the time are considered "scoundrels with a Torah license." The reluctance to give this permission to eat meat is evidenced by the prohibition against eating blood.

> *Only flesh with the life thereof, which is the blood thereof, shall ye not eat. (Genesis 9:4)*

To have to remove the blood in order to be Kosher is a way of making flesh-eating more difficult and a reminder of the compromise in permitting meat-eating. Even while allowing the eating of meat and not the eating of blood, the Torah gives a suggestion for respecting the life of t he animal. There is also a "catch 22" quality to this Kosher law because the physiological reality of the Kosher commandment not to have the blood of the animal is impossible to fulfill. Although one can drain blood from the arteries and veins, it is not physiologically possible to drain it from the capillaries. From the scientific point of view, the only way to be fully Kosher is to be vegetarian. In Genesis 9:5 it says:

> *And surely, your blood of your lives will I require…*

Directly related to the temporary concession to the carnal desires of humanity, we see an immediate result in a decreased life span. Humanity is forced to pay for its blood lust. Within one generation of the Genesis 9:3 statement to Noah, the life span decreased to one third of its previous length, from approximately 900 years to 300 years, and then eventually to 70 years. Our current medical research has documented that a flesh-centered diet has a detrimental effect on health. This is the physiological modern-day fulfillment of "your blood of your lives will I require."

During Exodus, it appears that God tried to make the Jews return to vegetarianism by just giving them the manna in the desert. Again, however, the flesh lust of the people made them rebel from the diet. They demanded flesh food from God.

> *And the mixed multitude that was among them fell a lusting; and the children of Israel also weeped on their part, and said, "Would that we were given flesh to eat." (Numbers 11:4)*

Although Moses was frustrated with the lust of the people, God granted their request by providing them with quails blown in by the wind. But God's anger at their rebellion and their flesh-eating desires brought a plague to the people who ate the quail.

> *While the flesh was yet between their teeth, ere it was chewed, the anger of the Lord was kindled against the people, and the Lord smote the people with a very great plague. (Numbers 11:33)*

> *Many died and the place where this took place was called the "Graves of Lust"; there they buried the people that lusted. (Numbers 11:34)*

It is hard to interpret this concession of eating the quail as supportive of a flesh-centered diet. It is far easier to interpret this incident as evidence of God's direction that the people be vegetarian and that the consequences of meat-eating would be poor health and a shortened life span.

The Torah consistently describes vegetarian foods in a positive light and as a reward. The Divine bounty and the Song of Songs is described in terms of fruits, vegetables, and other vegetarian cuisine. There is a blessing before eating vegetarian food such as fruit of the vine and the bread of the earth, but there is no specific blessing for eating flesh food…

Although there is not enough information to absolutely prove that some of the prophets were vegetarian, such as Isaiah, Jeremiah, Amos, Hosea, Daniel, and Ezekiel, there are certainly quotes from their teachings that suggest they taught against the killing of animals and animal sacrifice. These quotes also suggest that they taught a vegetarian lifestyle, as they do not say that people should raise animals to slaughter and eat their flesh. As these were true prophets, one can only assume they lived their teachings. Examples of those teachings are:

> *…and the fruit thereof shall be for meat, and the leaf thereof for medicine. (Exekiel 47:12)*

> *He who kills an ox is like him who slays a man. (Isaiah 66:3)*

> *Please test your servants for ten days, giving us legumes to eat and water to drink. Then compare our appearance with that of the youths who eat of the king's food. (Daniel 1:12-13)*

> *For I desire goodness, not sacrifice; obedience to God, rather than burnt offerings. (Hosea 6:6)*

> *When they present sacrifices to me, it is but flesh for them to eat; the Lord has not accepted them… (Hosea 8:13)*

> *I will restore my people to Israel. They shall rebuild ruined cities and inhabit them; they shall plant vineyards and drink their wine; they shall till gardens and eat their fruits. (Amos 9:14)*

> *Thus said the Lord of Hosts, the God of Israel, to the whole community which I exiled from Jerusalem to Babylon: Build houses and live in them, plant gardens and eat their fruit. (Jeremiah 29:4-5)*

And then from The Tasty Economical Cookbook-Volume II, the Islamic Holiness M.R. Bawa Muhaiyaddeen, an Islamic saint and vegetarian says:

> A true human being must have compassion toward all lives. There are so many ways to eat good clean food, without killing or tormenting other lives, and without eating the flesh and bones or other lives…If a man eats meat, he will take on the qualities of the animal he eats.

The qualities of all these animals can be imbibed by eating their flesh…And once those qualities enter, the man's anger, his hastiness, and his animal qualities will increase. The animal's blood will intermingle with his blood…These animal qualities are what causes one man to murder another, to harm and torment another.

From an unpublished discourse, Bawa Muhaiyaddeen clarified vegetarianism as the result and natural consequence of the development of spiritual consciousness:

When a man's mind attains a state of completeness in wisdom and when he reaches a state where he will not hurt any life within himself (in one's own mind), then he will not harm anything on the outside either. Inside he will not intend any harm or pain to any other life. Nor will he do anything harmful or eat any life on the outside. This is a state of wisdom, clarity, and the light of God. This is Sufism.

Man is such a dangerous animal, and it is only when he changes his behavior that he becomes a good man, a true human being. When he changes into a good man, he will no longer have within himself the thoughts of killing or gaining victory over another life. He will not have within himself the qualities of distressing other lives, of wanting to harass or ruin other lives. If he does not kill anything on the inside, then he will not kill anything on the outside.

Once a person has the wisdom, the potentialities, and the qualities of the true human being, once he attains that liberation, he will have reached the exalted state of God. The darkness in him will have been dispelled and he will love his neighbor as he loves himself. Once he attains the quality of loving every other life as he loves his own, he will never kill another life. Nor will he ever cause pain to another life. Because he feels that the other life is also his own flesh, he will never eat flesh.

According to Bawa Muhaiyaddeen, in the past, The Prophet came and told them, "Do not kill. It is a sin. You are taking another life." But because people were not able to follow this teaching, Mohammed then had to limit, but ultimately allow, the eating of flesh because the people were not of the consciousness that allowed them to go beyond their blood lust.

As in Judaism, the killing of animals was limited by laws that were very difficult to follow. These laws are called qurban, involving the slaughter of animals after certain prayers are recited and while one looks the animal in the eyes.

As with the Kosher laws, the Koran lists forbidden foods rather than the foods one must eat. These forbidden foods center on meat. There are elaborate regulations for preparation that limit the amount of animals one is able to kill and therefore make meat eating considerably more of a burden than eating a vegetarian diet…

In the Talmud, Rabbi Yishmael said,

> From the day that the holy Temple was destroyed it would have been right to have imposed upon ourselves the law prohibiting the eating of flesh. But the rabbis have laid down a wise and logical rule that the authorities must not impose any decree unless the majority of the members of the community are able to abide by it. Otherwise the law and those who administer it get into disrepute.

Perhaps this is the crux of the issue for why meat-eating has been allowed by many of the major religions, including Judaism, Christianity, and even Buddhism. Out of compassion for the limitations of their followers, the essential compassion for all life found in all religions needed to wait until the people were ready. I wonder if we have been waiting too long.

That evening for dinner, I would half-heartedly eat chicken for the very last time, and my dear friend would gift me Dr. Cousens' book because I couldn't put down. The next day at lunch, I had a salad with black beans, guacamole, and lots of salsa. When I arrived home that evening, I had a baked potato with coconut oil and garbanzo beans for dinner. The day after that, I gave the rest of the chicken drumsticks and chicken sausages in my freezer to a friend because I couldn't bring myself to cook them, let alone eat them. I took it day by day because that's the only way I could fathom it. When I felt the yearning for steak or chicken wings, I returned to Chapter 17 in Conscious Eating for spiritual support, which quickly extinguished my "blood lust". Over the course of the next three weeks, I managed to not have a single serving of meat, instead I turned to wild caught smoked salmon and pickled herring in wine, when I felt I was going to lose my mind.

Three weeks after swearing off of chicken and other land-dwelling animals, I came home from work to the most tragic scene in my life. My daughters were visiting my parents for the summer and had been gone for about six weeks already. My husband was deployed to Afghanistan, so it was just me and our flock of now thirty hens hanging out for the summer, twenty three newbies almost ready to start laying their eggs. Three weeks after honoring my daughter's wishes from just a few months before and beginning a life of not eating our pets' relatives, I came home to find our yard littered with motionless mounds of feathers. Where little heads normally pecked at the grass and scratch feed I had just thrown down about six hours ago, nothing but the grass moved in the breeze. I screamed in terror, over and over again as I looked out the window and hoped and prayed that if I stared long enough, I would see maybe just one moving about. Nothing.

As I walked through the yard that evening, counting little bodies that I was digging graves for, I'm certain my wails could be heard on the busy street in front of our house, and for at least a hundred yard radius. I don't know if I've ever cried so much or felt so much heartache. When I came across one of my older babies whose chest feathers had been ripped out by her attacker, her flesh looked exactly the breast packaged neatly in the meat section of the grocery store, and I screamed over and over again that evening between the *Why?, Never again! Never again will I put your flesh near my mouth!* That was pretty much the final day I would ever think of chicken as food again. But I was far from home-free.

It was a social event almost a month to the day I first opened up *Conscious Eating*, that would try my willpower and faith, and succeed. Fourth of July, barbequed pulled pork: any North Carolinian could relate. I tried to ignore it for about an hour into the gathering, happily enjoying the California Potato Salad I had brought along, when I could resist no more. I imbibed like a lush with about four ounces of the contraband and immediately felt the remorse. It would be about four days after that that I would really feel the meat was out of my system. So much for being able to "digest it so easily", since I have type-O blood and all. Three months later, at yet another social event hosted by the same couple, I fell for it one last time- pulled pork sandwiches as the appetizer to my vegetarian entrée (I was trying!) You would think if I was going to step outside the lines I would be a little more selective and try not to consume the most questionable meat around. Apparently not.

That really was the last time though, October 12, 2013, that meat would make its way onto my plate. And I'm happy to say that in the late spring of 2014, when my eldest daughter informed me that she would also no longer be eating fish, I said, "That's a good idea. I think we're all going to join you." I've fallen off that wagon once recently by ordering salmon at a business dinner at the end of June, but I'm ready for it to be the last. So, today, I am amazed to say that I cannot bring myself to provide you with even one meat recipe. I'm not trying to convince anyone to give up meat, I simply can no longer promote its consumption. But I'm certain there are plenty of Paleo cookbooks out there that can give you more than enough recipes to pair with the ones in this book, where the beef isn't.

Suggested Reading:

Conscious Eating, Gabriel Cousens, MD

Survival in The 21st Century: Planetary Healers Manual, Viktoras H. Kulvinskas, MS

Pottenger's Cats: A Study in Nutrition, Francis M. Pottenger, Jr., MD

Animal Machines, Ruth Harrison

Diet for a Small Planet, Frances Moore Lappé

Appendix B
Restocking Your Pantry

Gutting your diet of grains, soy, poor quality oils, and dairy, inevitably means your going to have to gut your pantry as well. The following staples can be found on line and in the interest of helping you gather your ingredients sooner rather than later, you can find all of these items in the SatFatRox Amazon store on our website, www.SatFatRox.com/the-store.

In the chart below you'll fiind your grocery list. The list of flours are pretty much the only ones you'll need to bake everything from Focaccia to Chocolate Chip Cookies. Buy them in bulk and split the cost with a friend who might want to join you on your journey.

Flour/Baking	Necessary	Fats and Oils	Dry Beans	Jar Fare
garbanzo bean	pink salt	coconut oil	lentils	applesauce
coconut flour	salt-free organic herb seasoning	palm shortening	chickpeas (garbanzo beans)	tomato products (paste, sauce, etc)
tapioca starch		red palm oil		
potato starch	garlic granules	cocoa butter	black beans	olives
Potato flour	raw cacao powder	California extra virgin olive oil	pinto beans	sauerkraut
xanthan gum			black-eyed peas	curry paste
grain-free baking powder	powdered peanut butter	high quality grapeseed	lima beans	roasted sweet red peppers
			navy beans	
cinnamon	canned coconut milk	Herbs/Spices	red beans	tahini (sesame seed paste)
baking soda		oregano	kidney beans	
cream of tarter	pitted dates	basil	Banza Pasta	Bragg's Coconut Aminos
vanilla extract (alcohol free)	raw honey	parsley	Super Foods	artichokes
	organic molasses	dill weed	raw cacao nibs	Dijon mustard
ground vanilla bean	Stevita stevia powder	turmeric	dry Goji berries	balsamic vinegar (no color added)
shredded coconut	Stevita or Sweet Leaf Liquid	cumin	Akea Fermented Superfoods and Probiotics	Bragg's Raw Apple Cider Vinegar
		ginger		

Where to Buy

www.NCSuperFood.com
Akea Fermented Superfoods Supplement

shop.mercola.com/catalog/food-beverage,47,0,0.htm
coconut flour, cacao nibs, coconut oil

www.CyberCucina.com
Traditionally fermented olives, artichokes, and more

www.BulkApothecary.com
Cocoa butter

www.CinnamonVogue.com
Ceylon cinnamon

www.TropicalTraditions.com
Bittersweet chocolate chips, organic applesauce, organic palm shortening, gold label coconut oil, expeller-pressed coconut oil, jarred organic tomato products, and more.

www.WildernessFamilyNaturals.com
Organic Soy-Free Mayonaise, cacao, dried fruit and other safe bets!

www.TeaMotions.com
Organic, hand-blended adaptogenic teas

www.EatBanza.com
Banza Pasta Made From Chickpeas!

Amazon.com
Everything you could possibly imagine. Especially Pur Gum so you can stop chewing artificially- sweetened gum.

www.SincerelyNuts.com
Dates in bulk. Don't buy ANY dry fruit that has been treated with SULFUR DIOXIDE, it's on the Proposition 65 list of cancer-causing chemicals.

A few days in my Akea life…

Monday, July 21st, 2014

Breakfast (7:30 am):
Smoothie: 1 cup Strawberry Akearita Mix, 1 banana , 1 avocado, ½ cup organic frozen wild blueberries, 6 organic frozen whole strawberries (chopped), 2 scoops Akea Fermented Superfood powder. Blended on high with an immersion blender until smooth. Cracked in 3 raw organic eggs, blended gently for about 10 seconds.

Lunch (1:00 pm):
3 SatFatRox Biscuits, sliced and warmed in toaster oven.
Guacamole: 1 ripe avocado, mashed with a fork, 3 cloves organic garlic (crushed and chopped), 1 organic tomato (chopped into 1/3 inch squares), ½ red onion (chopped into 1/3 inch squares), ¼ tsp pink salt, 1 tsp organic no-salt herb seasoning.

Dinner (7:30 pm):
2 medium size pre-baked organic russet potatoes, diced and warmed on low-medium heat in 2 tablespoons coconut oil, seasoned with pink salt and organic no-salt herb seasoning (aka Country Fried Potatoes).

Green salad with 1 whole organic romaine heart, 1 organic tomato (cut into bite size pieces), ½ cup sliced organic cucumbers, ¼ cup chopped roasted red peppers. Dressed with pink salt, organic no-salt herb seasoning, California Olive Ranch olive oil and organic balsamic vinegar.

Tuesday, July 22nd, 2014

Breakfast (9:00 am):
Smoothie with 1 cup Strawberry Akearita Mix, 1 banana, ¼ cup raw organic cacao powder, ¾ cup organic frozen wild blueberries, 6 organic frozen whole strawberries (chopped), 2 scoops Akea Fermented Superfood powder, 6-8 drops liquid stevia drops. Blended on high with an immersion blender until smooth. Cracked in 2 raw organic eggs, blended gently for about 10 seconds.

Lunch: Didn't have time but never felt hungry until around 5:30 pm

Dinner (6:30 pm):
2 cups Panang Curried Lentils with ½ chopped organic raw onion, on top. 4 SatFatRox Biscuits (baked earlier in the day) dipped in 1/4 cup California Olive Ranch Extra Virgin Olive Oil mixed with 1/8 cup organic balsamic vinegar and ¼ teaspoon organic no-salt herb seasoning. I ate all of the dipping oil. ALL of it.

Bedtime snack (11:30 pm):
1 medium-sized baked organic potato with 1 tablespoon organic virgin coconut oil, pink salt, organic cayenne pepper powder, 2 raw organic garlic cloves, crushed.

Wednesday, July 23rd, 2014

Breakfast (9:30 am):
Smoothie with 10 ounces Strawberry Akearita Mix, ¾ cup organic frozen wild blueberries, 6 organic frozen strawberries (chopped), 2 scoops Akea Fermented Superfoods powder, 6-8 drops liquid stevia drops. Blend on high with an immersion blender until smooth. Cracked in 3 raw organic eggs, blending on lowest speed of immersion blender for about 10 seconds.

Lunch (2:30 pm):
1 Medium-sized Country Fried Potato, ½ cup Roasted Red Pepper Hummus and 2 sliced, lightly toasted SatFatRox Biscuits.

Dinner (6:30 pm):
2 cups Potato Green Bean Soup. 4 SatFatRox Biscuits (baked earlier in the day) dipped in 1/4 cup California Olive Ranch Olive Oil mixed with 1/8 cup organic balsamic vinegar and ¼ teaspoon organic no-salt herb seasoning.

Snack (11:30 pm):
1 Whole grapefruit and 1 Banana

Thursday, July 24th, 2014

Breakfast (8:00 am)
Smoothie: 12 ounces Strawberry Coconut Milk, 2 scoops Akea Fermented Superfood powder and 2 raw organic eggs, blended on lowest speed until smooth.

Lunch (1:30 pm)
2 medium-sized freshly baked organic russet potatoes with 2 tablespoons organic virgin coconut oil, ½ chopped organic onion, 1 diced organic tomato, ¼ tsp pink salt, ½ teaspoon organic no-salt herb seasoning.

Afternoon snack (3:30 pm)
2 Bananas, sliced, sprinkled with 1/3 cup finely shredded unsweetened coconut, and 1/8 teaspoon cinnamon

Dinner (6:30 pm)
3 Organic eggs, cooked in coconut oil, sunny-side up with yolk very runny, seasoned with pink salt and organic no-salt herb seasoning. 1 Avocado, sliced

½ cup mixed olives, Kalamata and Castelvetrano. 4 SatFatRox biscuits and 2 tablespoons California Olive Ranch extra virgin olive oil and 2 tablespoons organic balsamic vinegar.

Friday, July 25th, 2014

Breakfast (9:30 am)

Smoothie with 1 banana, ¾ cup organic frozen wild blueberries, 6 organic frozen strawberries (chopped), 2 scoops Akea Fermented Superfood powder, 6 drops liquid stevia. Blend on high with an immersion blender until smooth. 2 SatFatRox Banana Muffins with 1 tablespoon Coconut Peanut Butter

Snack (1:30 pm)

1 Coconut Cream Pie Lara Bar
1 scoop Akea Fermented Superfood powder in 6 ounces organic orange juice.

Dinner (7:00 pm)

Large bowl Black-eyed Pea Gazpacho
2 SatFatRox Garlic and Herb Biscuits

As you glanced over this food journal you might have noticed a couple of patterns developing. Firstly, every single morning starts with a smoothie that has at least 3 things in common from one day to another: 2 scoops Akea Fermented Superfood powder, raw eggs, and organic berries. As regimented as that sounds, I feel it has contributed immeasurably to the healing of both my body and mind. I cannot leave the house for the day without having some version of that smoothie, I will add 2 scoops of Akea Fermented Superfood powder to about 10 ounces of my Strawberry Ake-arita Mix, crack in my raw eggs and shake everything up the blender bottle I can take with me. That foundational shake gives me the peace of mind that I have put more nutrition into my body in one meal than many people consume in days, possibly even weeks.

Notes